Midwifery: Best Practice

For Books for Midwives:

Senior Commissioning Editor: Mary Seager
Development Editor: Catherine Steers
Project Manager: Joannah Duncan
Cover Design: George Ajayi

Midwifery: Best Practice

Edited by

Sara Wickham RM MA BA(Hons) PGCE(A)
Senior Lecturer in Midwifery, Anglia Polytechnic University

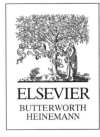

ELSEVIER
BUTTERWORTH
HEINEMANN

EDINBURGH LONDON NEW YORK OXFORD PHILADELPHIA ST LOUIS SYDNEY TORONTO 2003

Dedication

This book is dedicated to the memory of Maggie Smith, a midwife who was truly with women. Some of Maggie's most remarkable work was with women who had suffered sexual abuse and she published three articles on abuse in *The Practising Midwife* in 1998. These articles are republished in this volume.

Since Maggie's death in February 2001, a fund has been set up in her memory. 'Maggie's Fund' will be used to help midwives who wish to study or travel to improve practice areas close to Maggie's beliefs: the experience of vulnerable women, communication, relationships around childbearing and woman-centred care.

For more information on 'Maggie's Fund', write to:
Maggie's Fund
46 Tennyson Road
Lutterworth
LE17 4XA
Telephone: 0114 2229707 (day)

Acknowledgements

We would like to thank all those who have written articles for *The Practising Midwife* in the past, and especially those authors whose work is reproduced in this volume:

Jo Alexander, Tricia Anderson, Kirsten Baker, Sue Battersby, Maureen Boyle, Susan Burvill, Bridget Candy, Sarah Clement, Pauline Cooke, Jeremy Dearling, Lorna Davies, Jo Desborough, Jenny Edwins, Angelina Fellows, Valerie Finigan, Chloe Fisher, Caroline Flint, Jenny Fraser, Jo Garcia, Vivette Glover, Jenny Green, Jo Hartley, Lesley Hobbs, Deborah Hughes, Hannah Hulme Hunter, Sally Inch, Elizabeth Jones, Linda Kimber, Maggie Kirk, Sandy Kirkman, Sheila Kitzinger, Krystina Kweik, Fiona MacVane Phipps, Sally Marchant, Sally McGregor, Kath McKay, Maureen Minchin, Mary L. Nolan, Judith Ockenden, Michel Odent, Kate Olsen, Myra Parsons, Karen Ramsey, Becky Reed, Joyce Reid, Mandy Renton, Andrea Robertson, Jane Rogers, Jilly Rosser, Khadj Rouf, Jim Sikorski, Michele Simpson, Maggie Smith, Stephen Andrew Spencer, Ci Ci Stuart, Jean Sutton, B. Gail Thomas, Kenneth Wade, Benna Waites, Kate Walmsley, Alison Ward, Chris Warren, Frances Wedgwood, Sara Wickham, Jenny Wilson and Juliet Wood.

Special thanks to Sally Inch, Linda Kimber and Mandy Renton for their permission to reprint photographs from their personal collections.

Choice

Do we all have a right to make informed choices about our bodies, our pregnancy and birth experiences and our babies? And, if so, why is this still so far from being a reality for some women? Few midwives will be surprised that this section includes evidence which highlights – again – the lack of real choice which some women experience, and the effect that this powerlessness can have on their self-esteem. The issues are complex, and midwives are seeking to throw light onto them in order to improve practice.

B Gail Thomas argues that the concept of 'risk' has had a major effect on midwifery practice and attitudes to birth over the last few years and has ultimately fed into women's disempowerment. This is reiterated through the experience of Benna Waites, who wanted to choose to give birth to her breech baby vaginally. The article by Kirsten Baker on teenage pregnancy challenges our perceptions about which women are making informed choices. She asks us to consider whether the real issues for midwives are in trying to affect and inform women's decisions, or dealing with potentially more important issues such as poverty.

The 'choice' debate becomes more complex every time a new technology becomes available. Midwife Angelina Fellowes reflects on her experience as a woman and the enormity of the decisions which have to be made by women who choose to have even 'routine' antenatal screening tests. Pauline Cooke discusses enabling women with Group B streptococcus infection to make informed choices, while paediatrician Frances Wedgwood also reflects from her perspective as a woman making decisions about HIV screening. While these articles are about women making the very different choices that are right for them, they all reflect the enormity of these decisions for women and the burden of knowledge and technology upon these choices.

The inclusion of articles written by women who are also involved in the maternity services as professionals is a reminder that so many of us are potential or actual users of these services as well as working within them. How do our own experiences affect our professional lives? And how do our professional lives impact on our own experiences? How can we ensure that we use these experiences in a positive way in practice, without unintentionally allowing our own experiences to shape the way we deal with women making choices?

Recently, I discussed the issue of antenatal HIV screening with a group of midwives, some of whom were being judged by the number of women they were seeing who decided to have this test. While the midwives themselves felt that women should be given all of the information and enabled to make a free choice about this, they also felt pressure from employers to recommend that women had the test, in order to meet Government and local targets in this area. How did this happen? How did we get to a place where midwives are evaluated not by the proportion of women who feel they have been given adequate information and supported in their decisions, but by the number of women they persuade to accept a particular intervention which is perceived by someone else to be a good thing?

With choice becoming more of a political issue than ever, midwives need to take a wider view of these issues, as well as working with women on an individual basis. We should take the opportunity to think hard about what is being asked of us, and how we can truly be 'with women', whatever they decide to do.

The disempowering concept of risk

B Gail Thomas

Risk is a word which has been used increasingly over the past decade in relation to childbirth. While in the 1984 edition of *Mayes Midwifery*,[1] the word risk is used only to identify the fetus who may be compromised by 'fetal distress' or hypoxia, in the 1997 edition,[2] the concept of risk appears much more frequently and in relation to a whole variety of situations: amniocentesis, breech presentation, shoulder dystocia, preterm labour and Caesarean section as examples.

This change in the midwifery literature highlights a general trend in maternity care; we are much more focused on (and therefore constrained by) the concept of risk. The terms 'risk management', 'antenatal screening for risk of abnormality' and 'risk criteria for midwife-led care' surround us. We now label far more women 'at risk' than in the past; what impact does this labelling have on both women and midwives?

It is clear that one of the fundamental roles of the midwife is to identify potential or actual complications of childbirth, to implement relevant supportive measures and to refer appropriately to the obstetrician, GP or paediatrician. The multiprofessional approach to maternity care provides a safety net for women and babies; the professionals with the most appropriate skills in a given situation take responsibility for providing expert care. On the surface this seems quite clear cut; in reality, there is a large grey area which is referred to as the 'at risk' situation. The potential of complication (at risk) rather than its actual presence (diagnosed complication) blurs the lines of professional responsibility.

Impact of risk on women and midwives

Different groups of people see childbirth from different perspectives. The medical/obstetric model of pregnancy defines pregnancy as 'a potentially pathological condition requiring medical intervention'[3] leading to the view held by most doctors that pregnancy can only be considered as normal in retrospect. This example of the 'medicalisation of childbirth'[4,5,6] provides the context in which midwives are currently practising in the Western world, even though many would not agree with its emphasis. While individual midwives are not in a position to change this global context, they must understand it in order to be able to support women effectively. This means that they must question 'advances' in practice which, although developed with the intention of improving care for women, may also lead to their disempowerment.

The purpose of a risk-scoring system is to 'permit classification of individual women into different categories, for which actions can then be planned'.[7] Since the publication of *Changing Childbirth*,[8] the issues of choice and control for women have been powerful considerations in the provision of the maternity services. How then does this concept of identifying women as being 'at risk' fit with them being in control of the childbearing experience?

The example of risk in antenatal screening is given here to illustrate the possible negative effects of this concept on both women and midwives.

Risk in antenatal screening

Most women begin their pregnancies full of anticipation and excitement and they value midwives who help them to feel special and unique.[9] This positive feeling, however, can quickly change when, at the booking appointment, the woman is introduced to the concept of risk. As part of her introduction to antenatal care, she will be offered screening tests which will help to determine whether her baby is normal. It may never have crossed her mind that the baby would be anything but normal and she has to try and make sense of the meaning of being 'at risk'. Instead of feeling like a unique individual, she may feel more like a statistic; a member of an at-risk population simply because she is pregnant.

If she chooses to undergo the tests on offer, she will be presented with figures which are difficult to comprehend. The midwife is key in helping her to decipher this quagmire and, because of this, the midwife herself must understand and be able to articulate these complex concepts clearly. Women often need help in coming to grips with how significant a particular risk really is for them.

Individual decision-making

Decisions in daily life are constantly influenced by weighing up risks. Many people watch the weather report every morning in order to judge the risk of their getting wet in the rain, and to give them the information they need to make a decision about what to wear and whether to take an umbrella to work with them.

It is an interesting exercise to ask a group of students, when introducing the concept of risk, to decide on their individual cut-off point. The majority do not feel the need to take an umbrella when the chance of rain is 10%; most would take one for a 90% chance. The situation is usually equivocal for a 50% chance; some would and some would not. There are, however, always a few who don't fit into the usual pattern; those who always carry an umbrella 'just in case', and those who like walking in the rain and don't mind getting wet, so never carry an umbrella. There are also those who choose a different means of keeping dry like a jacket with a hood on it.

This activity is useful on a number of counts; it highlights to students how individual the response to the concept of risk is; it shows how difficult it can be to determine a cut-off point which is acceptable to the individual; and it identifies that there are always different ways of seeing things.

The students can then apply this idea of decision-making based on risk in the context of presenting antenatal screening tests to women. If the maternity service in which she/he works offers serum screening for neural tube defects and Down's syndrome, women will be considered to be at high risk of having a Down's fetus if the result shows a risk of 1:250.[10] In percentage terms, this would mean 0.4%, a far lower figure than that at which the majority would have left their umbrellas at home. Clearly, the impact of a child with Down's syndrome cannot be equated with getting wet in the rain, but the process of determining the significance to the individual is similar. The reality is that, unless the chance of rain is 0%, they all run the risk of getting wet at some point in the day. As the background risk of carrying a fetus affected by Down's syndrome is higher than 0% for all age groups, every pregnant woman runs the risk of having an affected baby.

It is the individual cut-off point of acceptability which is important for the midwife to explore with the woman, so she can make informed choices about whether to have screening tests. At which point does a woman still feel safe that she will not get wet in the rain or have an affected fetus: 1:500, 1:250, 1:100, 1:10? How does that compare with the background risk at her age? Will the results of serum screening give her information which is useful to her in the light of this? Is she able to cope with the uncertainty that the whole process entails or does she want to cover every eventuality like the person with the jacket and hood? If so, she may consider diagnosis rather than screening (but in this case she must be made aware of the statistical risk of miscarriage (1:100) which amniocentesis carries).

Information and understanding

Midwives are considered to be vital mediators in childbirth;[11] this mediation starts at the beginning of pregnancy when midwives help women to make sense of the services offered to them. This means being able to translate difficult concepts like the statistical risks involved in screening into something meaningful to the individual woman in her personal, social and cultural situation. It also means supporting the woman's choice once she has made sense of the best option for her as an individual.

In a recent survey by the NCT, it was found that some women felt that their rights to choose not to have antenatal screening were undermined by professionals who did not accept their decision to forgo any testing.[12] Midwives must reflect on their personal values and beliefs and work through these, so they do not influence the way in which they support women. In order for midwives successfully to treat women as 'special', they must be able to understand both the conceptual basis of the tests they are offering and the impact results may have on women. Women can be disempowered by lack of sensitive awareness as well as by lack of appropriate explanation. They cannot take control of something which they do not understand.

Prenatal screening tests have the effect of making all women potential cases of risk. When women choose to undergo serum screening, many will be told that they are at higher than average risk of carrying an affected fetus. There is evidence that, even if they are subsequently given the all clear, they still have anxieties about the pregnancy;[13] it seems likely that this anxiety may well carry on to the relationship with the baby once it is born. Once a women is defined as high risk (even though a complication has not been diagnosed), midwives might feel that her care is outside their province, and the doctor takes over responsibility.

The concept of 'risk' is increasingly dominating antenatal care in this country. This has a significant, if subtle, effect on the relationship between woman and midwife; it is likely both to compromise the autonomy of midwives and to disempower women.

Implications for practice

With the best of intentions, current developments in antenatal care increasingly undermine women's belief in their ability to produce 'normal' offspring without intervention. Women may feel compelled to participate in tests which are offered to them, believing that professionals know best. When a woman undergoes serum screening, she will automatically be given a risk factor; this is clearly a potential and not proven risk. However, the mere term risk denotes potential complication which may then move the woman's experience from the realm of 'normal' (i.e. with the support of the midwife) to complicated (i.e. under the management of a doctor). The lines become blurred; the token choice of 1:250 to be considered as high risk in the case of serum screening for Down's syndrome is based on statistics and does not take into account the woman's individual values and life circumstances.

The words 'at risk' create a negative impression, leading women to question both their own ability to procreate and the midwife's role as a source of support in a situation of possible complication. If we return to the earlier description of the medical approach to pregnancy as a 'potentially pathological condition' we are precariously close to considering all pregnancies as at risk (i.e. complicated) and no longer within the scope of midwifery practice.

Midwives can be disempowered by this label of 'at risk' as significantly as women can. It would seem that the way forward may be twofold. First, midwives need to demonstrate their ability to practise autonomously in the absence of a diagnosis of a complication. The label 'at risk' should not automatically lead to the midwife relinquishing responsibility to medical management and to the use of interventions which may be unnecessary. In the case of a confirmed complication, a collaborative approach to management, which includes the woman as an active participant in the decision-making process, is appropriate.

This leads to the second point; women need to understand what is happening to them and the options which are open to them. Midwifery should be about 'guiding women through unfamiliar territory',[14] providing them with the tools to make decisions which will lead to a fulfilling childbearing experience. Midwives must be able to explain complicated concepts (like risk in antenatal screening) in terms which are meaningful to women.

This challenge is open to all midwives. Constraints on time mean that very difficult issues must be explained clearly and succinctly, in order for women to be able to make truly informed choices. Perhaps most importantly, this means that midwives themselves must have a clear understanding of the concepts they are explaining.

Women deserve complete information, so that they are not frightened into complying but are able to decide for themselves which option suits best their individual and 'special' situation.

REFERENCES

1 Sweet B. Mayes Midwifery. 10th edn. London: Baillière Tindall; 1984.

2 Sweet B. Mayes Midwifery. 12th edn. London: Baillière Tindall; 1997.

3 Bryar R. Theory for Midwifery Practice. Basingstoke: Macmillan Press; 1995.

4 Davis-Floyd RE. The technological model of birth. Journal of American Folklore 1987; 100:479–95.

5 Oakley A. Who cares for women? Sciences versus love in midwifery today. Midwives Chronicle and Nursing Notes 1989; 102(1218):214–21.

6 Purkiss J. The medicalisation of childbirth. MIDIRS Midwifery Digest 1998; 8(1):110–12.

7 Enkin M, Keirse MJNC, Renfrew M, et al. A Guide to Effective Care in Pregnancy and Childbirth. 2nd edn. Oxford: Oxford Medical Publications; 1995.

8 Department of Health. Changing Childbirth: The Report of the Expert Maternity Group. London: HMSO; 1993.

9 Hutton E. What women want from midwives. British Journal of Midwifery 1994; 2(12):608–11.

10 Kennard A, Goodburn S, Golightly S, et al. Serum screening for Down's syndrome. Midwives 1995; 108(1290):207–10.

11 Kitzinger S (ed). Why women need midwives. In: The Midwife Challenge. London: Pandora; 1988.

12 Dodds R, Newburn M. Stress tests. New Generation 1997; 16(2):20–21.

13 Statham H, Green J. Serum screening for Down's syndrome: Some women's experiences. British Medical Journal 1993; 307:174–76.

14 Farmer E. My personal framework for practice. Unpublished essay submitted in partial fulfilment for the Diploma in Professional Studies Midwifery. Thames Valley University, London; 1996.

Young, pregnant... and pleased

Kirsten Baker

Sex comes before Maths and after French on Tuesdays, and the Government wants there to be more of it. Why? Because Britain has the highest teenage pregnancy rate in the European Union, and we need to be brought into line with our Continental cousins. Being young and pregnant is a Bad Thing, and improving sex education in schools is seen as a way of reducing its incidence.

Planned pregnancy

Sam had had her three children by the age of 21, and she has now been sterilised. 'I was 16 when my first daughter was born and she was planned, definitely. I don't have any regrets about having the kids – but I wish I hadn't let myself be talked into being sterilised. I want to get it reversed, but it'll cost me £2,000 and I haven't a clue how I'm going to get that sort of money together.'

Sam's youngest child is now five, and she still comes to the 'Young Mums' group' run by midwife Helen Minns in Oxford. Some of the other women there suggest – only half joking – raising money for Sam's operation by having a car boot sale. Like Sam, many of them first came to the group when they were young and pregnant, and still attend as mothers in their twenties. It has evolved into a loosely structured ante- and postnatal support group, and a topic which comes up regularly is the experience of the women on their journey there. Jayleigh describes it wearily: 'Yeah well, sometimes it's just looks, you know – looking at the children and then at me disapprovingly. Sometimes it's a tut-tutting kind of thing, as if I'm actually having sex under their noses on the bus. You get used to it.'

Helen Minns has not got used to it. 'I really worry about what this new focus on teenage pregnancy is going to do. There are some pregnancies which would be best avoided, clearly, particularly for very young girls who are just children themselves. But the Government's Social Exclusion Unit has just sent out a consultation document,[1] the whole thrust of which is on prevention. It's a pathologising approach, and I see that as dangerous. It reinforces this culture of disapproval – and their self-esteem is often not very high in the first place.'

Difficult to persuade

Why do young women become pregnant against this background? Many of them talk about 'falling pregnant' – letting it happen – rather than planning it. Sam and Jayleigh are no less articulate than women of any age about why they had children when they did: 'We felt ready for it – to have something of our own. I don't think I had a clue what it would be like though, the stresses and that. I had a completely unrealistic picture of what it would be like.'

The gap between the fantasy and the reality of childbearing may well be wider for young women, and particularly for those for whom life is not very promising. The incidence of pregnancy is certainly higher amongst young women who are poor, are achieving poorly at school, or are in care. It may indeed be difficult to persuade some women that not having a baby is preferable to having one, however 'accidentally'. Women who were themselves born to teenage mothers are also more likely to have babies at a young age, possibly replicating what is for them normal. One researcher found women of 17 worrying that they had left theirs 'too late' compared with their peer group.[2] The perspective from within this group of women is very different from how they are viewed from the outside. But being so viewed may cause these young women more problems than simply being disapproved of on the bus – uncomfortable and unacceptable though that clearly is.

Not high risk

Young women's experiences of antenatal care are coloured by the prevailing belief that being young and pregnant is undesirable. Women under 17 are often seen as being obstetrically 'high risk', and are therefore referred for an obstetric opinion. This may entail a long and expensive trip to a regional hospital where, as Helen says, 'they are often treated like naughty children when they get there. I have to explain that it makes all women feel like that!'

The evidence for categorising early teenage pregnancies as 'high risk' does not, on closer examination, seem to exist. The majority of studies on the physiology of teenage pregnancy located through a MIDIRS literature search found no correlation between age alone and poor obstetric outcome. The following summaries are typical of many:

'With the exception of an increased risk for preterm labor, it appears that pregnancy, labor and delivery do not pose enormous obstetric and medical risk to the very young adolescent primipara.'[3]

'The seemingly poorer birth outcomes of teenage mothers appear to result largely from their adverse socioeconomic circumstances, not from young maternal age per se.'[4]

The good results accomplished in our centre could be attributed to the free and readily available prenatal care and the quality of support from the family and welfare agencies that are involved with the care of teenage mothers.'[5]

These findings are borne out by the women's own experiences. Sam was at school when she first became pregnant, and planned initially to carry on with her studies. 'To begin with it all went really well, and they let me have time off to see the midwife and everything. But in the end it got too much and I left; I didn't have anyone to leave the baby with anyway, so I couldn't have carried on.'

Poverty

Becci brings another perspective to the issue. 'I was in care when I fell for my first, and because I was 15 they wouldn't house me, so I had to go to foster parents. When I was 16 they put me in bed and breakfast, but it was a really scary situation. I used to put my chest of drawers over my door at night cos there were these men in the building who used to prowl around... With my second baby she [the midwife] told me I ought to rest more, and I didn't have enough iron for the baby or something, so I was supposed to eat better. But the kitchen was on the floor below me, and I couldn't leave little'un, so I just ate stuff in my room. Anyway sometimes I only had a few pence for food before my benefit was due – I just nodded and said I'd try.'

Becci would say that her main problem was not that she was pregnant but that she was poor. Poverty, poor nutrition and poor housing have all been shown to be associated with poor outcomes in pregnancy – unlike age

alone. If the Social Exclusion Unit were to address some of the underlying issues which impact on women and families of all ages – benefits entitlements, flexible school and work, social support, access to suitable childcare – they would need to tackle a much more complicated task than persuading women of a certain age not to have children.

History lesson

The Government's latest approach has historical precedents. Ever since pregnancy and childbearing have been matters of national concern, a particular slant has consistently been adopted. For example, at the beginning of this century, concern over the standard of health of recruits for the Boer War drew attention to their development before birth and soon after birth. At around the same time, repeated social surveys indicated that poverty was having a major impact on families' health. However, responding to this underlying cause would have meant acknowledging that wages and benefits were inadequate, and opening a whole can of class worms. This would have had enormous implications. It was cheaper and more politically expedient to focus instead on the quality of mothering. In 1913, when Britain was in the grip of severe economic depression, the Medical Officer for Health for Finsbury said that the problem of infant mortality was 'mainly a question of motherhood and ignorance of infant care and management.'[6]

It now seems absurd to have selected such an individualistic approach to the social problems of poverty and their solutions. But arguably, it is essentially the same approach which the Government is taking today; by judging women to be suitable or unsuitable mothers on the basis of their individual characteristics, we fail to focus on a whole range of factors which affect all mothers' capacities to be good or bad parents. That, perhaps, is the pitfall of the hapless midwife who suggested dietary improvements to Becci without checking out her living conditions. Such lifestyle advice, whether about becoming pregnant or about behaving in a certain way once pregnant, is far easier to give than to follow, for a whole number of complex reasons. What is more, such advice arises from a very narrow understanding of health and is, therefore, inherently weak.

Smoke screen

Helen Minns is careful about what assumptions she is prepared to make about her client group. 'I think the only safe thing to say about teenage pregnancy is that it happens. It isn't always a good thing, and in some instances it would be better if it didn't happen – sometimes because of the circumstances which bring it about. But by lumping everyone together – a vulnerable

13-year-old and a supported 17-year-old – we can end up throwing a smoke screen over where the problems really lie.'

It can also lead to some quite absurd situations. For example, in one instance a 16-year-old girl had a partner of 14 who was going to be a father. He, for some unfathomable reason, was excluded from school – perhaps to prevent the infective spread of young fatherhood. Helen wonders whether there isn't a huge fear of teenage sexuality which lies at the root of some of the stigmatisation.

Sex, for sure, has a part to play, but the precise relationship between young people, sexual intercourse, contraception, abortion, pregnancy and parenthood would be hard to plot. Intervening as the Government proposes doing may be especially problematic, as Germaine Greer robustly points out:

*'If sex is to be preached at them, and if they are to be taught how to do it as they are taught how to dissect rabbits and compose nourishing meals, correct f***ing becomes an extension of the orthodoxy. Their sexuality is given up to the scrutiny of the older generation and the excitement is lost.'*[7]

Of course, what young people learn about sex at school will inevitably only be a fraction of what they actually assimilate about sex and sexuality. Their peer group, the media, their immediate family, and broader social and cultural influences will all have a part to play in how they behave. Health education in any area, whether information about contraception, smoking, bottle feeding, or eating soft cheese, is not the sole basis on which people make decisions, and this can be difficult for the educators. Feeling ignored and aggrieved when clients go against our good counsel can be profoundly uncomfortable.

But for education to truly educate, we need to recognise where the responsibility for learning lies. This may entail a more fundamental shift than changing some of the details of how we educate. For very vulnerable young women, it may be impossible to perceive how making a particular choice or adopting a particular lifestyle – such as pregnancy – is in her best interests. But if we fail to acknowledge that the agenda of those we seek to 'teach' may be different from our own, we are doing little better than those who purse their lips as Jayleigh struggles on to the bus with buggy and children in tow. It's a challenge, but we can do better than that.

REFERENCES

1 Social Exclusion Unit Consultation Document, Cabinet Office, October 1998.
2 Phoenix A. Teenage motherhood – 'insider' and 'outsider' perspectives. In: Phoenix A, Woollett A, Lloyd E (Eds) Motherhood: meanings, practices and ideologies. London: Sage; 1991.
3 Perry RL, Mannino B, Hediger ML, et al. Pregnancy in early adolescence: are there obstetric risks? Journal of Maternal/Fetal Medicine 1996; 5(6):333–339.
4 Reichman NE, Pagnini DL. Maternal age and birth outcomes: data from New Jersey. Family Planning Perspectives 1997; 29(6):268–272, 295.
5 Lao TT, Ho LF. The obstetric implications of teenage pregnancy. Human Reproduction 1997; 12(10):2303–2305.
6 (Cited in) Lewis J. The politics of motherhood. London: Croom Helm; 1980:65.
7 Greer G. Sex and destiny. London: Secker & Warburg; 1984.

Into the breech

A consumer's point of view

Benna Waites

I found out when I was 37 weeks pregnant that my baby was breech. The consultant confirmed this with a scan, told us the baby was an extended breech, and asked me how I felt about a Caesarean. I had been looking forward to giving birth to my baby and major abdominal surgery, if avoidable, seemed worth avoiding. My partner, having watched a series of birth videos in our antenatal classes, passed out after the Caesarean video, so he was not terribly enamoured of the prospect either. However, we were also of the opinion that Caesareans undoubtedly had their place – I would never have hesitated to have a Caesarean, and deal with the physical and emotional consequences for me, had someone provided me with convincing evidence that it was best for my baby. But, feeling as I did, I needed that evidence. My question was simple. Would it be safer for my baby to come into the world by Caesarean?

Major offensive

My consultant did not answer this question directly, but told me it was quite possible to have a vaginal delivery, though he would want to see my pelvimetry prior to making a decision. I asked how many women had their breech babies vaginally at my local hospital, and he told me that very few first babies were born vaginally, although some second babies were.

The week that followed saw me start a major baby turning offensive – which included acupuncture, homeopathy and positioning – all to no avail. Christine Hall, an acupuncturist who offered us considerable support and help in starting to think through our options, put us in touch with Annie Francis, a trainee midwife who had had two breech babies of her own. She gave us a copy of the MIDIRS leaflet on breech birth,[1] which became our bible for the following three weeks. It is disappointing that these high-quality, balanced and enabling leaflets do not seem to have found their way

into patient antenatal care. The conclusion reached by the review of research that formed the basis of this leaflet was that, although there was a shortage of good quality, large-scale research, there was no good evidence to contraindicate vaginal birth, and that the option of vaginal or Caesarean birth was therefore open for discussion with the woman herself. It made it clear that a significant percentage of breech births attempting vaginal delivery end in Caesarean. It also pointed out the higher incidence of congenital abnormalities in breech babies. This was the first point at which the sense of loss about a breech baby really hit me. Not only had my whole preparation for labour become fraught with complex information assimilation and decision making, but more importantly every new parent's worst nightmare – that of there being something wrong with the baby – was being highlighted as a real possibility. I did a lot of crying at this stage, feeling, perhaps rather petulantly, that it was all horribly unfair and that I had somehow been cheated of my final weeks of rest, relaxation and happy anticipation.

Birth positions

On the question of positioning in labour the MIDIRS leaflet was non-committal, saying that in some centres expertise was being developed in standing breech, in the belief that this increased the chances of a normal spontaneous delivery, but that this belief has not been evaluated. This was to be our next question: was there any reason to compromise my hopes of giving birth to my baby in a position of my choosing? When we had discussed positions for labour in our antenatal class, I had instinctively felt that I wanted to be on all-fours. I had a strong sense that I did not want to be on my back as I thought this might increase the pain, and it seemed sensible to be working with, rather than against, gravity. All-fours also seemed less of a strain on my thigh muscles than other active birth positions. I was encouraged that in all three of my pregnancy and birth books, two of which were generalist (one by Miriam Stoppard, hardly famed for her anti-establishment stance), there were pictures of women giving birth to breech babies in a standing position, with explanatory notes about how sensible it was to use gravity in this way in the birth of a breech.

At our appointment with my consultant the following week he had the results of my pelvimetry, which were good. I asked whether I would be supported in giving birth in a position of my choosing such as standing, all-fours or laterally. He smiled and said benignly, 'You can assume whatever position you wish, my dear.' I was impressed by his permissiveness, but this was too important an issue to be fudged: one of my biggest fears was being in labour and having to fight my way through the birth.

'So just to clarify', I said, 'are you saying that the medical team will support me in delivering the baby on all-fours, for example?'

He replied, 'Well, for second stage, of course, we will need you to be in lithotomy, so that we can use forceps – it is terribly important to control the birth of a breech'. I also asked who would be present at the birth, hoping that perhaps there might be some way of ensuring someone with experience of breech could be there. 'The medical team' was as specific as he was willing to be.

At this point we became deeply troubled. To start with, the plan for stage two that had been outlined to me did not feel quite like I was being given the opportunity to give birth to my baby myself. Forceps, like Caesareans, have their place, but without convincing evidence that they were routinely necessary, I was very reluctant to proceed on the basis that they would be used, come what may. To those new to the business of birth, being confined on one's back with one's feet in stirrups has a rather appalling mediaeval quality to it. We had also read a paper by Caroline Flint on breech birth which stated that 'the greatest danger to the baby seems to be the trauma caused by the person delivering the baby being over anxious and too rough in their delivery techniques'.[2]

We were concerned that there was no guarantee that the medical team would contain anyone with more than a handful of breech birth experiences at best (particularly in light of my local hospital's tendency to perform Caesareans for breeches), and that this inexperience and the anxiety that it could engender could be actively harmful for our baby. The MIDIRS leaflet states, 'If a woman chooses to have a vaginal delivery, skilled and supportive practitioners should be available.' This gave us invaluable strength and determination to proceed with attempting a vaginal delivery and to look into finding skilled practitioners elsewhere. The same day

(now at 38 weeks pregnant) we booked an appointment with my community midwife and started to discuss the possibility of transferring. She confirmed that the vast majority of breeches were delivered by Caesarean at my local hospital, and that if vaginal delivery was attempted this would be in lithotomy with forceps and an epidural would almost definitely be used. It is interesting that epidurals appear to be common practice in vaginal breech delivery, despite the MIDIRS research review stating that there is no evidence that it is indicated and 'may be associated with the prolongation of the second stage'.

Transfer of care

Although the thought of transferring hospitals at this stage in my pregnancy felt like an enormous and highly unsettling upheaval for both of us, we were fairly optimistic that the birth we wanted would not be too difficult to find within the NHS. It was one of those moments when I feel grateful for the range of options that having London on my doorstep provides. My midwife was supportive and suggested a referral to a teaching hospital not too far away that she thought had more experience in vaginal delivery of breeches and took a more flexible approach.

In addition to transferring for the birth, I was also hoping to find somewhere that had experience of offering external cephalic version (ECV). Having read about this in the MIDIRS leaflet, which recommended ECV after 37 weeks of pregnancy, I was surprised that it had not been mentioned at my first appointment. A week later, at the end of my second appointment, I brought it up, assuming that the experience was not available at my local hospital and that I could perhaps be referred elsewhere for the procedure. Instead the consultant looked surprised and said he would try it there and then. He did not carry out a scan to check the position of the placenta, as I had expected, and it took two minutes for him to decide that it was not possible as the baby was extended and engaged. I was left with the nagging sensation that I had been fobbed off, but felt unable to request a referral elsewhere as my consultant clearly felt he had dealt with the issue.

My midwife said that the only way she could see of me having another try at ECV was if I transferred my entire care. I have found out subsequently that ECV is not offered routinely by my local hospital. I have a friend who had a similar experience in another part of the country. Indeed, my friend was initially told that ECV was dangerous and was no longer done. It seems that some maternity units have not caught up with more recent research supporting ECV. Since experience correlates with success in ECV it would seem appropriate for maternity units to be considering both training (or retraining) their obstetricians and adopting a policy on referring elsewhere while skills are being relearned. Clearly ECV is an option only; some women may not wish to have it. But at this stage in my pregnancy I was desperate to try anything safe that would help my baby return to the normality of having his head down.

After an initial false start at transferring my care (during which a midwife at the teaching hospital told me impatiently on the phone that it was impossible to transfer my care so late on as they had been booked up for months, leaving us utterly despairing), the Director of Midwifery at this hospital called me to say she had had a fax from my GP and had made an appointment with one of the doctors there. In conversation about positioning for labour, she told me of a small audit they had done some years previously of standing vaginal breech deliveries in which three of their 25 babies had suffered poor outcomes. This sent us reeling with shock. We had never wanted to do anything risky, and though small scale, and I believe unpublished, this evidence came closest to convincing me to have a Caesarean.

Although it was clear from our discussion that Caesarean was favoured by this hospital I felt it was worth attending the appointment to hear what the doctor had to say, and to discuss the possibility of being referred for ECV. The senior registrar we saw stated categorically that, 'Caesarean is best for baby'. When I asked him about the conclusion of the MIDIRS leaflet, he said he was not familiar with the leaflet and so could not comment. He said it would not be politic to take me on for ECV alone without my consultant's referral.

Independent midwives

At this point we reached the conclusion that the birth we wanted was not available in the NHS and started to explore the possibility of independent midwifery. I do not have time to pay tribute to the warmth, support and information that was provided by the network of people I spoke to. I met someone recently who had had a similar experience to mine, although her baby had turned at the last minute, who had spoken to some of the independent midwives I had, and we were both amazed by the amount of gratis consultation they provide. I had the opportunity to talk through my concerns about standing breech delivery and learn that this was indeed a controversial area, but that nothing like the same controversy surrounded other positions, such as all-fours, perhaps due to the more moderate and controllable use of gravity. I was given Donald Gibb's name at King's College Hospital and so started trying to contact him, while also trying to find an independent midwife in case my attempts to transfer to King's proved as unsatisfactory

as they had with the previous teaching hospital.

I wanted to have my baby in hospital, so the independent midwife with whom I had provisionally agreed to work started looking into getting an honorary contract with a hospital reasonably close to me. She had worked with various hospitals locally before and did not anticipate any problem with this. However, in the following days it emerged that hospitals that had previously given her a contract were not willing to do so with a breech. Their policy on breech was that it was managed by the medical team and that vaginal breeches were always delivered in lithotomy with forceps. This would, in short, override any input the independent midwife might wish to make.

The right hospital

While this was happening, I spoke to a midwife at King's who made me an appointment to see Donald Gibb, but said she could not promise anything. We were the last appointment of the morning clinic: seen in Mr Gibb's lunch hour. I described briefly how it was I had come to his clinic and what I was hoping for. To our immense relief and overwhelming happiness it rapidly emerged that Mr Gibb was a man with a mission. I suspect he is a man with many missions, but the one so acutely relevant to us was his sense that the skills to deliver breech babies were being lost unnecessarily, and that vaginal breech delivery, if carried out by experienced professionals, is a safe and viable option. Perhaps partly because of his experience with breech, and perhaps also his more open-minded attitude to things, he was also willing to attempt stage two in a position that suited me, such as all-fours, though was not willing to try a standing breech due to the current controversy about this. He was keen not to use an epidural, and was not willing to induce me – preferring to opt for a Caesarean if I was very late. He stated that he would be present at the birth, and that if he was out of the country he would arrange for another consultant with some experience of breech and a similar attitude to attend. This commitment, which was immensely reassuring, also made me realise how fortunate I was that he was taking me on, since doing so would take up a significant part of his time, and perhaps intrude into his personal life. He made it clear that if my labour did not progress favourably, he would proceed with a Caesarean, which I had known from the beginning was a very real possibility.

I felt that I had at last found someone who would deliver my baby vaginally if it were possible, and whom I could trust to make the right decision about a Caesarean. He attempted ECV using ultrasound and monitoring the baby's heart rate afterwards which took approximately 15 minutes. Although this was unsuccessful, and for the record very painful, I was glad that I had at last had a proper try. The sizing scan suggested my baby was 8lb, which he felt was the upper limit that he would be happy delivering, though with my favourable pelvimetry, he was happy to proceed.

It is hard to describe the relief and elation this consultation brought us. We knew where we were going to have our baby, and I slept better that night than I had done for a long time. At last, we were being supported by someone within the NHS system, which had the effect of shifting our sense of being bolshie, demanding militants, not caring for the health of our baby, to being quite normal people with a quite normal understanding of the research, with perhaps an abnormal determination to find the birth we wanted. We could at last stop the struggling and get on with looking forward to the birth of our baby.

In a sense, this should be where my story ends. I have conveyed, I hope, the agonising decision making, high speed information assimilation and enormous stress that comes with a breech baby. The axe I have to grind is that some of the agony is part and parcel of having a breech baby, but some of it does not need to be. It concerns me that although I eventually managed to find what I wanted within the health service, I had a lot on my side helping me to do this. Research shows that white, middle class, articulate people stand a better chance of succeeding at this kind of thing than others. I had a highly supportive partner and family. I was lucky enough to get connected with an amazing network of people, who provided a wealth of information and support. I work in the health service and am quite accustomed to negotiating with the medical profession. I was not hampered by the belief that 'doctors are always right'. Doctors are human and do not always manage to be absolutely up to date with latest research, and like the rest of us may muddy the line between evidence and subjective opinion or judgement. I imagine there are few things more traumatic than being at a birth that goes wrong, yet decision-making about breech needs to be based on the bigger picture rather than individual doctors' experiences. They may be slow to respond to popular pressure to change because it is easier to stay with what is known.

The birth

Of course, an account of a pregnancy could not possibly end without an account of the birth. I went into labour two days before my due date. My contractions started at 11.30am and, apart from the odd period early on when they slowed down a bit, increased in intensity and length as first stage progressed. I felt all my contractions in my back alone, and so found it unbearable to be on my back

during a contraction. I stood, was on all-fours or lay on my side when I was very tired. I had a TENS machine on, tried gas and air briefly but did not find it particularly helpful, and did not use any other pain relief. Mr Gibb was called at home, and, despite it being a Sunday evening and him not being on-call, he came in when I was approximately 9cm dilated. Second stage started somewhere between 10 and 11pm. Present were the consultant and a midwife, and an SHO and a registrar who were invited to come in and observe. At some point during second stage a paediatrician joined us.

At first I found it difficult to push any longer than the contractions helped me to, and there was a period in the middle of second stage when we seemed to get stuck. The baby's bottom would crown in the middle of a contraction and then slip back again to where it had been before. The possibility of a Caesarean was muttered about but fortunately Jasper's heart rate remained strong throughout. After the ravages of first stage, I could literally feel my strength returning as the minutes passed and my pushing got stronger and stronger. I was given an episiotomy and shortly afterwards Jasper was born at quarter past midnight in one massive contraction lasting 40 seconds. At the beginning of the contraction his bottom had started to emerge but was barely out, at the end his head came out, helped I believe by the consultant using the Moriceau-Smellie-Veit manoeuvre. He was healthy and weighed in at 8lb 7oz. It was the most incredible experience of my life and yet, compared to the weeks before, felt remarkably straightforward.

Luck or evidence?

My GP told me at my six-week check that I had been lucky, that I had taken the high-risk option and got away with it. I mentioned the research and the MIDIRS leaflet and he dismissed it saying that research studies of sufficient size had not been carried out but even a small risk in his view was simply never worth taking. He may have a point: small risks will only emerge in large-scale research, and it remains possible that giving birth to breech babies vaginally is slightly riskier. But I am not convinced. Another woman from my antenatal class had a breech baby by Caesarean at our local hospital. Her son came out with fluid on his lungs which was so severe that he spent a week recovering in the neonatal unit. Single cases do not prove anything, but it is my impression that the risks of Caesarean to both mother and baby have come to be under-represented in the breech debate.

Since getting connected up with the breech issue, it has become clear to me that my experience of trying to negotiate for a labour I wanted is standard fare for women with breech babies. Many women are told that the only option is Caesarean, and many are so appalled by the thought of lithotomy and forceps that they opt for Caesarean. What I was shocked by was the way in which obstetric practice seems to lag behind both research evidence and women's views. With cephalic babies, my local hospital's modern maternity unit appeared to be really qute progressive, possessing active birth equipment and encouraging women to think about positions for labour. It felt as if having a breech catapulted me into somewhere very different, where my baby was to be carefully managed out of me. I would stress that I am no opponent of intervention in birth when it contributes to the health of the baby. However, in breech birth it seems that sometimes intervention is justified on the grounds of convention rather than evidence.

I want to stress that considerations about the health of my baby were of the highest importance throughout the whole process. Sometimes disputes between women and the obstetric profession are characterised as representing the rights of the woman on the one hand and the safety of the baby on the other. This seems to me to be a false dichotomy – I for one would never wish to champion my right to choose over the safety of my baby. As well as being a mother with a breech birth experience I am also a clinical psychologist employed by the NHS. I have a rigorous research training, and am used to basing decisions on research evidence. I felt that there was insufficient evidence to back up the course of action that many professionals I encountered were advising.

Need for change

It is clearly impractical for every woman who wants the opportunity to try for a vaginal delivery without forceps to be referred to Donald Gibb or the small number of consultants like him. I appreciate that changing the way the NHS responds to breech requires a major attitudinal shift, as well as a change in training to ensure that experience with vaginal delivery of breeches does not die out. If vaginal breech birth is as safe as Caesarean breech birth then it has to make sense to make it easier for women to take up this option if they choose to.

Emotionally I am so very happy to have had the wonderful experience of birth that I did. Economically, even taking into account the cost of training and paying someone with breech birth experience to be present at vaginal deliveries, the relative cost to the NHS of Caesarean and the subsequent levels of maternal morbidity must be worse. The system is in urgent need of change. From a purely selfish point of view, I hope that if my next baby is breech I will not have the exhausting struggle I had this time, and will be able to get on with the comparatively straightforward process of giving birth.

REFERENCES

1 Breech presentation – options for care. Informed choice leaflet for professionals. Bristol: MIDIRS; 1997.

2 Flint C. Babies presenting by the breech. Obstetrics and Gynae Product News 1989; summer:21–23.

Painful choices

A midwife's personal experience of antenatal testing

Angelina Fellowes

Antenatal screening tests are carried out to detect or exclude any fetal abnormalities. As a midwife, I am well aware of this. As a pregnant woman, I also looked to these tests to provide me with reassurance – peace of mind that all is well. However, I, like others,[1] have often wondered at the value of the triple test. It seems to me strange that the only information we can gain from the test is the probability of a problem being present. It could give needless extra worry if you screen positive but are carrying a normal healthy child, or give a false sense of security if you screen negative – after all, even if the chances of a problem were 1:5000, that would be no consolation if you were that one!

Confidence

It was with this in mind that, when I was in my third pregnancy, I decided against further tests beyond the routine scans and AFP tests. Having had two healthy children with uneventful pregnancies, I embarked on this pregnancy with some degree of confidence that all would be well. Of course, as with any pregnancy there is always that small nagging feeling that a problem may arise, but never for one moment did I really believe that a major problem would develop and apply to my baby; that is the sort of thing which happens to other people.

At my routine antenatal anomaly scan at 20 weeks' gestation, I found that the nagging feeling could be ignored no longer. The radiographers could not visualise the chambers of our baby's heart and, while initially this was thought to be due to the position of the baby, it soon became apparent that there could be a real problem, and further investigation was necessary. After a swift referral to our area fetal cardiology specialist centre, our worst fears were confirmed – our baby had a major cardiac anomaly. The extent of the anomaly was difficult to assess on scan alone.

Suddenly, the pregnancy was no longer exciting; fear and uncertainty were constantly with us. We were left with choices which we did not even want to consider. As another mother who experienced this commented: 'This is a mockery of the concept of choice. A lesser of the two evils choice, a devil and the deep blue sea choice, the no choice choice. An only choice where the other choices are yet more horrible, too horrible to choose.'[2]

No more tests

We decided that the pregnancy must continue, our baby must be given every chance of survival. We also chose not to have any further invasive tests, in case they revealed an even worse tragedy which would leave us with no hope to cling on to.

It was our hopes and prayers and the immense support from family, friends and colleagues that carried us through the pregnancy. While the pregnancy continued we lived in a kind of limbo which went on and on, all the while wishing we were blissfully unaware that there was a problem or that we were ignorant of what might lie ahead. Why should we have all this worry when we couldn't do anything about it? All we could do was wait.

The only way I could get through the pregnancy was to live in a state of denial – that surely this was not happening to us. The whole picture was too traumatic for me to contemplate all at once, so I only allowed a fraction of reality in at a time – just enough to cope with. I did extra shifts at work, getting lost in other people's lives (ironically, most often by delivering their healthy babies). Sharing their joy helped, especially as I too had experienced it with the birth of my two sons. While I was so busy I did not have to think of my own personal situation. At home with my husband and sons, life was invariably hectic and if there was time to spare I painted my plain pine furniture until my family were convinced that nothing was safe from my painting and stencilling.

I also lived in the hope that maybe, just maybe, they had got it wrong. Deep down I knew this wasn't the case, as time and again more scans revealed that all was not well. As the weeks passed we were being prepared for the future, as much as anyone can be prepared for such events. At last the day arrived for the pregnancy to be induced. The relief was immense, the painting had to stop! However, as one nightmare ended, another one began.

Intensive care

At least now something could be done. Now we were grateful for the knowledge of our baby's condition, glad of this inside information which would give him every possible chance of life. The time and place of delivery was planned, the paediatric intensive care unit with all its doctors, nurses, cardiologists and surgeons were ready to receive this baby, ready to do their best. I was delivered in a centre of excellence for the treatment of children with heart defects. Our admiration for their skills knew no bounds; if anyone could save our baby, they could.

The first few days of my son's life passed in a daze. Luke was diagnosed as having a hypoplastic right ventricle, double inlet left ventricle, aortic stenosis, pulmonary stenosis and transposition of the great arteries. This was one of those times when having some nursing and midwifery knowledge was not helpful – his problems seemed insuperable. When the details of his operation were fully explained, the surgeon's tasks seemed too complicated to even contemplate. However, against the odds, Luke survived.

After three weeks in hospital Luke was allowed home together with his brothers (who had taken all this trauma in their stride), and we could be a family again. The past months merged into the distance like a bad dream.

Luke has since had further heart surgery and has come through it without any major complications, and he will need further surgery in the future. So far we are delighted with his progress and ever grateful to all those involved in his care – too numerous to mention, but all remembered.

Happy child

Although Luke has had some delay in his development (which we hope is temporary), he is a cheerful, happy little boy who is a cherished part of our family. His brothers love him to bits and delight in his baby ways. They are also proud that their brave brother has overcome so many problems. He loves playing peek-a-boo, listening to nursery rhymes and watching Teletubbies. He enjoys being around other children, especially when they give him extra attention. In short – we wouldn't be without him.

We have been changed by these events. A whole new world, that we weren't aware existed, has opened up to us. We have seen how some people spend their lives, for weeks, even months, on the cardiac wards with their child's life hanging in the balance, going from one flicker of hope to the next. We have seen the courage of these children and their parents and the dedication of the staff. We are aware that we are the lucky ones, but we are still cautious of the future, as we don't know what it may hold.

Two-edged sword

When the prenatal diagnosis was first made, we were faced with a two-edged sword. Staying ignorant would have saved us a lot of worry and pain during my pregnancy, but having some knowledge allowed us to prepare for Luke's arrival and to give him the best possible chance of survival by ensuring he received optimum care. This may well have saved us the suffering of losing a baby whom we weren't aware had a problem – until it was too late. Despite all the heartache, we made the right choice.

REFERENCES

1 Massey-Davies L. A woman's right not to choose. The Practising Midwife 1998; 1(7/8).

2 Katz Rothman B. The tentative pregnancy. 3rd edn. London: Pandora; 1994.

Difficult decisions

Group B streptococcus and intrapartum antibiotics

Pauline Cooke

One of the many challenges to midwives in this post-*Changing Childbirth* era is that of helping women to make informed choices. Choice goes much further than consent, as the latter implies simply the acceptance or refusal of an intervention or treatment proposed by a health professional. The *International Code of Ethics for Midwives* deals with this difference, and states that:

'*Midwives respect a woman's informed right of choice and promote the woman's acceptance of responsibility for the outcome of her choices... Midwives work with women, supporting their right to participate actively in decisions about their care and empowering women to speak for themselves on issues affecting the health of women and their families in their culture/society.*'[1]

The key concepts here are i) respect for the right of choice, ii) the promotion of the woman's responsibility and iii) support for their active participation in decision making. These are fundamental to sensitive, women-centred midwifery practice.

Rather than discuss the theory, I would like to illustrate these concepts by telling the stories of two women's pregnancies and births. Hannah and Rachel, both carriers of the group B streptococcus (GBS), were part of my caseload last year.

Hannah

Hannah was 24 weeks pregnant with her first baby when we first met. She was 29 years old, a medical registrar and married to Gary, a neonatologist. At 21 weeks, she had referred herself to the hospital with possible ruptured membranes. No liquor was seen on speculum examination but, because of a vaginal discharge, a high vaginal swab (HVS) was taken, which yielded both candida and GBS. She was treated with antibiotics (inappropriately) and a further HVS one week later was negative for GBS. However, GBS is known to be transitory and antibiotics during pregnancy are neither indicated nor appropriate.[2] At this time, one of the medical staff recommended intrapartum antibiotics for Hannah and a note was made in her records: 'GBS – antibiotic cover during labour'.

Having had an interest in GBS for some years, I had previously searched the literature and knew of both a Cochrane Library review[3] and information from Group B Streptococcus Support on the internet.[4] The information from this support group is helpfully packaged into a six-page summary aimed at professionals, a 16-page booklet entitled *For women who carry GBS* and a 33-page document entitled *GBS: The Facts*.

When she was 35 weeks pregnant, I shared the information from GBS Support with Hannah and, following a discussion with Gary, she confirmed her decision to have intrapartum antibiotics. In preparing Hannah for labour, we discussed coping strategies and the advantage of staying at home for much of the labour. This needed to be balanced against the recommendation that intravenous antibiotics should be given at the onset of labour or at least four hours pre-birth.[4]

At 41 weeks, Hannah went into spontaneous labour and when I saw her at home at 8am she was contracting mildly every three minutes and using TENS. The baby's head was two-fifths palpable above the pelvic brim and on vaginal examination her cervix was posterior, thick, 1cm long and 1cm dilated. I then left Hannah to go to speak at a study day. She was well supported by Gary, her mother and her mother-in-law.

Hannah's labour progressed rapidly over the next three hours and at about 11am Gary bleeped me to say he was bringing Hannah into hospital. As I had not quite finished my teaching session a colleague welcomed them onto the delivery suite and by 11.50am Hannah was contracting strongly every three minutes and her cervix was anterior, thin and 4-5cm dilated. I arrived soon after and a venflon was sited. Augmentin 1g was prescribed and given intravenously at 12.30pm. Hannah began experiencing rectal pressure at 14.00 and some 20 minutes later her membranes ruptured spontaneously revealing fresh meconium-stained liquor. At 14.45, I confirmed full dilatation and Hannah had a strong urge to push. After just 15 minutes of pushing, the fetal heart rate decelerated to 80bpm with slow recovery. I called for medical help and the decision was made to perform a ventouse delivery under pudendal block. Hannah gave birth to a baby girl at 15.22, weighing 3.830kg, needing no active resuscitation.

Apart from Hannah's GBS carriage, there were no other factors present to increase the risk of transmission to the baby (Table 1.5.1). Hannah stayed overnight in hospital, her baby was examined carefully by a paediatrician, and the family was transferred home the next day. Both parents were fully aware of the signs of infection in the baby and I continued postnatal care until day 27, by which time Hannah was breastfeeding with confidence and her baby weighed a healthy 4.6kg!

Rachel

Rachel was 21 weeks pregnant with her second baby when we met. She was 37 years of age, an accountant, married to Richard, a computer consultant. Her first child, Rebecca, had been born in 1994 after two missed abortions in 1992 and 1993. Rebecca was born by forceps delivery, weighing 3.148kg. Following the birth, Rachel had prolonged bleeding and dyspareunia. Her GP took an HVS which yielded GBS and the following year, Rachel underwent a revision of her episiotomy incision. In 1997, Rachel became pregnant again but an amniocentesis revealed Down's syndrome and the pregnancy was terminated.

In the early part of her current pregnancy Rachel wanted to delay any antenatal appointments until prenatal diagnosis had taken place, so until that time we talked over the phone. Rachel underwent a nuchal fold translucency scan followed by an amniocentesis which showed normal karyotyping.

During our first meeting, I reviewed Rachel's history and noted her GBS carriage. At 27 weeks, Rachel told me that she was considering a home birth and we revisited our discussion about GBS. I gave Rachel the GBS Support leaflet for women[4] and discussed with her the recommendation about intrapartum antibiotics and the potential for this complicating a home birth.

By 36 weeks, Rachel and Richard had decided on a home birth. They were fully informed that intrapartum antibiotics would reduce the risk of the baby developing a GBS infection from 1:400 to 1:8000.[4] We reviewed possible side effects from the antibiotics including a rash and, rarely, a severe allergic reaction. After a few days of thought, Rachel informed me that she wanted her baby

Table 1.5.1 Recognised factors which increase the risk of neonatal GBS infection

Maternal GBS carriage
Previous baby with GBS infection
Preterm labour (<37 weeks' gestation)
Preterm pre-labour rupture of membranes
Prolonged rupture of membranes (more than 18-24 hours before birth)
Raised temperature during labour (37.8°C or higher)
GBS urinary tract infection at any time during present pregnancy

to be born at home with no antibiotic cover during labour. I was convinced that this was a fully informed decision and that they understood the implications of their choice.

I discussed Rachel's decision with her affiliated consultant who advised that I should take an HVS when labour began and ask for an urgent result. Rachel was happy with this and we awaited the start of labour. Rebecca had been born at 39 weeks and once this stage had been reached, Rachel became increasingly impatient! Three days later, one Saturday afternoon, Rachel asked me to come and assess her cervix and sweep the membranes. The baby was very active and the head was three-fifths palpable. Rachel's cervix was central, thick, 1cm long and 1-2cm dilated. I swept the membranes, but had little confidence in its effectiveness! However, Rachel woke at 2am the next morning with contractions. I arrived just after 3am when she was contracting every five minutes. Her cervix was fully effaced, thin and 3cm dilated. I took an HVS and left to collect some more equipment.

When I returned, Rachel was obviously in established labour, feeling nauseous and kneeling by the side of the bed. By 4.30am she was experiencing some rectal pressure and her membranes ruptured spontaneously just after, releasing clear liquor. Soon afterwards, a colleague arrived to support me. At 5.10am, Rachel's cervix was fully dilated with the presenting part at the level of the ischial spines. Rachel was actively pushing, in an all-fours position, supported by Richard and watched by her daughter Rebecca.

Despite superhuman effort, the vertex did not become visible and I rechecked both the descent and the position of the baby at 5.45am. The station was 1cm below the spines and the baby's position was direct occipito-anterior with no increase in moulding or caput. At 6.00am we discussed possible transfer to the hospital and encouraged Rachel to stand for pushing. Fifteen minutes later, the fetal heart decelerated to 80bpm and my colleague called an ambulance to attend. The heart rate remained between 100 and 110 bpm between pushes and by 6.25am Rachel proudly announced that she could really feel the baby's head coming down and it was visible on pushing. The ambulance crew arrived and was asked to wait downstairs. At 6.40am the baby's head was born. As the shoulders did not follow with the next contraction, I asked Rachel to get on her knees again on the floor. Gentle traction with the next contraction still did not achieve delivery of the posterior shoulder so Rachel was helped onto her back on the floor while my colleague gave suprapubic pressure over the posterior aspect of the anterior shoulder. To our great relief, the baby's body was born at 6.44am, four minutes after the head. Stimulation was given: the baby's heart rate picked up to over 100bpm in less than one minute and the baby responded quickly and was soon breathing.

The ambulance crew was dispatched and the family welcomed their new son and brother, while the two midwives got their breathing and heart rates back to normal! Baby Joseph weighed 3.950kg and fed beautifully on the breast. Before I left the house, we reviewed the signs to look for in the baby which might suggest GBS infection. I particularly mentioned grunting, tachypnoea, poor feeding and lethargy. I knew that Rachel and Richard would observe their baby very closely and call me immediately if they were concerned. I returned that evening to find the baby pink, warm, with good muscle tone and a normal respiratory rate. He had been mucousy during the day, but was now feeding well at the breast.

I was called the next day by the laboratory who had found the HVS positive for GBS. In a sense, this did not change the situation as Rachel and Richard had been vigilant in observing their baby and would continue this for as long as necessary. We knew the important period was 48 hours, after which the risk of the baby developing an infection decreases.

On day four, Rachel was relaxed and happy with Joseph's progress. At ten days I handed over care to my colleague who had supported me at the birth, while I went on annual leave. Joseph now weighed 4.200kg and was thriving. I called in to see Rachel after my holiday and we reviewed the birth and her decision to decline antibiotics. She was convinced this was the right decision for her and was especially happy to have had the baby at home, supported by her family and a midwife who knew her well.

If she ever has another baby the decision about antibiotics for GBS carriage will be less difficult than the decision about a home birth in the light of a history of shoulder dystocia!

Discussion

One of the most helpful discussions in *Changing Childbirth*[5] centres around the issue of safety. Barely a week goes by in either my midwifery practice or in my teaching when I do not think about or quote what is stated about this concept:

'Safety is an underlying principle of the maternity services. No one cares more about achieving a safe and happy outcome to a pregnancy than the pregnant woman and her partner. ... Safety is not an absolute concept. It is part of a greater picture encompassing all aspects of health and wellbeing. Each woman should be approached as an individual, and given clear and unbiased information on the options that are available to her, and in this way helped to balance the risks and benefits for herself and her baby.' (p9-10)

Hope comments that 'individuals differ both in what they value and in their propensity to take risks'.[6] Hannah and Rachel's stories offer good, real-life examples of this because although they were both carriers of GBS and had access to the same information, they made very different decisions. The decision was, at its heart, about balancing risks and benefits.

For Hannah and Gary, the risk of the baby developing an infection outweighed the risk of an adverse reaction to antibiotics and a more complicated labour with a venflon causing discomfort.

For Rachel and Richard, the benefit of birth at home without antibiotics outweighed the small risk (1:400) of an infected baby.

Hope[6] examines three components of choice:

1 Information

This refers to the quality and quantity of information available and the way it is presented. The emphasis is on the process of being informed. In other words, the receiver of the information must be able to understand and make use of it.

2 Education

This second component refers to the context in which the information can be understood. Hannah and Rachel's choices depended not simply on information but on how that information was understood. Written information may help to provide knowledge, but there also needs to be an opportunity for discussion and consultation. Continuity of carer appears to offer an ideal framework for such education.

3 Power and involvement

The first two components by themselves are not sufficient for choice. Women need the power to exercise such choice and midwives need to relate to women in such a way as to welcome and encourage their clients' active participation and involvement in decision making.

Conclusion

This article has sought to demonstrate important principles of women-centred care in relation to decision making. Approaching women as individuals and respecting their autonomy are fundamental aspects. A more complex issue is that of promoting responsibility for the outcome of choices. Midwives often comment that it is easy for women to accept responsibility when all goes well, but what if it doesn't? What if Rachel and Richard's baby had developed a severe infection and needed treatment in neonatal intensive care? This is not an easy question to answer, but such a scenario should be discussed as part of the decision-making process. And if baby Joseph had become seriously ill, apportioning of blame and being made to feel guilty should have no place in the support of his parents. Difficult decisions, yes, but they are inevitable in the promotion of choice and the provision of women-centred care.

REFERENCES

1 International Confederation of Midwives. International Code of Ethics for Midwives. London: ICM; 1993.
2 Feldman R. The group B streptococcus. The Practising Midwife 1998; 1(1):20–22.
3 Smaill F. Intrapartum antibiotics for Group B streptococcal colonisation (Cochrane Review). In: The Cochrane Library, issue 4. Oxford: Update Software; 1998.
4 Group B Streptococcus Support on the internet: http://www.gbss.org.uk
5 Department of Health. Changing Childbirth. Part 1: Report of the Expert Maternity Group. London: HMSO; 1993.
6 Hope T. Evidence-based patient choice. London: King's Fund Publishing; 1996.

HIV screening choices

Frances Wedgwood

Ruby's mother, Lola, wasn't happy. Nor was Ruby's GP. When I saw her in the paediatric rapid referral clinic I agreed. Something wasn't quite right with Ruby. Unlike her four older siblings, Ruby wasn't thriving – the glands all over her body were swollen and at eight months she still wasn't sitting. I called in the consultant and we discussed the possible diagnoses but we knew what was to follow. We had seen it before. Ruby's HIV antibody test was positive and viral PCR confirmed the presence of virus in her blood. A few weeks later a positive viral culture left the diagnosis in no doubt. Ruby was in the early stages of AIDS.

Childhood HIV is a ghastly business. Its repercussions spread far beyond the child itself. Lola had been in her current relationship for three years. She had not known her partner was HIV positive. Now she was too. Fortunately Ruby's older sister Olivia, a bright and chatty two-year-old, was not. Nor were her three half siblings. When pregnant with Ruby, Lola remembered the midwife mentioning HIV at the booking visit but, having four children in rude health, she didn't think it was important. To cap it all she was pregnant again.

But of course it didn't end there. Ruby's father left, unwilling to accept the diagnosis. It looked as if the family would fall apart. But Lola kept it together. Ruby started on drug therapy and made startling progress, regaining her motor milestones very quickly. It now looks likely that she will live into adulthood.

Lola took AZT throughout pregnancy and had an elective section. She had enjoyed breastfeeding her older children and it was with sadness she decided to bottle feed Ruby's baby brother Edwin. But repeated viral PCR and viral culture tests proved negative and six months after Edwin's birth we were able to confirm that he was free of HIV.

I spent a year working as a paediatrician in an HIV unit in London. In that time I saw a steady stream of children just like Ruby. The presentations were all too familiar: pneumocystis pneumonia, tuberculous meningitis, staphylococcal septicaemia, disseminated chickenpox. Some of them are now dead. One or two had newly-born siblings at the time of their own diagnosis who, when tested, were also positive. All the children we diagnosed on our unit were born in the UK after the introduction of AZT for HIV infection in pregnancy. None of their mothers had known their HIV status when they were pregnant. At a time when other countries, such as France, were seeing a steady decline in paediatric AIDS following the introduction of universal screening in pregnancy with consent,[1] it all felt so unnecessary.

Unbelievably, when I first became pregnant my midwife tried to dissuade me from being tested. I felt that I was high risk enough. During the course of my career I had had at least five needlestick injuries. Once, as a house officer, I had been sprayed with blood by an AIDS patient with haemoptysis. I would not have been able to forgive myself if I had stuck my head in the sand at the one time in my life when I could choose to make a difference. When I persisted, the midwife looked at me as if I were somehow disreputable.

An informed choice

I had no illusions about the consequences for my partner and me if I tested positive. I also knew the options for my baby weren't clear cut. The absolute safety of AZT is not established. Amongst the tens of thousands of babies born to mothers who have taken AZT there have been eight cases of mitochondrial dysfunction, a rare, often fatal, condition.[2] Most research has suggested an added 14% risk of transmitting HIV through breastfeeding[3] (but this may not be the whole story, according to a recent study which found that exclusive breastfeeding carried no more risk than artificial feeding[4]). Moreover, given the huge benefits of breastfeeding, is formula feeding the best alternative for HIV-infected women? Some authorities have suggested as alternatives to bottle feeding a shorter total duration of breastfeeding, more emphasis on exclusive breastfeeding, heat treatment of the mother's own expressed breastmilk to kill the virus, donations of breastmilk by non-infected mothers, milk banking or wet nursing and use of modified animal milks.[5]

Having HIV raises questions about many of life's choices, not least the opportunity to breastfeed and to have a natural childbirth. I wouldn't have relished an elective section. But I knew that studies suggest that elective Caesarean helps prevent transmission.[6] However, despite the different statistics flying around and the differing levels of success reported, the bottom line stayed the same. If I chose to be tested I could make a difference. Whether intervention reduces transmission to 0.8% as suggested by French data or 2.2% as the most recent British data suggests,[7,8] I could choose to up my baby's chances significantly. If the worst came to the worst my decision to have a test would be the most positive choice I could have made. I could choose to avoid Ruby's fate.

Two years on, after a negative test, a vaginal delivery and 14 months' happy breastfeeding, I find myself pregnant again. On this occasion the midwife didn't bat an eyelid when once again I asked to be tested. Quite frankly I found it a much easier test to accept than the nuchal translucency scan or the triple test. Unlike the screening tests for Down's, screening for HIV meant that I could choose life.

It all suggests the climate is changing. Yet a few weeks later the High Court ruled that a baby girl be compulsorily tested for HIV,[9] a case which must have sent very negative messages to the community. There couldn't be a more powerful argument to dissuade pregnant women from being tested than the spectre of the involvement of the law if you don't do as you are told. Many women will conclude after that High Court ruling that an HIV test is an open invitation to the State to take away your choices over how you raise your child. Certainly, having HIV takes away many hopes and dreams. But for me, making a well-informed decision to be tested was a positive choice. An opportunity to save a life.

Names have been changed to protect identities.

REFERENCES

1 Nicoll A. Antenatal screening for HIV in the UK: What is to be done? Journal of Medical Screening 1998; 5:170–1.
2 HIV in pregnancy and early childhood. Drug and Therapeutics Bulletin 1999; 37(9).
3 Dunn DT, Newell ML, Peckham CS. Risk of HIV-1 transmission through breastfeeding. Lancet 1992; 340:585–8.
4 Coutsoudis A, Pillay K, Spooner E. Influence on infant feeding patterns on early mother-to-child transmission of HIV-1, South Africa: A prospective cohort study. Lancet 1999; 354:471–6.
5 Latham MC, Greiner T. Breastfeeding versus formula feeding in HIV infection. Lancet 1998; 352:737.
6 The International Perinatal HIV Group. The mode of delivery and the risk of vertical transmission of HIV-1. N Engl J Med 1999; 340:977–87.
7 Mandelbrot L, Le Chenadec J, Berrebi A, et al. Perinatal HIV-1 transmission, interaction between zidovudine prophylaxis and mode of delivery in the French perinatal cohort. JAMA 1998; 280:55–60.
8 Trinh Duong, Ades AE, Gibb DM, et al. Vertical transmission rates for HIV in the British Isles: Estimates based on surveillance data. BMJ 1999; 319:1227–1229.
9 Judgement in the matter of C (a child) and in the Matter of the Children Act 1989. Before Mr Justice Wilson, Royal Courts of Justice, 3 September 1999.

The midwife 2010

Exploring the impact of genetics on the future of midwifery

Sally McGregor   Maggie Kirk

TEN YEARS FROM NOW

Information overload

I am exhausted. Last night it was my turn to staff the 'Midwife Direct' line – you know, the one with the slogan 'We aim to deliver!' Four hours of answering questions, thinking and generally being on your toes. Mind you, I would rather be doing this as my sub-speciality than ultrasound scanning.

I find people are well informed but so anxious. I had a couple last night on the video link – Andrew and Erica. She is 36 weeks pregnant. They had watched the episode of Coronation Street where Tracey Barlow demands a Caesarean section on the grounds that the pain of labour would interfere with the bonding process. The possibility really worried them, so they downloaded a ten-page document from the Internet on the pros and cons of different types of pain relief and then gave me a ring. People still want your opinion, but you have to be so sure of your facts. Everyone has access to so much information that sometimes when I do Midwife Direct, I feel like I am sitting an exam!

One of the problems is there are too many choices. Gone are the days when you just had to reassure people that decisions would be shared between themselves and the professionals. Since the advent of the Life-Long Learning agenda ten years ago there are Internet access stations everywhere. You can't even nip into Tesco's without being confronted by one.

Pregnancy planning

I'm off to my Predictive Planning class later. We run them at the Citizen Health Resource Centre (not allowed to call it a GP practice these days). The classes were difficult to get off the ground initially, but since the focus of care has changed from 'diagnose and treat' to 'predict and prevent', people are more motivated to take an active part in their own health. There are pregnancies that are unplanned, but the majority try to do things 'properly'. There is so much pressure on couples now – from a variety of sources – to produce the perfect child.

There are two key aspects to predictive planning classes: discussing couples' expectations of screening, and getting them to maximise their preconceptual health based on their genotypes. I encourage people to bring their Smart Cards, which hold all their health information. During the classes people look at their individual risk, and then calculate their combined risk (with their partner) of passing on a particular gene to their offspring. The calculation takes into account environmental and lifestyle factors, and their age. My role is to act as a resource – as midwives we have made a conscious decision to move away from being directive. People tend to be very well motivated to modify their behaviour if they believe it may benefit their offspring or influence their insurance premiums. Mind you, there are always those, usually the ones that have a passion for chocolate or cigarettes, that use the excuse 'My addiction is in my genes so there is nothing I can do…'.

The number of screening tests available is amazing. It is important to explain what is available commercially and what they can get through the NHS. In the NHS we only do susceptibility testing, to calculate the lifetime risk of developing common things, like diabetes, cardiac disease and Alzheimer's.

Geoff came in with his partner Angela and wanted to know if the baby could be tested for the 'intelligence gene' as soon as Angela got pregnant. I told them that sort of test was not available on the NHS – but you can get anything on the Internet. I am worried about the availability of such tests where there are no regulations. Angela was tested privately and told she didn't have the 'mothering gene'! She was quite distraught: 'What is the point of continuing?' she asked, 'I will never make a mother, the baby will be taken away from me'. There is no support or counselling before or after these tests. It's usually left to professionals like myself in the NHS to pick up the pieces.

We try to do all bookings from home. It doesn't take long, as people generally have their own Smart Cards and I can always link to the hospital database with my lap-top. As midwives we are responsible for validating family history and checking all the databases for potential health problems. Now we have the computer software to undertake these tasks it makes life so much easier. You have to be so litigation-conscious these days. I have found that having the tele-link between the Resource Centre and the Clinical Genetics Centre is very reassuring both for my clients and for myself. Not having to travel miles and wait for hours in clinics is a real bonus for people. I have learnt so much by taking an active part in the consultations. Just as well really, as clients always think of things they meant to ask once the tele-link has been closed down.

I run my antenatal clinic from the Resource Centre. Today I had to refer two newly-booked women to the Healthy Lifestyle Facilitator, as one has been identified as being at risk of stress incontinence and the other of gestational diabetes. We can do so many investigations from here. The emphasis antenatally is on fetal screening, using DNA chip technology. We use maternal blood for the majority of tests, so it is much less invasive than it used to be. Any suspicious results are e-mailed to the specialists at the Clinical Genetics Centre. We can set up a video consultation to discuss the best plan of action and it means the prospective parents get a realistic picture about the outcome from all parties. Mind you, I have had to develop my skills in facilitation!

High expectations

With all this technology, expectations are really high. I delivered a baby called Lucy the other day. Her parents believed that she had been screened for every conceivable disease. When Lucy was born it was obvious that she had some sort of syndrome. As you can imagine, people don't expect mistakes to happen with the new technology. The couple are very angry and I know the mother is finding it really difficult to cope. The father sits and holds Lucy but the mother will not have anything to do with her. I will go and see them later, but it is so difficult to know what to say to them. I understand they are thinking of suing.

I really enjoy doing my postnatal visits. Later, I am going to see Alison and Roger and their new baby. I have known them since they came to the predictive planning classes I ran last year. Less and less of my work is done in the postnatal period as now the emphasis is on the preconceptual and antenatal periods. I miss the contact with the mums and babies. The amount of time we have to spend providing information and getting informed consent for all the tests available is getting ridiculous. Our breastfeeding rates had really begun to suffer, until we formalised the arrangement with the National Childbirth Trust, who now go in and assist with all breastfeeding.

Alison and Roger were anxious from the minute she conceived. They were convinced that there was something wrong with the baby. She had every antenatal test going and had ultrasound scan after scan. I really don't think they enjoyed the pregnancy at all. Anyway, I have had all the results back from the postnatal screen and everything is normal. But I just know that they will be worrying about something else now and will want to know if any more screening tests are available.

Limits to choice

This evening, at our local health group meeting, we will be discussing Donna, one of the women that I delivered about a month ago. Donna didn't come to prediction planning classes – she said she wanted to let nature take its course. Her little girl has Down's Syndrome. Donna loves her to bits and is delighted with her. The little girl will probably need quite a lot of medical and social intervention over the years and there is a debate about the funding. The health authority is arguing that as it has provided all the resources and technology to screen for potential disabilities, people have an obligation to take what is offered. As Donna chose to decline all screening services she must accept the consequences. The health authority argues that it cannot be expected to pay for the error of judgement that Donna has made. I expect part of the discussion will be about whether to introduce mandatory testing for a number of diseases. The debate will probably get quite heated.

I'll speak up for Donna, but I'm just one member of a large team. I wish we had debated these issues years ago. But then, few of us really believed that advances in genetics would have the impact that some were predicting. We thought it was all part of 'Millennium Fever'. Seems so long ago now – well, like last century!

BACK TO THE PRESENT

Where we are now

The desire for a healthy child is natural. The current high expectation of a 'successful' outcome has been fuelled by the high standard of care given to pregnant women during pregnancy and childbirth. The wide range of screening tests offered to women to assess maternal

Table 1.7.1 Points for discussion

Public access to information
Predictive planning and preconceptional care
The midwife's role in maximising health
Introduction of susceptibility testing within NHS
Communication of 'risk'
Availability of genetic tests through commercial avenues
Non-invasive technology to screen the fetus
Video consultations
Mandatory screening
Professional participation in debate

wellbeing, fetal development and fetal abnormality leads prospective parents to believe that any problems with the baby will be identified.[1] In the neonatal period, newborns are tested for a range of conditions such as PKU, hypothyroidism, cystic fibrosis and (in Wales) Duchenne Muscular Dystrophy. It is argued that knowledge about the likelihood of a child developing a disease or having an abnormality provides the opportunity for parents to plan for the future.[2]

The Human Genome Project (HGP) is well underway. It aims, by the year 2003, to identify the position of all the genes on a chromosome ('map') and to identify their chemical structure ('sequence').[3] Once the position of a gene for an inherited disorder has been located on a chromosome, tests can be developed to indicate an individual's risk of having that gene. When the gene itself has been identified, then a diagnostic test can be developed to detect the defective gene in the individual. It is anticipated that this will have a significant impact on clinical medicine and public health, as all the major genetic factors associated with human disease will be identified.

Breakthrough is close

It is already possible to identify the genes that predispose individuals to single gene disorders such as Huntington's disease and cystic fibrosis. The HGP has shifted attention now onto the common disorders such as cancer and diabetes. Increased understanding of the genetic component of these diseases means that in the near future it will be possible to:

- develop a new system of classification for diseases, based on an understanding of mechanisms as opposed to clinical appearance

- detect the onset of disease at an earlier stage than is currently possible. Predictive testing of asymptomatic individuals will help identify the lifetime risk of developing a particular disease, whilst the testing of symptomatic individuals will allow more accurate diagnosis and prognosis
- increase the opportunities for preventing the onset of disease – as knowledge increases about the interaction between genes and the environment it may be possible to predict and prevent the onset of disease by the modification of risk factors[4]
- provide new, better targeted and more effective treatment – ultimately, gene therapy.[5]

The impact on midwifery

The progress likely to be made in genetics and new technologies, driven by the Human Genome Project, may have a profound impact on midwifery practice m terms of:

- the emphasis on taking accurate family histories and understanding the implications of the data collected
- the number of screening tests offered to prospective parents, pregnant women and neonates
- the new taxonomy of disease and identification of subtypes leading to targeted care and treatment for pregnant women and their offspring.

With genetic advances will come dilemmas – for would-be parents, for prospective parents, for new parents and for midwives. With greater autonomy may come the 'burden' of choice. Midwives will need to develop further their knowledge of and skills in:

- genetic literacy
- understanding the advantages/disadvantages associated with testing
- understanding and communication of risk
- models of decision making and the psychology of decision making.

The scenario presented above seeks to explore some of the challenges that genetics and new reproductive technologies may pose for midwives in the millennium. Although speculative, it is based upon a review of the current literature, and it also incorporates some of the hopes, fears and concerns of professionals currently engaged in clinical practice and research. It is hoped that the scenario will be thought provoking and that it will stimulate professionals currently engaged in the delivery of care to women and their families to take part in the debate associated with genetic advances.

REFERENCES

1 Marteau T, Michie S. Genetic counselling: some issues in theory and practice. In: Marteau T, Richards M (eds). The Troubled Helix: Social and psychological implications of the new genetics. Cambridge: Cambridge University Press; 1996: 104–122.
2 Mahony C. A painful legacy. Nursing Times 1999; 20(95):26–27.
3 Zimmern R. The human genome project: a false dawn? BMJ 1999; 319:1282.
4 Bell J. The new genetics in clinical practice. BMJ 1998; 316:618–20.
5 Richmond M. The implication of genetics and genomics for health care and the pharmaceutical industry. London: University College London; 1999.

Reflecting on choice

- What are the barriers in your practice area to women 'getting their way' about informed decisions they have made? Are there ways in which some of these barriers could be overcome?
- What is your risk 'cut-off point'? (See this discussed in B Gail Thomas' article.) How does your concept of risk differ from that of your colleagues and friends? How might this impact on your practice?
- Are there any groups of 'minority' women in your area? Are there barriers to their making informed choices? What would be needed in order to break down these barriers?
- All midwives occasionally experience situations where a woman makes a decision that they feel is 'wrong'. How do you deal with this? How do you meet your professional obligations in these situations while remaining an advocate for the woman? How do you meet your own needs in debriefing and reflecting on these experiences?
- Have you ever been put in a situation where you are expected (either explicitly or implicitly) to 'persuade' women to make a particular choice? How have you dealt with this? What can you do to address any issues raised by this type of situation?

Group exercise

One of the things many midwives do over time is to develop 'spiels', or verbal packages of information about different choices (e.g. third stage management, vitamin K, antenatal screening tests) which they give to women at the appropriate time. Once developed, we tend not to vary these too much.

Fill a bag with index cards which have different topics written on them. Each midwife or student picks a card from the bag and writes on the card what she would say to a woman who needed to make a choice about that issue. (Writing this down makes it anonymous, although this can also be done verbally if the group is comfortable with this.) The cards are replaced in the bag and each can be pulled out and discussed.

There are two main questions that should be asked in relation to each spiel:

- Is this information as unbiased as it could be, or does it reflect the midwife's preference or opinion?
- Is this information based on current evidence, or does it need updating? (This updating could be undertaken by the group, who might then choose to develop information summaries for women and/or midwives.)

Pregnancy

If the principles of antenatal care came about as the result of poor health of men in the early part of the twentieth century, are these principles still relevant to the care and experience of pregnant women almost a hundred years on? How much of what we do is of real benefit to women and babies, how much is based on up-to-date and sound evidence, and how does what we do affect pregnant women and their babies? If women were asked to design their ideal antenatal visit with a midwife, how closely would it resemble what we actually offer women at this time?

One of the first things that happens at a 'booking' meeting between a woman and her midwife is the calculation of the date the baby is expected to arrive. For most midwives, this is a two-minute task, yet its effects are profound. The date which is chosen (and perhaps later amended) affects important issues which arise later in pregnancy, such as the possibility of induction and women's expectations about when pregnancy will end. Perhaps more importantly, the discourse which surrounds this calculation can either empower a woman in valuing her own knowledge about her body, or teach her that her knowledge is not as valuable as that offered by a cardboard circle or a machine. Tricia Anderson and Jilly Rosser explore the issues surrounding the calculation of a woman's expected date of delivery, and suggest ways of making this more accurate in the light of current evidence, including women's knowledge. Their articles act as a reminder that we often need to revisit the most fundamental issues in striving to improve practice.

Bridget Candy and colleagues also consider one of the most entrenched aspects of midwifery practice; the antenatal visiting schedule. These researchers note that, although one of their fears was that hypertensive disorders may be missed with a reduced schedule of visits, this fear was not borne out by the results of the research. We should remind ourselves that, although antenatal care is one of the mainstays of the system of 'midwifery care' which is offered in the UK, the physical checks which are carried out during visits are a relatively unevaluated set of screening tests, the use of which may or may not improve maternal and child health. In the case of pre-eclampsia, a number of diagnostic tests are also used and interpreted by midwives, and Kath McKay's article offers an overview and explanation of these.

Whatever the evidence on the effectiveness of screening tests, another important issue concerns our approach to women when carrying these out, and our understanding of how women are affected by what we say and do. Kate Olsen carried out a small study on abdominal examination, reflecting on her observations of other midwives and changing her own practice as a result. Midwives often comment that, once qualified, there is little opportunity to observe the practice of other midwives. As a result, we often develop routines in practice (which save valuable time) and become used to our own ways of doing and saying things. How often do we get the chance to observe our own or other midwives' practice from the perspective of an outsider, or the pregnant woman?

In analysing the effect of stress in the antenatal period on the health of babies, Vivette Glover shows that the evidence supports midwives' beliefs that a correlation exists between the two. Although Vivette's aim was not to explore sources of stress in the antenatal period, this is an issue which midwives also discuss. It is not as simple as looking at internal and external issues in women's lives outside of their contact with us, although this remains extremely important. In the context of our increasingly 'pick and mix' society, we are offering women a tremendous number of choices to make from their first contact with us. How much less stress is caused to women when we are enabled to carefully think out our words and actions?

Issues of sensitivity, choice and communication are also highlighted in Jenny Edwins' qualitative research with women who gave birth to babies with a diagnosis of Down's syndrome. One woman says that she and her partner were perceived as if 'we were from another planet' because they did not want to terminate the pregnancy. The implications which Jenny drew from her study are not only relevant in relation to the experience of these women, but can also be applied to many other situations where women are making difficult choices in pregnancy.

How to calculate an EDD

Tricia Anderson

In modern maternity care, the EDD (expected date of delivery) has become a critical piece of information. It determines whether the fetal size is 'right for dates', whether the pregnancy is premature or postmature, which place of birth is advisable and at what point induction of labour might be recommended. An inaccurate EDD on a woman's notes can expose her to inappropriate interventions and may alter her entire experience of pregnancy, labour and motherhood.

Working out the EDD

Calculating an EDD is more complex than it first appears. Given the tremendous implications for women and babies of even being a few days 'out' with an EDD, it behoves us to calculate the EDD as accurately as possible, based on a woman's full individualised history.

Taking a history

Taking a woman's history is an art. It relies on establishing a genuine dialogue between the woman and her midwife in an atmosphere of trust so that the woman will feel able to share intimate facts about her body and sexual life with someone she has never met before. In order to calculate an EDD the following points need to be discussed:

- Her menstrual history
- Any contraceptive history
- Physical signs of pregnancy, assessment of uterine size
- The woman's own knowledge of when ovulation or conception took place.

The woman may know exactly when sexual intercourse took place or when she ovulated, and this knowledge should be respected, whilst reminding her that conception can take place several days after intercourse. However, a woman's knowledge of her own body should never be dismissed; ovulation has been known to occur twice in one month and some women may have a sense that they became pregnant at a certain time. Looking at a calendar and going through family events, weekends, special occasions and so forth, may help a woman work out when conception is likely to have occurred.

Menstrual history

Ask the woman about the normal length of her cycle and the number of days her menstrual period usually lasts. The average length of a woman's menstrual cycle is 28 days, with ovulation taking place 14 days before menstruation. However, in a woman with a cycle longer or shorter than 28 days, ovulation will still take place 14 days before menstruation. For example, in a woman with a regular 35-day cycle, ovulation will take place 21 days after the LMP. Similarly, ovulation will take place ten days after the LMP in a woman with a 24-day cycle.

The commonly-used length of pregnancy is based on a regular 28-day cycle. Therefore it is essential that the EDD is adjusted according to the length of each woman's menstrual cycle. Women with cycles shorter than 28 days should have the difference subtracted from the EDD; women with longer cycles should have the difference added to the EDD.

This is an essential part of the calculation, which should be clearly documented in the notes. Simply reading an EDD from a plastic gestational calculator without making the appropriate adjustments for a woman's individual cycle will result in an inaccurate EDD. Sadly, many hospital notes do not include space for the justification behind the calculation to be explained, making it difficult for subsequent caregivers to confirm. Without such an explanation, a carefully calculated individualised EDD may be simply crossed out and replaced with one based on a 28-day cycle read from a gestational calculator by a midwife or doctor without the time to take a careful menstrual history.

Small, difficult-to-read gestational calculators are often inaccurate and may alter a woman's EDD by several days.[1] In maternity units where induction of labour is offered routinely at ten days post-term, even one or two days' difference can make a significant impact on the woman's care. Only large, clearly printed wheels should be used as an aid to calculating the EDD. Throw those small ones away!

Length of pregnancy

The woman should be asked for the date of the first day of her last normal menstrual period (LMP). It is important to ask specifically about the last normal period; if there is any doubt, ask her to describe her last two periods.

Was her most recent period at all unusual for her? A lighter and slightly earlier than usual bleed could be an implantation bleed. This occurs when the fertilised ovum embeds into the decidual lining of the uterus at five to seven days following ovulation, rather than being a full menstrual period. This means true menstruation will have occurred approximately three weeks earlier and thus the EDD needs to be calculated from the previous LMP date.

A light or unusual period might be the result of a missed abortion, especially if accompanied by diminishing physical symptoms of pregnancy. Immediate follow-up with an ultrasound scan or referral to a doctor or specialist early pregnancy clinic should be offered.

Jilly Rosser's article (reprinted as chapter 2.2 here) explains that the average pregnancy actually lasts longer than we thought. Naegele's rule consists of adding one year to the LMP, subtracting three months and adding one week. Some midwives may have been taught to add nine months plus seven days to the LMP. This in itself means the EDD will vary if the short month of February is included in the pregnancy.

However, Naegele's rule has now been challenged. A more accurate average length based on recent studies has been calculated to be 283 days (i.e. 40 weeks plus three days) from the LMP. Adding these three extra days will reduce the number of inductions for post-term pregnancy and makes EDDs based on an accurate menstrual history just as accurate as those based on ultrasound scans. Midwives might like to raise this issue at the appropriate multidisciplinary clinical practice meetings within their trust.

If the woman does not know her LMP, has a very irregular cycle or has not had a normal period since stopping the contraceptive pill or since her previous pregnancy (particularly if still breastfeeding), it will be impossible to calculate an accurate EDD. In this instance the use of ultrasound technology for an early dating scan may be advised.

Contraceptive history

Barrier methods of contraception or the non-hormonal interuterine device (the coil) do not affect the EDD. Women using natural family planning methods are likely to be able to tell you exactly when they ovulated. It is women who have just finished the oral contraceptive pill (either the combined pill or the progesterone-only pill) or the injectable or implanted hormonal contraceptive whose menstrual history will be affected. If they have just finished taking the pill within the last three months, their most recent vaginal bleeding may not have been a true menstrual period but a 'break-through' bleed. If a woman is not sure that her normal menstrual cycle has re-established since coming off the pill, then she may be advised to have a scan in order to be sure of her EDD. Women who have hormonal implants in situ will need referral to a doctor to discuss removal.

Signs of early pregnancy

These can be a useful double check to reaffirm how many weeks pregnant the woman is and may include:

0-8 weeks
- amenorrhoea
- breast changes, tenderness/tingling, increase in size or pigmentation of areolae
- nausea and vomiting
- tiredness

10-12 weeks
- enlargement of the uterus, just palpable above symphysis pubis
- fetal heart sounds first heard with hand-held fetal monitor
- frequency of micturition.

Other factors

It has been suggested that race, maternal height and parity have a bearing on the length of normal pregnancy (see chapter 2.2 in this book). We do not yet have enough information available to work out separate formulas for calculating EDDs in each of these groups. However, midwives might like to bear these issues in mind when advising individual women about induction of labour; a tall, white primigravid woman is likely to have a naturally longer pregnancy than a short, Afro-Caribbean multiparous woman.

Conclusion

Calculating an accurate EDD is a basic midwifery skill that must not get lost in a whirl of technology. With the detailed, modern knowledge of menstruation and ovulation and more accurate information about the length of normal human pregnancy now available to us, midwives can help women work out when their baby is due with just as much precision as by ultrasound technology.

The practice of crossing out a woman's own EDD (based on her knowledge of her own body and her own sex life) and replacing it with a date calculated by a machine can now be limited to those occasions when the LMP is not known with certainty. Dare we hope that the money wasted on routine dating scans will be diverted to fund resources which can really make a difference to the health of women and their babies?

REFERENCE

1   McPharland P, Johnson H. Time to reinvent the wheel. Br J Obstet Gynaecol 1993; 100:1061–1062.

Calculating the EDD
Which is more accurate, scan or LMP?

Jilly Rosser

There are many aspects of modern maternity care about which midwives feel uncomfortable – but foremost among them must be 'correcting' the expected date of delivery (EDD) of a woman who is sure of the date of her last menstrual period (LMP). We do this when an early ultrasound scan (USS) gives a different date to that calculated from her LMP, because research shows that dating by early USS is the more accurate of the two techniques.

Good news for uncomfortable midwives everywhere. What the research actually shows is that USS is only more accurate when the dating by LMP is done according to Naegele's rule. USS is no more accurate when dating by LMP is done with a formula based on more recent, large-scale research, which reveals that Naegele's rule is out by two to three days. It is just as accurate to calculate gestational length by adding three days to Naegele's formula and using the LMP, as it is to use an ultrasound dating scan.

A brief history

The precept that pregnancy lasts 280 days from the LMP is attributed to Aristotle (384-322 BC). Naegele's contribution (1778-1851) was to get around the irregularity of the Christian calendar by adding a rule of thumb for the practising midwife; to the last day of the LMP add seven days and nine months.[1] This is Naegele's rule. Depending on whether the shorter month February is included in the pregnancy, or whether the two consecutive long months July and August are included, whether it is a leap year etc., this corresponds to adding between 280 and 283 days, most commonly 280 days and on average 281 days. Naegele's rule has not been substantiated by any large-scale research.

It is curious that Naegele's formula has persisted into modern times as the gold standard, as there are a number of studies which show that it is not the most accurate.

The most robust of these is an observational study undertaken in Sweden, based on over 400,000 births.[2] This found that the average duration from LMP to birth is 283 days (according to the mode*).

Anecdotal evidence also lends credence to the practice of adding 283 days to the date of the LMP. In Denmark, older midwives report that their practice before routine ultrasound was introduced was to use Naegele's rule but with the modification of adding ten days instead of seven days. Although this practice is not described in Danish obstetric books, the old midwives explain that adding ten days was something they had learned from experienced midwives in the community.[3]

Post-term pregnancy

The only evidence-based benefit of routine ultrasound scans in early pregnancy is that they date the pregnancy more accurately and therefore lead to fewer inductions for post-term pregnancy than dating by LMP.[4]

But what would be the effect if dating by ultrasound scanning were to be compared with dating by LMP plus 283 days? This would not only make dating by LMP more accurate than it is now, it would make it just as accurate as dating by USS.[5] This is because, in the only study which has compared the actual date of delivery to EDD based on LMP and EDD based on a scan, it was found that the EDD based on a scan was, on average, two days late.[6]

Thus a clinically practical and accurate way to estimate the day of delivery is by LMP plus 283 days. Changing to this practice would reduce the number of inductions for post-term pregnancy, and thus remove the one benefit of routine scanning in early pregnancy.

The same rule for everyone?

What is still not clear is whether 283 days is the average length of pregnancy for all women, or whether gestational length is influenced by social, racial or obstetric factors. The evidence on this is sketchy.

Maternal height seems to be relevant – in the North West Thames region in 1988 the proportion of pregnant women undelivered by their EDD was strikingly influenced by maternal height. Less than 40% of women of a height less than 145cm, but more than 60% of women of a height more than 175cm, were undelivered by their EDD.[7]

A small US study found that the average length of pregnancy (median) for primigravidae was 288 days and for multigravidae 283 days.[8] A much older study (1867) estimated that the average pregnancy duration for a first birth was 284 days and for subsequent births was 281 days from LMP.[9]

In a comparison of black and white women of similar economic background, it was found that black women had an average (mean) gestational length 8.5 days less than for white women.[10] It has also been found to be shorter – 278 days – in Japanese women.[11]

The large study referred to above calculated that women aged 35 and over tended to give birth two days earlier than those below 35.[2]

None of this evidence is sufficiently robust to guide practice. More research is needed – a nice midwifery study crying out to be done.

When the LMP is uncertain

Not surprisingly, when the LMP is not known with certainty, the woman has recently used oral contraception, or her periods are not regular, then dating by USS is more reliable than using the LMP. The earlier in pregnancy the scan is done, the more accurate the result.

Conclusion

The widely held belief that USS is more accurate than LMP for dating pregnancy is based on an archaic method of calculating the length of gestation. It is time for Aristotle to move over, Naegele's rule to be rewritten, and three days to be added to the formula for calculating EDD.

An appropriate name for the resulting new formula would be Clausen's Guide, after Jette Clausen, the Danish midwife who has pioneered understanding in this area. And she wouldn't want it to be called a rule – she knows that the predicting of a date for delivery, even by the best way known to woman, is at best a guide.

- There are three types of average: median, mean and mode. In this case, because the distribution of the data is skewed to the left (owing to the number and timing of premature births) and the shape of the distribution graph is quite sharply peaked, the most appropriate average to use is the mode. (Personal communication. Tim Peters, Reader in Medical Statistics, University of Bristol.)

Acknowledgement: Much of the information on which this article is based is the work of Jette Aaroe Clausen, Danish midwife and Ole Olsen, Danish statistician.

REFERENCES

1 Naegele K. Lehrbuch der Geburtshilfe für Hebammen. Heidelberg, Germany; 1830.
2 Bergsjø P, Daniel W, Denman III, et al. Duration of human singleton pregnancy: A population-based study. Acta Obstet Gynecol Scan 1990; 69:197–207.
3 Personal communication. Kirsten Blinkenberg (Danish midwife since 1954).
4 Neilson JP. Routine ultrasound in early pregnancy (Cochrane Review). In: The Cochrane Library, Issue 4, 1999. Oxford: Update Software.
5 Olsen O, Clausen JA. Routine ultrasound dating has not been shown to be more accurate than the calendar method. Br J Obstet Gynaecol 1997; 104:1221–1222.

6 Backe B, Nackling J. Term prediction in routine ultrasound practice. Acta Obstet Gynecol Scand 1994; 73:113–118.
7 Saunders N, Paterson C. Can we abandon Naegele's rule? Lancet 1991; 337(8741):600–601.
8 Mittendorf R, Williams MA, Berkey CS, et al. The length of uncomplicated human gestation. Obstet Gynecol 1990; 75:929–32.
9 Ahlfeld F. Beobachtungen über die Dauer der Schwangerschaft. Monatsschrift für Geburtskunde und Frauenkrankheiten. Berlin: Verlag von August Hirschwald; 1869:266 305.
10 Henderson M, Kay J. Differences in duration of pregnancy. Arch Environ Health 1967; 14:904–11.
11 Saito M, Yazawa K, Hashiguchi A, et al. Time of ovulation and prolonged pregnancy. Am J Obstet Gynecol 1972; 112:31–38.

Antenatal visits

Bridget Candy   Sarah Clement   Jim Sikorski   Jenny Wilson

Ten years ago, pregnant women in Britain at low risk of developing complications in pregnancy and labour could expect to have about 13 antenatal check-ups. Now, the number of scheduled visits a woman receives often depends on where she lives. In 1997, the Audit Commission carried out a sample of hospital trusts and found that the recommended schedule of antenatal checks for women with uncomplicated pregnancies varied, with different trusts recommending different numbers of checks.[1] This variation may be the result of differing levels of awareness of the research evidence and recommendations, or it could be due to different interpretations of the evidence.

From its inception in the late 1920s, the UK pattern of four-weekly antenatal visits from booking to 28 weeks, then fortnightly to 36 weeks and weekly from then on, has rarely been questioned. But in the 1980s, Marion Hall and her colleagues in Aberdeen undertook a retrospective study and found that, when a reduced schedule of antenatal visits was introduced, it seemed to be as safe as the usual, higher, number of visits.[2] In 1982, the Royal College of Obstetricians and Gynaecologists recommended that maternity providers review the number of antenatal visits for low-risk women.[3] However, this recommendation was never widely implemented until it was repeated a decade later in the Department of Health's report, *Changing Childbirth*.[4] At this time, there was a clear need for more evidence about the effectiveness and acceptability of reduced antenatal visit schedules.

Although randomised controlled trials (RCTs) cannot answer all health research questions, they are generally considered to be the best research design for comparing effects of different interventions, such as antenatal visit schedules.[5] A well-conducted RCT has several important advantages over other types of studies. Controlling for bias and confounding permits an RCT investigator to compare like with like (in this case two groups of women) more reliably than any other research

methodology, as the results are less likely to be affected by different characteristics between the groups.

The Antenatal Care Project

The first British, or indeed European, RCT that compared a reduced schedule of antenatal visits with a traditional schedule was undertaken in South East London. This project, known as the Antenatal Care Project, has been reported in full elsewhere.[6] The schedules compared were 13 visits, referred to as 'traditional care', and a reduced schedule of seven visits for nulliparous women or six visits for multiparous women, referred to as 'new-style care'. Information was gathered from the women's clinical notes and from postal questionnaires sent to the women antenatally and postnatally. 2,794 women participated (26% declined: the most common reason for not taking part was that they did not want to have fewer visits). 73% of women who took part completed at least one of the two study questionnaires. The number of visits a woman received was more similar than intended for the two groups; those in the traditional group had on average 11 as opposed to the intended 13, and those in the new-style group had nine, as opposed to the intended six and seven visits.

A wide range of clinical maternal, fetal and newborn outcomes was assessed. Probably the greatest concern to the researchers was that pregnancy-related hypertensive disorders (PRHD) would be detected late, or missed, resulting in increased morbidity. The incidence of Caesarean section for PRHD was considered to be a reasonable proxy measure for this morbidity.

The group of women allocated to the traditional schedule was compared to those allocated to the new-style schedule. For all clinical outcomes, no statistically significant difference between the two groups was found. The Caesarean section rate for PRHD was 1% in the traditional group and 0.8% in the reduced schedule

Table 2.3.1 Clinical outcome of reduced antenatal care visits versus standard antenatal care visit schedule

	No. in sample	No. of visits achieved in standard schedule	No. of visits achieved in reduced schedule	Clinical outcome
Walker et al (US, 1997)	81	11	8	Same
Sikorski et al (UK, 1996)	2,794	11	9	Same
McDuffie et al (US, 1996)	2,764	15	12	Same
Munjunja et al (Zimbabwe)	15,994	6	4	Better
Binstock et al (US, 1995)	549	11	8	Same

Table 2.3.2 Acceptability and psychosocial outcomes outcomes of reduced antenatal visits versus standard antenatal visits schedule

	Acceptability	Psychosocial outcome
Walker et al (US, 1997)	Better	Same
Sikorski et al (UK, 1996)	Worse	Worse
McDuffie et al (US, 1996)	Same	–
Binstock et al (US, 1995)	Same	–

Table 2.3.3 Keypoints from RCTs

In general the studies have shown that, for low risk women, a small reduction in the number of antenatal visits does not appear to affect the clinical safety of women or babies.
There remains an unproven risk that very rare, but dangerous, outcomes may be missed.
It would appear, in the long term, that reduced schedules do not have a negative effect on psychosocial outcomes, but they may result in women being less satisfied.

group (this is not a statistically significant difference). There were, however, some differences in process outcomes. Those in the traditional schedule had more day admissions and more ultrasound scans, and were also more often suspected of carrying a fetus that was small for gestational age. This suspicion was unfounded as no difference was found between the groups in the number of babies of low birth weight. The project, therefore, concluded that the two schedules appeared to be equally safe for the physical outcomes examined.

Other RCT results

There are four other published RCTs that have explored the effect of reducing antenatal visit schedules for low risk women.[7-10] Clinical outcomes measured were similar to those measured in the ANCP, and included preterm delivery, low birth weight, Caesarean section, apgar score, number of days in neonatal intensive care and pregnancy-induced hypertension. The trials were not undertaken in Britain, and their conclusions are not entirely translatable to a British population. Table 2.3.1 summarises the sample size and intervention details, and compares their results and those of the ANCP for clinical outcomes of a reduced antenatal visit schedule versus the standard antenatal visit schedule.

Only one trial found a difference in clinical outcomes between a reduced and a traditional schedule of visits. In Munjunja's trial, women following the reduced schedule had fewer cases of hypertension.[9] The authors suggest that this is because there was less opportunity for measuring blood pressure and therefore small or transient rises were not noted. This may indicate, as the ANCP found for the measurement of gestational age, that more visits led to over-diagnosis. Alternatively, it may reflect a lower diagnostic rate but if it did, there is no evidence in either study of any detrimental effect on clinical outcomes. However, women in Munjanja's trial booked at a median of 28 weeks' gestation which may have had the effect of not including women who developed very early onset pre-eclampsia and eclampsia, a group with high perinatal and maternal mortality and morbidity.

Although, overall, clinical results for the trials were consistent, these trials varied in quality. Binstock's study, for example, did not use true randomisation.[7] Also, only one trial managed to achieve the intended reduction in the number of visits.[9] This is likely to be because more women booked later in this trial than the others, allowing less time for any deviation from the study's protocol.

Systematic reviews are a useful way of summarising RCTs undertaken in an area. They are reviews that incorporate strategies to minimise bias and to maximise precision, thus enabling an overall conclusion to be reached from all the research. All of the trials considered in this paper have been included in a Cochrane systematic review.[11] This review concluded that a small reduction in visits for low-risk women could be implemented without any adverse clinical perinatal outcome.

Rare dangerous conditions

Despite there being no reported adverse effects of reduced schedules, care must be taken in concluding that less antenatal care is just as safe clinically. The questions of how few visits would be clinically safe, and whether dangerous conditions could be missed, remain. Even though the RCTs in total involved over 20,000 women, this number is not large enough to detect small overall changes in perinatal or maternal mortality. Furthermore, even though the World Health Organisation is currently conducting a larger RCT in developing countries with well-established maternity services, this large trial is not expected to have sufficient power to determine any differences in maternal or perinatal mortality.[12]

Psychosocial outcomes

Antenatal services should be acceptable to the women who use them, therefore it is important to look at women's views. Antenatal care, as we know, also has non-clinical functions, such as providing information, support and reassurance. The ANCP, and all but one of the other RCTs, explored women's views about different antenatal care schedules. In the ANCP, seven of the eight questions used to assess maternal satisfaction showed that women receiving the traditional schedule were significantly more satisfied. The ANCP also explored a wide range of psychosocial measures. There was evidence of some poorer outcomes in women allocated to the reduced schedule. They were significantly less likely to feel listened to at antenatal visits, tended to describe their babies more negatively in pregnancy and postnatally, and were more worried during pregnancy about their baby thriving, and postnatally about coping with their babies. No differences were found between the groups in the incidence of depression.

The acceptability and psychosocial outcomes of the studies are more varied than the clinical ones (as shown in Table 2.3.2). This may reflect many factors. For example, as the studies were undertaken in different countries, there are cultural and social differences between the study populations. The maternity services will also be structurally different in each study site. As already mentioned, all studies suffered some methodological problems which may account for some of the variation in these outcomes.

In addition, unlike the clinical outcomes, the way different studies gathered women's views varied greatly. In the ANCP, for example, various scales and questions were used to assess depression, worry and anxiety, while the only other trial that explored psychosocial effectiveness[10] measured anxiety only.

In McDuffie's trial[8] women completed questionnaires in the clinic as opposed to in the privacy of their own home. People are much more reluctant to express dissatisfaction in a clinic. In the four studies that reported the numbers of women who declined, all found that a large proportion declined (26% in Sikorski's,[6] 30% in Walker's,[10] 33% in McDuffie's[8] and 52% in Binstock's[7]). If the most common reason women declined to take part was that they did not want fewer visits, it means that those who are more favourably disposed to reduced schedules are more likely to be over-represented in studies with high numbers of decliners.

The Cochrane systematic review also evaluated satisfaction. The authors concluded that the evidence of the four trials supported the policy of reducing the number of antenatal visits but that this policy is likely to lead to some women being somewhat disappointed.[11]

Long-term effects

The fact that women in the reduced schedule group were more worried about their babies and saw them more negatively led to concern about the possible long-term effects of reduced visit schedules. The Antenatal Care Project Follow-Up Study, designed to investigate this possibility, was completed in 1998.[13]

The study looked specifically at whether there were any long-term effects on the mother-child relationship, maternal psychological wellbeing and the woman's and her child's use of the health services. 1,117 women returned the questionnaire. After adjusting for women who were untraceable, this equates to a response rate of 61%. The questionnaires were completed on average 2.7 years after the birth of the child. The study found no differences in any of the outcomes assessed between those who were allocated to the new style of visits and those to the traditional schedule of visits. However, the results of this study should be viewed with some caution since about 40% of the original sample were lost to follow-up.

Other research and issues in this area

Women's expectations and dissatisfaction

Incidences of dissatisfaction found in the ANCP survey may be related to women's expectations; people tend to be happier with existing care than with new forms of care.[14] We do not know whether dissatisfaction would persist if new-style care became the norm. This possibility is supported by a small survey undertaken in Bedfordshire.[15]

The survey showed that when a reduced schedule of visits was introduced, the proportion of women who found it acceptable increased over time. Before the reduced schedules were introduced, 80% of women were against it. After the reduced schedules had been running a year, the number against it had fallen to 45%. However, around half the women who took part remained dissatisfied after the reduced schedule was established as the norm. Care must be taken in interpreting these results, as the response rate when women were questioned for the second time was relatively low, at 44%.

Nevertheless, dissatisfaction is not entirely determined by women's expectations, since the analysis of the ANCP data showed that women reporting no prior expectation about the number of visits they would receive were still dissatisfied with fewer visits.[16]

Styles of delivery of care

Although there are some concerns about the psychological effect of reducing the number of antenatal care check-ups, this may not mean that the standard number of visits should be retained. Women's psychological needs may be better met by other means. Research undertaken recently in Sweden found that reduced schedules were acceptable to women; although women were given every chance to have extra visits if requested, only a few did.[17] The researchers suggested that the need for self-initiated extra visits was limited because women had enough time with their midwife to meet their need for information and communication. Every woman had her own personal midwife and was encouraged to contact her whenever she wanted. Perhaps this type of care goes some way to fulfilling a woman's psychological needs, and could be classed as individualised care. Others have suggested the provision of drop-in clinics as a way to meet women's psychological needs.[18] In the ANCP it was found that 89% of women said they would welcome a drop-in clinic. However, these options may have disadvantages. Some women may not want the responsibility of choosing when to initiate extra care. Also, those most in need of high quality care are often the least likely to receive it.[19,20]

Conclusion

Research has not been able to provide a definitive answer to the question of what is the most appropriate schedule of antenatal visits women at low risk of complications should follow. All published RCTs have found that traditional and reduced schedules have similar clinical outcomes. In fact, a reduced schedule may be better clinically for some conditions as there appears to be less over-diagnosis of certain problems. On the other hand, there is still a possible risk that a serious problem may be missed.

The pooled results of research that explored non-clinical factors were less clear. It could be argued that the ANCP is the most relevant project to the UK, as it is the only one undertaken in this country. It was also the only study that used a wide range of questions and psychological scales to measure satisfaction, worry, anxiety and depression. It is reassuring that in its follow-up study, the negative psychological outcomes found amongst women following the reduced schedule were no longer apparent approximately two-and-a-half years later. It is possible that dissatisfaction is transient and may decrease as reduced schedules become the norm, as the Bedfordshire study suggests. Also, as the study in Sweden concluded, if women feel supported by having care more individually tailored and have open access to midwifery care, then a reduced schedule may be more acceptable.

Research is a useful guide in planning the most appropriate number of antenatal visits. Questions remain, but further research will bring us nearer to the answers.

REFERENCES

1   Audit Commission. First class delivery: Improving maternity services in England and Wales. Abingdon: Audit Commission Publications; 1997.
2   Hall M, Chng P, Macgillivray I. Is routine antenatal care worthwhile? Lancet 1980; 2:78–80.
3   Royal College of Obstetricians and Gynaecologists. Report from the RCOG working party on antenatal and intrapartum care. RCOG: London; 1982.
4   Department of Health. Changing Childbirth. London: HMSO; 1993.
5   Jadad A. Randomised Controlled Trials. London: BMJ Books; 1998.
6   Sikorski J, Wilson J, Clement S, et al. A randomised controlled trial comparing two schedules of antenatal visits: The antenatal care project. BMJ 1996; 312:546–553.
7   Binstock MA, Wolde-Tsadik G. Alternative prenatal care: Impact of reduced visits frequency, focused visits and continuity of care. Journal of Reproductive Medicine 1995; 40:507–512.
8   McDuffie RS, Beck R, Bischoff K, et al. Effect of frequency of prenatal visits on perinatal outcome among low-risk women. JAMA 1996; 275:847–51.
9   Munjanja SP, Lindmark G, Nystrom L. Randomised controlled trial of a reduced-visits programme of antenatal care in Harare, Zimbabwe. Lancet 1996; 348:364–9.
10 Walker DS, Koniak-Griffin D. Evaluation of a reduced-frequency prenatal visit schedule for low-risk women at a free-standing birthing centre. Journal of Nurse-Midwifery 1997; 42:295–302.
11 Villar J, Khan-Neelofur D. Patterns of routine antenatal care for low-risk pregnancy. Neilson JP, Crowther CA, Hodnett ED, et al. Pregnancy and Childbirth Module of the Cochrane Database of Systematic Reviews. In: The Cochrane Library, Issue 4, Oxford: Update Software; 1999.

12 Donner A, Piaggio G, Villar J, et al. Methodological considerations in the design of the WHO Antenatal Care Randomised Controlled Trial. Paediatric and Perinatal Epidemiology 1998; 12 suppl 2:59–74.
13 Clement S, Candy B, Sikorski J, et al. Does reducing the frequency of routine antenatal visits have long term effects? Follow up of participants in a randomised controlled trial. British Journal of Obstetrics and Gynaecology 1999; 106:367–370.
14 Porter M, MacIntyre S. What is, must be best: A research note on conservative or deferential responses to antenatal care provision. Social Science and Medicine 1984; 19:1197–1200.
15 Johnson G. Changing to 'new style' antenatal care. British Journal of Midwifery 1998; 9:564–7.
16 Clement S, Sikorski J, Wilson J, et al. Final report of the Antenatal Care Project, Department of General Practice and Primary Care, Guy's, King's and St Thomas' School of Medicine, 1994 (unpublished data included with permission from the authors).
17 Berglund AC, Lindmark GC. Health services effects of a reduced routine programme for antenatal care: An area-based study. European Journal of Obstetrics, Gynaecology and Reproductive Biology 1998; 77(2):193–9.
18 Lobo A. Too much of a good thing? The case for a reduced schedule of antenatal visits. The Practising Midwife 1998; 1(4):19–21.
19 Brown S, Lumley J. Antenatal care: A case of the inverse care law? Aust J Publ Health 1993; 17:95–103.
20 Hemmingway H, Saunders D, Parsons L. Women's experiences of maternity care in East London: An evaluation. London: Directorate of Public Health, East London and City Health Authority; 1994.

Maternal stress or anxiety during pregnancy and the development of the baby

Vivette Glover

We have recently carried out a study of 100 mothers at Queen Charlotte's Hospital, at 32 weeks' gestation, and shown that those who were most anxious had impaired blood flow through the uterine arteries. This may help to explain why the babies of very anxious mothers tend to be smaller or born earlier.

We have also shown that there is a strong correlation between plasma levels of the stress hormone cortisol in the mother and in the fetus. If the pregnant mother has raised cortisol, this may have a direct effect on the development of the fetal brain, and affect the child's later responses to stress.

Introduction

It is a common belief among both mothers and midwives that if the mother is stressed or anxious during pregnancy, this can affect the baby. However this has not yet had much effect on clinical practice. This is partly because we do not understand the scientific basis of any possible links. Also, there have been no controlled trials to establish what type of intervention would be best. Does anxiety early in pregnancy have the worst effect, or is it more important at the end? Would relaxation therapy be beneficial? All these questions need to be answered. We have recently been carrying out research to try to understand the biological basis of the mechanisms by which maternal mood might affect the development of the baby.

Background

Several studies have shown that the babies of stressed or anxious mothers tend to have significantly lower average birthweight for gestational age, and be born earlier.[1] This is a difficult area of research, with many possible confounding factors, such as parity, age, smoking, social class and so on. However, the more recent studies have controlled for these factors. One large, thorough study compared the outcome for mothers who had severe stress during pregnancy, such as the death of a close relative, with matched controls.[2] The babies in the stressed mother group were born with a smaller average head size and a worse neurological score. This study thus shows that maternal stress during pregnancy appears to affect the development of the baby's brain.

There was also an effect on birthweight. The effect on body size was comparable to that of maternal smoking: an average reduction of about 250g. Barker and his co-workers at Southampton have shown that lower birthweight, across the whole range, is in itself associated with health problems in later life, such as hypertension and ischemic heart disease.[3] Thus if mothers who are anxious have babies that are only somewhat smaller this can have implications for the later health of the population.

There are a few studies which have looked at the longer term effects of maternal antenatal stress or anxiety on the behaviour of the child. Although these studies have been retrospective and have not controlled for possible mediating factors such as alcohol or smoking, the evidence does suggest that there may be long-term effects on the children's behaviour. Stott assessed infant morbidity in a randomly-selected population and related this to maternal stress during pregnancy.[4] He found a highly significant correlation between the maternal stress and infant problems such as eczema, poor growth, late development and also early behavioural disorders. The infants of the most stressed mothers were described as restless, clinging and hyperactive. Meier studied the early behaviour of children born to mothers who were pregnant during the Six Day Arab-Israeli war with a similar group born one or two years later.[5] He found that the first group had significant delays in developmental milestones such as walking, and they were also more antisocial, tense and easily irritated.

Animal studies

The possibility that there may be long-term behavioural problems for the children needs to be taken seriously because of the very strong evidence from animal studies. Much research on both rats and monkeys has shown that stressing the mother during pregnancy can both reduce birthweight and permanently affect the behaviour of the offspring. If a monkey is stressed during mid to late gestation by exposure to unpredictable noise, the offspring themselves have a heightened response to stressful situations later, producing elevated levels of cortisol. They were less adaptable to novel situations. The authors say that the behaviour of these monkeys was similar to that of children classed as 'difficult'.[6]

Many effects of prenatal stress on the babies have been described in rats. The male rat offspring of stressed mothers have been reported to show feminised behaviour, and female offspring later show altered maternal behaviour, together with other changes in exploration and aggression.[7] A sexual difference in response to prenatal insults is a common finding, with males generally being the more strongly affected.[8]

Maternal stress has been shown to have a permanent effect on the corticosterone receptors in the rat fetal brain. This could explain the long-term alterations in stress responses. The fetal brain is in a constant state of development and, as we know, is readily affected by outside influences such as drugs. It appears that it can also be permanently affected by the hormonal environment.

Mechanisms

There are several mechanisms by which maternal stress or anxiety might affect the fetus. Raised hormone levels in the mother may be transported directly across the placenta. There may also be impaired blood flow to the baby through the uterine arteries. We have studied both these possible mechanisms in women.[9,10]

STUDY ONE

Placental transfer of hormones

It is generally thought that the placenta is a very effective barrier to chemicals, such as stress hormones, in order to protect the fetus. Indeed it is very rich in protective enzymes. However, few studies have been able to compare hormonal levels in both mother and fetus at the same time. We were able to obtain some extra blood when fetuses were being sampled for clinical investigation, and obtained maternal samples at the same time. Blood from abnormal fetuses was not used. We found that maternal levels of cortisol were about ten times higher than those in the fetus, but that there was a highly significant correlation between the two: $r = 0.63$ ($p<0.0001$). This is compatible with substantial (80-90%) metabolism of maternal cortisol during passage through the placenta, but as fetal levels are naturally much lower, a contribution of 10-20% extra from the mother could still double fetal levels.

This correlation between maternal and fetal cortisol may help to explain the mechanism by which antenatal maternal stress affects fetal development, especially the glucocorticoid system in the fetal brain.

STUDY TWO

Impaired uterine blood flow linked with maternal anxiety

The aim of this study was to test the hypothesis that anxiety in pregnant women is associated with abnormal blood flow in the uterine arteries. This was assessed by using colour Doppler ultrasound to measure the Resistance Index and the presence of notches in the waveform pattern. A notch indicates particularly high resistance to blood flow. These parameters have previously been associated with adverse obstetric outcome, particularly intrauterine growth restriction and pre-eclampsia.

One hundred non-smoking women, with no medical complications, were recruited at parentcraft classes. Immediately before their Doppler ultrasound examination at a mean gestational age of 32 weeks, the mothers completed a questionnaire. This was the two-part Spielberger, which measures both State Anxiety (how you feel right now) and Trait Anxiety (how you generally feel). Doppler recordings were obtained on videotape and later analysed by the same operator blind to the results of the questionnaires.

There was a significant association between the uterine artery resistance index and both State and Trait Anxiety ($rs = 0.31$, $p<0.002$ and $rs = 0.28$, $p<0.005$ respectively). When the groups were divided into two, using the predetermined cut-off of 40, women in the raised State Anxiety group had significantly worse uterine waveform patterns than those in the lower anxiety group. Using Trait Anxiety (>40), there were also differences between high and low anxiety groups, but they were somewhat less significant.

Of the more anxious group, 4 of 15 (27%) had a mean uterine artery resistance index (0.68 (a level of clinical concern) compared with 3 of 85 (4%) in the less anxious group ($p<0.01$). Those with a notch were also significantly more anxious.

This study demonstrated an association between anxiety and raised or impaired uterine artery resistance index, thus showing that the most anxious women had the worst blood flow to the baby. Whichever way we analysed the data, women with raised anxiety were more likely to have abnormal uterine artery blood flow parameters than those with lower anxiety. This association was more pronounced for State than Trait Anxiety. However, there were more women in the raised Trait than raised State group, and this study was not able to determine whether it was anxiety early in pregnancy or later that caused the abnormal blood flow.

Discussion

Impaired uterine blood flow is generally considered a chronic phenomenon, predominantly due to failure of placental trophoblastic invasion in early pregnancy. However, this may not always be the case. It is possible that later changes in uterine blood flow also occur – such as might be associated with transient maternal hormonal changes, as shown in animal models.

We do not know whether the associations we have demonstrated between anxiety and Doppler pattern are acute or chronic. Although in our study the associations were stronger for State than Trait, the top 15% with either score were largely the same patients, and they had similarly abnormal waveform patterns. Further work is needed to determine whether overall anxiety during pregnancy or even prior to or at conception, might affect uterine artery blood flow patterns, or instead, whether the association is only with the current emotional state. It is also possible that there is some underlying factor which causes both increased anxiety and diminished trophoblastic invasion.

It is unlikely that our subjects had any particular reason to be concerned about the progress of their pregnancy, as those with pre-eclampsia or intrauterine growth retardation, known before the Doppler scan, were excluded.

We do not know what causes the impaired uterine artery blood flow but an obvious candidate mediator is noradrenaline. High scores on the Spielberger State Anxiety questionnaire are associated with raised plasma noradrenaline levels. Also, infusion of noradrenaline decreases uterine blood flow both in pregnant sheep and guinea pigs. In sheep, reproductive tissues, including the uterus, were more sensitive to the vasoconstrictive effects of noradrenaline than other body tissues.

Although there are many contributors to fetal growth and birthweight, reduced blood flow through the uterine arteries could partially explain why women who are anxious during pregnancy tend to have smaller babies.

Conclusion

There is increasing evidence that if mothers are very anxious or stressed while pregnant it can have an adverse effect on the development of the baby. We have recently found two biological mechanisms by which these effects may be mediated. Midwives who have contact with women throughout their pregnancy should be in a good position to identify women at risk. Much more research is now needed to find out effective interventions for reducing stress and anxiety and improving outcome.

REFERENCES

1 Wadwa PD, Sandman CA, Porto M, et al. The association between prenatal stress and infant birth weight and gestational age at birth: a prospective investigation. Am J Obstet Gynecol 1993; 169:858-865.
2 Lou HC, Hansen D, Nordenfoft M, et al. Prenatal stressors of human life affect fetal brain development. Develop Med Child Neurol 1994; 36:826-832.
3 Barker DJP. Fetal origins of coronary heart disease. BMJ 1995; 311:171-174.
4 Stott DH. Follow-up study from birth of the effects of prenatal stresses. Develop Med Child Neurol 1973; 15:770-787.
5 Meier A. Child psychiatric sequelae of maternal war stress. Acta Psychiatr Scand 1985; 72:505-511.
6 Clarke AS, Schneider MI. Effects of prenatal stress on behaviour in adolescent rhesus monkeys. Ann NY Acad Sci 1997; 807:490-491.
7 Insel TR, Kinsley CH, Mann PE, et al. Prenatal stress has long term effects on brain opiate receptors. Brain Res 1990; 511:93-97.
8 Grimm VE, Frieder B. Differential vulnerability of male and female rats to the timing of various perinatal insults. Int J Neurosci 1985; 27:155-164.
9 Gitau R, Cameron A, Fisk A, et al. Fetal exposure to maternal cortisol. Lancet 1998; 352:707-708.
10 Teixeira J, Fisk N, Glover V. Association between maternal anxiety in pregnancy and increased uterine artery resistance index: cohort based study. BMJ 1999; 318:153-157.

Biochemical and blood tests in midwifery practice

1: Pre-eclampsia

Kath McKay

Pre-eclampsia continues to be a major complication of pregnancy. Hypertensive disorders,[1] of which pre-eclampsia is one, accounted for 20 direct deaths in the most recent triennial report (1994-1996);[2] the second largest cause of maternal death.

The midwife has an important role in the care of women with pre-eclampsia, both in the early detection of abnormal clinical signs and continuing care once a diagnosis has been made.[3,4] As part of this role, midwives should provide information to women and their partners and monitor the care prescribed by the medical team.

An important component of this care is the battery of tests ordered by the medical staff, often with little explanation to the women concerned. This article aims to explain the basis for such tests, clarifying the relationship between the test undertaken and the disorder of pre-eclampsia.

By understanding the rationale for a test and the significance of the result, the midwife is better equipped to provide information and monitor the appropriateness of the care provided. However, it must be always be borne in mind that the test results need to be viewed in conjunction with other clinical findings such as blood pressure (BP), urinalysis and the fetal condition. Midwives should remember that how a woman feels, and any symptoms she may have, are also important in providing information about her condition.

A brief description of the pathophysiology of pre-eclampsia is given first, to aid understanding.

Pathophysiology of pre-eclampsia

Pre-eclampsia is defined here as: 'A condition characterised by hypertension, proteinuria and evidence of systemic dysfunction'.[5] To date, the underlying cause of pre-eclampsia is uncertain.

In normal pregnancy, changes in the blood vessels at the site of the placenta prior to 20 weeks allow adequate placental perfusion. However, in women with pre-eclampsia these changes do not occur (or do not occur adequately) and there is consequently a reduced blood flow to the placenta. The resulting 'ischaemic' placenta is thought to produce a substance or substances that cause the systemic disease. This factor, Factor X,[6] then causes widespread constriction of capillaries and damage to their endothelial lining in several body systems. This theory helps explain why the delivery of the placenta following birth improves the woman's condition.

Hypertension and proteinuria are the commonest signs of pre-eclampsia, although rarely it presents without these signs.[5] However, because of the potential of the disorder to affect almost any body system, other tests are utilised to aid diagnosis and assess the progress of the condition. The biochemical and blood tests that follow are not a definitive list, but are frequently used to provide information on the systemic effects of pre-eclampsia.

Haematological tests

- **Haemoglobin (Hb)**: In normal pregnancy, an apparent decrease in Hb levels is observed, due to the dilution effect of an increase in the plasma volume.[7] In women with pre-eclampsia, the expected plasma volume increase is impaired,[5] consequently affecting the Hb estimation. Additionally, if the disease progresses, Factor X is thought to damage blood capillaries, which causes them to become 'leaky' and fluid moves from the blood vessels to the extravascular areas.[6] Consequently the blood becomes even more concentrated and the Hb result will reflect this. Therefore a raised Hb (expressed as g/dl) is considered a rough but useful indicator of reduced plasma volume. Sibai et al[8] found that plasma volume is normal in women with mild disease and decreased plasma volume is associated with severe disease.

Table 2.5.1 Blood indices – examples of normal ranges in pregnancy

Test	Range	Comments
Haemoglobin	11-13g/dl[16]	lowest Hb at 32/52, when plasma volume maximal[7]
Haematocrit	0.33-0.39(l/l)[16] 0.31-0.34(l/l)[7]	variations found in normal pregnancy[7]
Platelets	150-400x10⁹/l[16]	day to day variations[9]

- **Haematocrit (Hct):** This test also provides an indication of the level of haemoconcentration as a consequence of reduced plasma volume. A high haematocrit is suggestive of hypovolaemia and is associated with an increased incidence of adverse perinatal outcome,[9] perhaps because of the reduction in available blood volume for placental perfusion. No exact Hb/Hct level can define significant haemoconcentration. Dekker and Walker[9] suggest that serial measurements are useful for monitoring the course of the disease, as various factors can influence Hb levels, e.g. maternal smoking and iron deficiency.

- **Platelets:** Platelet consumption has long been recognised as a feature of pre-eclampsia – platelet levels

are thought to decrease because they are used in aggregation following damage to the endothelial cells of the capillaries. Significant thrombocytopaenia is taken as <100x10⁹/l and is associated with severe disease.[10] It is below such levels that effects on bleeding times have been found and associated with low grade disseminated intravascular coagulation (DIC).[11] As there can be day-to-day variations in platelet counts, serial measurements are considered more informative. Examples of normal ranges are provided. Results outside these may be considered 'abnormal' but should not be considered in isolation. This applies to all the ranges cited.

Liver function tests

Pre-eclampsia has the potential to affect most body systems and liver function tests can reflect any hepatic impairment. It has been suggested that hepatic involvement is common and has serious implications for the severity of the disease process.[9] The origins of the dysfunction are thought to be due to vasoconstriction of the blood vessels and endothelial damage. Altered liver function tests may be part of the HELLP (haemolysis, elevated liver enzymes, low platelets) syndrome.[12]

Table 2.5.2 Liver function tests – examples of normal ranges in pregnancy

Test	Range	Comments
AST	40u/l[15]	serum levels usually remain unchanged in normal pregnancy[13]
ALT	40u/l[15]	levels unchanged in normal pregnancy[13]
alkaline phosphatase	60iu/l – 1st trimester[15] 80iu/l – 2nd trimester[15] 140iu/l – 3rd trimester[15]	increase in 3rd trimester due to placental alkaline phosphatase[13]
total albumin	34g/l, decrease to 28g/l at term[15]	often performed in conjunction with total protein
total bilirubin	17µmol/l[15]	

Table 2.5.3 Renal function tests – examples of normal ranges in pregnancy

Test	Range	Comments
Plasma creatinine µmol/l	65 – 1st trimester[14] 51 – 2nd trimester[14] 47 – 3rd trimester[14]	large variations in values within 24 hour period limits use of the result[14]
Creatinine clearance mls/minute	130 – 1st trimester[15] 142 – 2nd trimester[15] 120 – 3rd trimester[15]	less useful as renal function test if pre-existing renal disease or reduced renal output[16]
Serum uric acid µmol/l	0.28 – 16/52[9] 0.39 – 36/52[9]	serial measurements more informative. level >350µmol/l = hyperuricemia[9]
Urea mmol/l	3.5 – 1st trimester[15] 3.5 – 2nd trimester[15] 3.1 – 3rd trimester[15]	values >4.5mmol/l, need to assess renal function further[14]
Total urinary protein	upper limit of 250mg in 24 hours[1]	>500mg 'abnormal'[14]

- **Aspartate transaminase (AST)**: This enzyme is involved in cellular metabolism, as part of aerobic respiration in the cells. It is found in high concentrations in the liver, heart, muscle, kidney, pancreas and red blood cells. Therefore if any of these areas are damaged, the blood levels of the enzyme will increase. As this enzyme is present in several tissues, the test is not specific for liver function.[13]

- **Alanine transaminase (ALT)**: This enzyme is involved in cellular respiration. However, it is found at low levels in other tissues, except in the liver. High levels are therefore considered relatively specific for hepatic damage.

The levels of both AST and ALT normally remain unchanged in normal pregnancy.

- **Alkaline phosphatase**: This enzyme is involved in cellular metabolism and is present in nearly all tissues. The serum alkaline phosphatase activity changes in many diseases affecting liver function. In pregnancy, the levels of the enzyme increase from the first trimester and reach up to 3 times female non-pregnant levels by late pregnancy, but this is due mainly to placental phosphatase.[13] In the care of women with pre-eclampsia, exaggerated increases in alkaline phosphatase activity may point to both placental and hepatic damage.[9]

- **Total albumin**: Plasma albumin is only synthesised in the liver and therefore is useful as an indicator of liver function. In normal pregnancy, the observed decrease in albumin levels is caused by an increase in plasma volume and not as a result of liver insufficiency. In pre-eclampsia, however, low levels of albumin may be the result of protein lost via proteinuria. A reduced albumin level may be clinically important, as serum albumin influences the movement of fluid within the blood capillaries and levels less than 20g/l have been associated with pathological oedema.[9]

- **Total bilirubin**: Serum bilirubin levels do not usually rise in pre-eclampsia, unless the condition is complicated by the HELLP syndrome.[9]

Renal function tests

- **Creatinine clearance**: This test provides information about the volume of plasma completely cleared of creatinine per unit of time, expressed in millilitres/minute. The clearance rate is used to assess the glomerular filtration rate (GFR), which gives an indication of renal function. It is usually assessed via a 24-hour urine collection, because variations are known to occur throughout the day.[14] In normal pregnancy, the creatinine clearance values mirror the changes in the GFR and increase until late in the third trimester.[15] In pre-eclampsia, creatinine clearance values may be reduced as a consequence of a fall in GFR, the extent of which depends on the degree of renal involvement.

- **Serum creatinine**: Creatinine is a waste product of protein metabolism and is excreted via the kidneys, by glomerular filtration. As it is linked to protein metabolism, the levels can be affected by the amount and timing of ingested protein, e.g. cooked meat, or a vegetarian diet.[14] In normal pregnancy, an increase in GFR is associated with a fall in serum creatinine levels, as it is excreted more efficiently. In pre-eclampsia, renal function may be impaired due to vasoconstriction and hypoperfusion (via Factor X), resulting in a reduced GFR.[16] The serum levels are usually estimated sometime within the 24 hours of the urine collection for creatinine clearance and will show raised levels if renal function is impaired.

- **Plasma uric acid (urate)**: This is the end product of protein metabolism. It is normally excreted by the renal tubule and has become used as a marker to 'diagnose' pre-eclampsia. Redman and Roberts[17] suggest levels are always raised in pre-eclampsia and elevated results may precede the appearance of proteinuria. High levels are also associated with poor fetal outcome.[12] Some healthy women may have high levels due to diet, and a single random measurement is of no use clinically.[14] Therefore serial measurements are used to monitor progress in women with pre-eclampsia.

- **Total urinary protein**: Even when the kidneys are functioning properly, low levels of protein will be measurable in a urine sample taken during pregnancy. The loss of excess protein from the kidneys (significant proteinuria) is thought to occur through damaged endothelial cells in the kidney. This process is sometimes referred to as 'leaky' capillaries. A total urinary protein value greater than 500mg/l in a 24-hour urine collection is considered to be clinically important, and is associated with severe disease.[10]

- **Urea**: Urea is a by-product of protein metabolism. Raised levels are indicative of impaired renal function, and provide additional information when assessing the extent of renal dysfunction.[10]

- **Electrolytes**: There is little evidence to support the use of electrolyte levels in diagnosing or assessing the progress of pre-eclampsia.[9]

Conclusion

In contemporary obstetric practice a variety of tests are ordered by medical staff to monitor the progress and severity of pre-eclampsia. The reference ranges vary and each maternity unit should have guidelines/protocols available to inform decision making. While all the tests have their limitations, they are useful in assessing a woman's condition and provide an important part of the information required by obstetricians when considering whether to intervene in a pregnancy to deliver the baby.

Results indicating hypovolaemia, hyperuricaemia, significant thrombocytopaenia and raised liver enzymes (see tables) are associated with severe disease and adverse outcomes for women and the fetus/baby.[9] However these need to be considered together with blood pressure levels, response to antihypertensive therapy, clinical symptoms and fetal condition.

With greater understanding of these tests, midwives will be better placed to provide women with accurate information and to monitor the care they receive.

REFERENCES

1 Davey DA, McGillivray I. The classification and definition of the hypertensive disorders of pregnancy. Am J Obstet Gynecol 1988; 158(4):892-898.

2 Sallah K. An introduction to the report on maternal deaths. Br J Midwifery 1998; 6(12):772-774.

3 Bennett P. Pre-eclampsia II: the midwife and detection. Mod Midwife 1994; 2(9): 20-22.

4 Bennett P. Pre-eclampsia IV: the midwife's role after diagnosis. Mod Midwife 1995; 3(1): 25-26.

5 Roberts JM, Redman CWG. Pre-eclampsia: more than pregnancy-induced hypertension. Lancet 1993; 341:1447-1454.

6 Walker JJ, Dekker GA. The etiology and pathophysiology of hypertension in pregnancy. In: Walker JJ, Gant NF (eds). Hypertension in pregnancy. Oxford: Chapman and Hall; 1997:39-75.

7 Letsky EA. The haematological system. In: Chamberlain G, Broughton Pipkin F (eds). Clinical physiology in obstetrics, 3rd edn. London: Blackwell Science; 1998:71-110.

8 Sibai BM, Anderson GD, McCubbin JH. Eclampsia II: clinical significance of laboratory findings. Obstet Gynecol 1992; 59:153-157.

9 Dekker GA, Walker JJ. Maternal assessment in pregnancy induced hypertensive disorders. In: Walker JJ, Gant NF (eds). Hypertension in pregnancy. Oxford: Chapman and Hall; 1997: 107-161.

10 Broughton Pipkin F. The hypertensive disorders of pregnancy. Br J Med 1995; 311:609-613.

11 Ballegar VC, Spitz B, Kiechen L, et al. Platelet activation and vascular damage. Am J Obstet Gynecol 1992; 166:629-633.

12 Mushambi MC, Halligan AW, Williamson K. Recent developments in the pathophysiology and management of pre-eclampsia. Br J Anaesth 1996; 76:138-148.

13 McIntyre N, Rosalki S. Tests of the function of the liver. In: Williams D, Marks V (eds). Scientific foundations of biochemistry in clinical practice, 2nd edn. Oxford: Heinemann; 1994:383-398.

14 Baylis C, Davison JM. The urinary system. In: Chamberlain G, Broughton Pipkin F (eds). Clinical physiology in obstetrics, 3rd edn. London: Blackwell Science; 1998:263-307.

15 Ramsay MM, James DK, Steer PJ, et al. Normal values in pregnancy. London: WB Saunders; 1996.

16 Tucker Blackbun S, Loper D. Maternal, fetal and neonatal physiology: a clinical perspective. Philadelphia: WB Saunders; 1992: 336-378.

17 Redman CWG, Roberts JM. Management of pre-eclampsia. Lancet 1993; 341:1451-1454.

From a different planet

Women who choose to continue their pregnancy after a diagnosis of Down's Syndrome

Jenny Edwins

Seven years ago, while working as a community midwife, I met a woman who decided to continue her pregnancy after the baby she was carrying was found to have Down's Syndrome (DS).

Despite the fact that approximately 50 couples make this choice every year in the UK, neither I nor any of my colleagues had first hand experience of a similar scenario. The literature virtually ignored the option to continue a pregnancy. One study from the US[1] surveyed parents who had continued their pregnancies after diagnosis of DS, but the paper didn't tell me how the parents felt about their experiences because the emphasis was on the role of amniocentesis and the likelihood of its uptake in future pregnancies. Watkins[2] offered anecdotal evidence relating to continuation of pregnancies with lethal abnormalities, but the couple that I knew were anticipating a lifetime for a child with special needs, not his death in infancy.

A mountain of research-based information exists about the difficulties that women face when they choose termination of pregnancy (TOP) for fetal abnormality, but it was as if other options were unthinkable.

This clear gap in the knowledge on this subject provided me with the rationale to undertake a qualitative study that asked the question: 'What is it like for women who choose to continue a pregnancy to term, knowing that their baby has Down's Syndrome?'

Methodology

Science and technology develop through quantitative research and the generation of 'hard' facts. This positivist paradigm should be balanced by qualitative inquiry that explores the impact of medical developments upon the individual. Nurse and midwife researchers began to adopt phenomenological methods of inquiry in the early 1980s[3,4] and this approach was the appropriate one for seeking answers to my research question.

Spiegelberg[5] defines phenomenology as 'A philosophical movement whose primary objective is the direct investigation and description of a phenomenon as consciously experienced, without theories about their causal explanation and as free as possible from unexamined preconceptions and presuppositions.'

In other words, phenomenology is a way of getting inside other people's heads and accepting their view of the world, without judgement. Edmund Husserl (1859-1938) is considered the founding father of phenomenology. He developed a method that used the concept of 'bracketing' to clear the researcher's mind of his or her everyday biases that might influence a study. Current-day qualitative researchers often reject bracketing as being too mechanical and difficult to achieve. Reflexivity has developed as an alternative, which accepts that researchers bring many aspects of themselves to any situation. If they stand back and reflect upon their own history, they can acknowledge any potential for distortion of the data collected and their subsequent analysis.[6] It seemed impossible for me as a researcher/practitioner to suspend many years of clinical experience and motherhood. I therefore relied heavily upon a reflexive approach to make my own feelings explicit.

Sampling

In the absence of an existing sampling frame for the women that I wanted to meet, I enlisted the help of the Down's Syndrome Association. Their newsletter published a short article outlining my proposed research project. Five women volunteered to help and I knew, from past experience, that this number would generate a considerable amount of information. As a small, non-probability convenience sample there was no potential for the generalisation of findings, but generalisation is not the aim of phenomenological inquiry. All of the women were educated and articulate, over 35 years of age and married. Their children with DS were between one and five years old, alive and well and living at home. Four out of the five had older siblings.

In view of their age, three women had chosen maternal serum screening (MSS) as a procedure that would help them to decide upon the necessity for amniocentesis. The decision to undergo amniocentesis after a high-risk result seemed to follow almost inevitably. The other two women declined MSS but accepted detailed ultrasound scanning (USS) in the second trimester as part of the 'package' they had experienced in previous pregnancies. Both were opposed to TOP for moral and religious reasons, but accepted amniocentesis as a means of finding out more about the health of their babies once USS had identified physical markers.

Ethics and interviewing

Ethics Committee approval was sought and gained from the University of Central England. Interviewing can create ethical problems and measures were taken to minimise risks for the participants. Long interviews can provoke an outpouring of suppressed emotion; while this may be healing, it can also cause unresolved conflicts to resurface. Patton's[7] advice – to debrief women after the interview with a telephone call – was followed.

Webb[8] analyses the relationship between the researcher and the researched from a feminist perspective, and concludes that it can never be equal. Although being reflexive is a strategy that social researchers use to work towards equalising their relationship with the women who participate in qualitative research, it became clear to me as the interviews progressed that fundamental inequalities remained. For instance, Barbara talked at length about her future and the difficulties she envisaged in coping with a child with special needs. I recognised her need to talk and made time for her to do so, but then used prompts to bring her back to the subject of her pregnancy. After the interview I felt uneasy at my ability to manipulate the course of events to meet my own needs as a researcher. Data had to be collected relating to a particular period of time and this focus drove me to meet my goal. The relationship between interviewer and interviewee can never be equal, but reflexivity and reflection were used to maintain awareness of the potential that the researcher holds to manipulate.

Findings

Analysis of the data resulted in an interpretation of the context of the women's experiences, which I then sought to link in with existing theories. This descriptive approach allowed the women to speak for themselves and for the reader to get a feeling for the diversity of experience, as well as the similarities. Each interview highlighted particular aspects of the decision to continue the pregnancy, and brief excerpts from the narratives will serve to draw out some of the key issues.

Alice used to work in a hospital laboratory and knew about the concept of risk in relation to MSS. Screening, for her, was an opportunity to acquire information rather than a route to the termination of a less-than-perfect baby. A high-risk result from MSS tipped Alice into a frenzy as she tried to find out all she could about DS to inform her choice if the amniocentesis proved positive. Her frustrations grew as her questions were dismissed during the scan following amniocentesis:

'When I asked about DS we were told 'don't worry, go home and forget about it – you don't need to find out anything yet – try to put it out of your mind'. It's not realistic to say that! You're at high risk so why not find out about DS now? If people ask for information they should give it. I was frustrated and angry.'

Kirkham[9] suggests that the false reassurance of telling women 'not to worry' is akin to telling them to 'shut up'. It undermines the individual and closes down channels of communication at times when the need for open discussion is greatest. Poor communication skills compounded feelings of isolation. Eve described a total lack of support:

'...because there just wasn't a system for us to fit neatly into now.'

Hospital staff caring for Diana displayed insensitivities that Buckman[10] describes as 'therapeutic impotence':

'The hospital saw the amnio as a choice. If it was good it was good – if it was bad it was gone. We were unique to them – everyone else had gone through with termination – we were from another planet.'

Ultrasound scanning played a large part in clinching the decision to carry on, as women sought information about the baby's physical health. Alice's account of a detailed cardiac scan illustrates the power of the technology in facilitating bonding. At the point of having this scan, she was undecided about her choice:

'I used to think 'he's dying', and part of me hoped that when I went for the cardiac scan there would be massive inoperable defects. Part of me hoped that nature had got it wrong but was going to finish the job off – it wasn't my decision really. And that was also the thing with the amnio, that if I have a miscarriage the decision would be taken out of my hands. So we went for the scan and he was really lively, really busy, fit and healthy. He looked fine. As I watched him I was surprised but pleased. He seemed very real after that scan and we were very protective. His name was B.'

Positive experiences from scanning were universal in

strengthening feelings of certainty that the decision to carry on with the pregnancy was right for each woman. This essence of certainty was also heavily supported through ethical and religious beliefs, age, or a difficult reproductive history. Certainty was strong enough to lock out any hint of guilt or regret in relation to decisions that had life-long sequelae for whole families. It could be seen as a mechanism that gave the women the conviction and inner strength to make a decision that runs contrary to the expectations of much of society.

Grieving and coping

Parents of children with disabilities often grieve for the loss of the 'normal' child that they anticipated at the beginning of pregnancy.[11,12] However, there is no visible death or the accompanying rituals such as sympathy cards and a funeral that bring acknowledgement of loss. The grief felt for the loss of the anticipated child is conceptual. He, or she, has been replaced by a different individual with very special needs. The initial shock and grief for the idealised baby turned to a lingering sadness for Barbara, as she contemplated the real difficulties that her child would have whilst growing up:

'Yeah, it's the death of the normal child you wanted so much, but this is not something you can go through within a short period of time. Since my mother died I've been learning how to cope with her death – it's something you have to do for the rest of your life. I'll be learning how to cope with A's special needs for the rest of my life, not only in practical terms but in emotional terms. Life will be very difficult for her and me.'

The realisation that life will be hard for the mother as well as the child leads on to a previously little acknowledged focus for grief:

'I'm grieving for myself actually. The whole of my future changed. I expected my children to leave home – I didn't expect it at this level – the whole of my life. I'm very sorry for myself – it's not what I saw for my future.'

Alice continues by describing how difficult it was to make her feelings known:

'I thought, why can't you tell what I'm feeling like inside? It was very unfair – I didn't give them any clues whatsoever. I hated this person that I was. I hate Down's Syndrome. I've been depressed ever since – I hate it.'

Society has a particular yardstick for the attributes that a 'good' mother possesses. This feeds the potential for psychological disturbance as the end product of unresolved guilt and grief.[13] Greater insight of a woman's grief for the changes in her own life might result in support that is more realistic and meaningful. Referral to skilled counsellors might be appropriate in helping some women to acknowledge and work through deep-seated and difficult feelings.

Coping strategies during the last half of a pregnancy were influenced by patterns of grieving. Some women moved on very quickly; grief was short-lived and adjustment focused upon looking forwards, making plans for meeting the special needs of the baby. Others were overwhelmed by the prospect of the many challenges that they would face for many years to come, and became depressed. These findings mirror a survey by Damrosch and Perry[14] who identified two types of adjustment in parents who unexpectedly had babies with Down's Syndrome. They describe a straightforward, linear adjustment that was more common in fathers, and a pattern of peaks and troughs of chronic sorrow that mothers seemed to experience more frequently. The women in my study reported both types of adjustment. The influences that determine which pattern a woman might follow could include the level of external support from family, professionals and the wider community and the intrinsic moral and religious beliefs of the woman herself. The nature of support varied enormously with examples of good and bad from professionals, family, and friends alike. Support was seen as effective when the woman's autonomy was acknowledged and her decision accepted without judgement:

'My GP was quite important for me. I'd decided to have the baby but was thinking about adoption. I was feeling guilty. She said 'I know a woman whose son had Down's Syndrome and she gave him for adoption because she couldn't cope. If you do it, it will be OK'. I thought that was so good.'

Criticism relating to professional support centred mainly upon 'the system'. When staff had no frame of reference there was lack of a clear plan of care and feelings of isolation were intense:

'You just seem to fall out of the system – there's nothing there apart from the underlying assumption that that one would terminate.'

'We were completely unique to them and they were ill prepared. Everybody else had gone through with a termination – we were from another planet. I tried very hard to find someone who'd had this experience and there was no one.'

Time to prepare

The period of time from diagnosis of DS to the birth day was identified as a valuable opportunity to prepare practically and emotionally. Even when grief was prolonged and difficult, positive aspects of knowing in advance were acknowledged – Chitty et al[5] came to the same conclusion in their study of parents who carried on with pregnancies after diagnosis of lethal fetal abnormalities.

Alice made plans for known midwives to deliver her son. She didn't want to be stereotyped as 'the Down's delivery in room 3'. When Eve's baby was transferred to a specialist hospital shortly after birth she felt that the period of preparation time helped her to cope with the separation. Diana rationalised that she and her husband were fortunate in knowing about DS in pregnancy and compared their position to that of other parents who wait for a diagnosis as their child grows over months or years:

'We've got a good idea of what the future holds for us. I feel privileged – we've had so much preparation time. She's lovely – we love her to bits.'

There is a powerful argument against denying women diagnostic tests unless they make a prior commitment to TOP. The parents valued the tests as a way of finding out about the health of their babies. Preparation time didn't appear, in this study, to have any negative aspects.

Summary and implications for practice

This study aimed to generate an understanding of a minority experience, using a phenomenologically-inspired approach. The experiences which these five women shared with me so generously can only be described superficially in this brief article. The findings are ungeneralisable, and further research into areas such as the quality and nature of professional support would be valuable. Despite these limitations, the study gives rise to some implications for midwifery practice:

- Most of the women had unfulfilled needs for support. Midwives are in a position to provide this and can improve 'the system' from within if they formulate support mechanisms that facilitate the processes of decision making, grieving and coping.

- The gold standard of truly autonomous and informed choice is the goal. An awareness of your own history and feelings about antenatal screening and disability can identify potential biases before you enter into counselling situations.

- To communicate sensitively it is wise first to identify a woman's beliefs and to know her reproductive history. She may be able to recount her rationalisation for decision making. Building up a bigger picture of what this choice means for an individual will help you to offer realistic support.

- Give women information when they want it. It should always be readily accessible. Think about the function of screening and diagnostic tests. Some women want to use tests to acquire more information about a pregnancy and not as a route to TOP.

- Identify a plan of care to prevent feelings of isolation. Continuity of midwife and consultant obstetrician carers will be valued. Look beyond the postnatal period and link with health visitors and other agencies sooner rather than later.

- Look at the service that your unit provides for women participating in screening. Scrutinise it and then be proactive in addressing shortcomings.

- Be aware of the differing facets of grief that may emerge, and support or refer appropriately.

- Ask yourself whether you know enough about DS.

The author acknowledges the assistance of The Smith & Nephew Foundation and also wishes to thank Sheila Hunt for her support.

REFERENCES

1 Palmer S, Spencer J, Kushnick T, et al. Follow up survey of pregnancies with diagnoses of chromosomal abnormality. Journal of Genetic Counselling 1993; 2(3):139-151.
2 Watkins D. An alternative to termination of pregnancy. Practitioner 1989; 233:990-992.
3 Oiler C. The phenomenological approach in nursing research. Nursing Research 1982; 31(3):178-181.
4 Omery A. Phenomenology: A method for nursing research. Advances in Nursing Science 1983; 5(2):49-63.
5 Spiegelberg H. Doing phenomenology. The Hague: Nijhoff; 1975.
6 Renzetti CM, Lee RM. Researching sensitive topics. California: Sage; 1993.
7 Patton M. Qualitative evaluation and research methods. California: Sage; 1990.
8 Webb C. Feminist research: Definitions, methodology, methods and evaluation. Journal of Advanced Nursing 1993; 18:416-423.
9 Kirkham M. Communication in midwifery. In: Alexander A, Levy V, Roch S (eds). Midwifery practice: A research based approach. London: MacMillan; 1993.

10 Buckman R. How to break bad news: A guide for healthcare professionals. London: Papermac; 1992.
11 Farnham R. Grief work with mothers. Issues in Mental Health Nursing 1988; 9:72-82.
12 Davis H. Counselling families of children with disabilities. In: Davis H, Fallowfield L (eds). Counselling and communication in healthcare. Chichester: John Wiley; 1991.
13 Jones M. Mothers who need to grieve: The reality of mourning the loss of a baby. BJM 1997; 1(4):478-481.
14 Damrosch SP, Perry LA. Self reported adjustment, chronic sorrow, and coping of parents of children with Down's Syndrome. Nursing Research 1989; 8(1):25-30.
15 Chitty LS, Barnes CA, Berry C. Continuing with a pregnancy after diagnosis of lethal abnormality: Experience of five couples and recommendations for management. BMJ 1996; 313(7055):478-80.

'Now just pop up here, dear...'

Revisiting the art of antenatal abdominal palpation

Kate Olsen

Some time ago, I asked a group of women in an antenatal class what they thought about abdominal palpation, and they told me in no uncertain terms that they didn't enjoy it at all! They said that being palpated was not in general either a pleasant or a positive experience. A few women did find the examination reassuring in some way, but the majority of women I asked told me how impersonal, intimate and even painful the procedure was. They also described how the communication styles of midwives and doctors often left them more worried than reassured.

Their comments surprised me; midwives think of abdominal palpation as a routine assessment that we carry out daily at every antenatal appointment or admission to the labour ward. Yet from a woman's point of view it is an intimate, physical and often unpleasant examination she experiences at least a dozen times during the course of her pregnancy, over which she has little choice or control.

After reflecting on these comments, I decided to spend several mornings observing an antenatal clinic. This is what I found.

The examination

Each midwife had her own little 'catchphrase' which she used to ask the woman to lie on the examination couch. 'Can I get you to hop on my couch?' 'Can I get you to jump up?' 'Now just pop up and lie down here for me, dear.' No explanation was offered concerning what they were about to do, or why they wanted to do it. Neither were women given any sort of option to decline.

The women all complied with the request to lie down on the couch without demur. Some immediately revealed their bare abdomens, without being asked to do so, even when the midwife was still on the other side of the room. The majority lay waiting for the midwife to tell them what to do, and looked a little awkward when asked to reveal their naked abdomens.

'Let's just have a look then.' 'Can I see your tummy?' One woman replied 'If you must!' a little sarcastically. This slight discomfiture was apparent in women even in the last few weeks of pregnancy, when they had been palpated many times before.

None of the midwives asked if the woman needed to empty her bladder before the abdominal examination, as is recommended practice.[1] None washed their hands before or after the examination. Most made no attempt to check that the woman was comfortable, nor did they try to minimise exposure/maximise modesty by covering the woman's legs.

During the palpation, the midwives gave little feedback. Many faced away from the woman whilst doing the palpation without giving any eye contact. No attempts were made to check whether they were feeling too firmly or were making the woman uncomfortable in any way. Yet as they were having their abdomens palpated, the women wore expressions of puzzlement, concern and occasional discomfort. None of them smiled.

At some stage during the palpation, the midwives asked the only question, 'Feeling baby move?', and then said 'Let's listen to baby's heart, shall we?' At the end, they said 'All right – you can sit back down now'. During the palpation, women looked towards the midwife's face with an enquiring expression, but did not ask any questions or volunteer any unsolicited information.

The midwives all then wrote up their findings in the women's notes, using common professional abbreviations, without explaining to the women what they were writing.

The midwives

I asked a group of community midwives how they thought the women found the experience of being palpated. They, like me, had assumed that it was an enjoyable part of the antenatal consultation.

Women said...

I like hearing the baby's heartbeat, especially for the first time

Some of the hospital doctors and nurses are really rough – I felt quite bruised afterwards

I felt very vulnerable, especially when it was someone I didn't know

I didn't really like anyone touching me or my baby

I never really knew what they were looking for

They always say 'it's fine'; but you never know what's really happening

I suppose it's reassuring to know the baby's OK

It's nice to know which bump is what!

I always ask which way the baby is lying

You get used to being prodded and poked by the end of it all

It felt quite impersonal – you know, next bump please...

I don't really like showing my rolls of fat to anyone

When they push down for the baby's head, it really hurts – they really dig in

They kept on saying that the baby was going to be a good size... that worried me

It's a bit personal, isn't it – you know, they pull your knickers down and dig in

The midwife always has cold hands – and some of them have really long nails – one of them scratched me

Midwives said...

I think women like to know how the baby's doing

They like to hear the heartbeat, don't they

They like to know what position the baby's in

It's reassuring for them

I don't know – I've never thought about it

A woman-centred approach

My observations suggest that we need to think about it, as there seems to be a significant difference of opinion between what midwives percieve and what women experience. So how can we make our practice of abdominal palpation more woman-centred?

Following my small investigation, I have tried to alter my practice to be more woman-friendly by thinking what I am trying to achieve during a palpation. Midwifery textbooks give the following clinical aims of abdominal examination, with which we are all familiar:

- to observe signs of pregnancy
- to assess fetal size and growth
- to assess fetal health
- to diagnose the location of fetal parts

- to detect any deviation from normal.

But, as well as these clinical aims, a woman-centred approach to palpation can also provide the opportunity to:

- establish trust between a woman and her midwife
- promote bonding between a woman and her baby
- support a woman's belief in her ability to grow and nurture her baby, and in the normality of birth
- encourage a woman to respect, marvel at and delight in her own body
- acknowledge a woman's expertise in her baby's health
- show respect for and further a woman's belief in herself as an independent, autonomous adult.

Choice

The first issue is one of choice. I had never offered women any choice at all as to whether they wanted to have an abdominal examination (which is, if we think about it, a fairly inaccurate screening test of sorts!). I had developed the habit of using closed questions which left no room for answers or discussion. If informed choice is to become a part of maternity care, who decides the areas in which it is suitable for women to exercise 'choice'? And is it acceptable to perform any care as 'routine'?

So now I start by acknowledging that the woman is the expert in her baby's wellbeing – it is, after all, growing and moving inside her body – and ask her how the baby has grown since her last antenatal appointment and what position it is in. Small but important changes in the phrases I use hopefully communicate that I am trustworthy and respect her: 'Would she like me to feel the baby?' 'May I touch...?'. I wait for her answer before beginning. This seems particularly important when feeling in the pubic region for the engagement of the fetal head. I try to be more attentive to a woman's comfort and privacy, making sure I offer her the opportunity to empty her bladder.

When actually performing the palpation, I watch the woman's reaction and ask her to stop me if it is too hard or uncomfortable. I describe what I am feeling as I go, and use my finger to draw an outline of the baby on her abdomen. I tell her that now the baby is so many inches long, and how long its thigh bones are (this information is printed on my gestational calculator so I don't have to remember it!). I talk to the baby as well, to acknowledge its unique existence. I ask the woman if she would like to feel for herself, and take her hands so that together we feel the various parts of the baby. Partners and other children often get involved as well.

Would she like me to listen to the fetal heart and, if so, would she prefer I use a Pinard or Sonicaid? Throughout, my intention is to make the woman feel completely in control and the orchestrator of what is happening. I want her to go away with the impression that midwives are people who respect women and who can be trusted.

Communication

Abdominal palpation is intended by the midwife to confirm normality, and she may believe it to be reassuring. However, the very act carries with it the underlying message that things might not be going well, for why else carry out an examination? If women are made to worry about their ability to grow and give birth to a healthy baby by this simple examination ('I worried about it after that'), then we need to develop sensitive communication skills to reassure them.

The language we use is crucial. Phrases such as 'A big baby', 'Growing really well', or 'On the small side' can frighten women and significantly dent their belief in their ability to give birth successfully. I've opted for 'Not too big; not too small – just perfect'! I try to use lots of positive words and phrases as recommended by Caroline Flint.[2] I have also incorporated optimal fetal positioning[3] into my practice and so we talk a lot about the importance of fetal position, how it changes near term and how a woman can influence it if she understands the dynamics of her body.

When I document my findings, I always show the woman what I am writing and explain any terms I have used such as '2/5s palpable'. I haven't gone as far as writing 'head down' instead of 'cephalic', but maybe I should?

Positive change

Abdominal palpation is an integral part of midwifery care and the temptation is to carry it out by rote. It is also, as Elizabeth Davis says, 'A very pleasurable and important part of midwifery practice'[4] and something which I think many midwives enjoy doing. But it also offers a creative opportunity to develop a positive relationship with a woman and her baby; the manner in which it is done has implications for the whole of her pregnancy and birth.

Re-visiting how I carry out this intimate examination and realising that many women find it quite unpleasant and uncomfortable has altered my practice. The changes I have made are only small and they take up no more time, but I think they have made a significant improvement on my relationship with the women I care for.

REFERENCES

1 Thomson V. Antenatal care. In: Bennett VR, Brown LK (eds). Myles textbook for midwives. Edinburgh: Churchill Livingstone; 1989.
2 Flint C. Sensitive midwifery. Oxford: Heinemann; 1986.
3 Sutton J, Scott P. Understanding and teaching optimal fetal positioning. Tauranga: Birth Concepts; 1996.
4 Davis E. Heart and hands – a midwife's guide to pregnancy and birth. Berkeley, CA: Celestial Arts; 1998.

Reflecting on pregnancy

- How can we focus on the knowledge women have of their bodies, pregnancies and babies, in the midst of technology which purports to know more and better? How can we use this knowledge to assist us in practice?
- How can we help women to value the knowledge they carry in their own minds and bodies? Can we use the work which is being carried out in other fields on body wisdom and emotional anatomy to enable women to become more in tune with their own pregnancies, feelings and needs?
- Can midwives make opportunities to observe colleagues' practice and reflect on this experience?
- What is the purpose of each of the basic screening tests that we carry out as part of the 'antenatal check' (e.g. blood pressure, urinalysis, abdominal examination)? Is there evidence to support the use of each of these interventions? Do they carry risks? How can we present these as informed choices for women, rather than foregone conclusions?
- What is in place locally and nationally to support women who are making 'unusual' choices? Are you able to point women in the direction of support groups or organisations that can help talk through the decisions women face during pregnancy?
- How are you calculating women's expected dates of birth? How much weight is put on the woman's knowledge and her individual cycle? Is there provision in the area where you work to consider the latest evidence in this area and – if appropriate – to modify the tools used? How can this be put on the local agenda?

Group exercise

This exercise requires a brave student or midwife (!) and a supportive environment. Set up a role-play where one midwife carries out a 'booking' discussion with a woman (played by another midwife or student). To make this as realistic as possible, use whatever records or notes are used locally to trigger questions and record information gathered from the 'woman'. Observers can take notes of what is said and reflect upon how the drama unfolds. Discussion afterwards can focus on how far the woman's needs and choices were met, and how both the 'midwife' and 'woman' felt during the experience.

If no one wants to begin as the 'midwife', another way of doing this is to go through the records and discuss how you would phrase questions to women in order to gain the necessary information, and offer options without making your own feelings about the 'best' choice obvious.

Focus on:

Antenatal education

SECTION CONTENTS

Early pregnancy sessions
A formative evaluation

Alison Ward

An evaluation of team midwifery in Newcastle[1] found that women were of the opinion that they did not receive sufficient antenatal care in early pregnancy. In response to these views, early pregnancy classes were established to meet the needs of some women who felt they required early contact with midwives for the purposes of being given advice, support and information in the first trimester of their pregnancy. This paper discusses the planning, implementation and evaluation of these early pregnancy classes.

Although there is no single accepted definition of team midwifery[2] the Newcastle Team Midwives are responsible for a defined caseload of women registered with identified GP practices. The midwives take responsibility for the majority of their care during the antenatal, intrapartum and postnatal periods. The Gosforth Team covers four general practices with a caseload of 140 and 160 women per annum. The whole of the team midwifery service was evaluated in 1997 and included users' views of midwifery provision.[1] This evaluation highlighted a shortfall in the provision of midwifery contact and access by women to information and advice in the early part of their pregnancies.

The need to provide advice about health and behaviour in the early part of pregnancy had already been identified in an Audit Commission report.[3] The executive summary to this report stated, 'the views of the service users should be taken into account when planning services'. Service user involvement in service planning and evaluation is now a central tenet of all NHS policy.

Clearly a shortfall in early antenatal provision in Newcastle was mirrored across the country. These findings inspired us to develop early pregnancy classes.

Although antenatal education programmes are widely established,[4] research evidence regarding their effectiveness is not clear-cut. Antenatal education has been the focus for research for many years[5] and in the late 1970s and early 1980s there was a plethora of published work on antenatal education looking at efficacy and effectiveness[6,7,8] and most is not particularly positive.[9]

However, it appears that due to the complex nature, often disparate aims and a shift in emphasis, it is difficult to make generalised statements regarding antenatal education as a single entity without consideration of every attendee's individual needs.

Literature about early pregnancy advice and support to women is even sparser. The few articles found were mainly in North American literature.[10-13] This literature advocates the importance of early pregnancy classes but offers no evidence about their usefulness.

Development of sessions in Newcastle

Women on the team caseload were invited to attend a first class by individual letters and posters displayed within their general practices. The initial class and all subsequent classes have been held in the local health centre, providing a safe, secure and comfortable environment. The first class was offered to women up to and including the first 20 weeks of gestation. As the frequency of classes increased, women were offered attendance following booking, and enabling access from earlier stages of their pregnancy. For the first class a loose programme was devised to include the following topics:

Health promotion: wellbeing in pregnancy, nutrition and diet, fetal growth and gestational stages, exercise in pregnancy, aquanatal information, pelvic floor exercises, care of the back, relaxation, hazard information i.e. smoking, alcohol, drugs.

Psychological: emotions, expectations, fears, body image, clothes, sexual feelings and stress.

Antenatal care: why? Health professionals involved, relevance of procedures such as urine testing, blood pressure recording, abdominal palpation and auscultation of the fetal heart.

Screening: why? What is involved, blood tests, scans, risk assessments.

Minor ailments: what, why and how to cope i.e. nausea and simple remedies.

Miscellaneous: maternity benefits, working whilst pregnant, leisure time and preparation for their baby.

The teaching methods selected included resource-based learning, involving teaching aids i.e. visual images of intrauterine growth, printed information leaflets, quizzes and discussion with minimal amounts of formal, didactic teaching.

We decided to develop the sessions so that the content would build on the topics that women in the earlier classes identified as useful, and the methods adopted to deliver the session were selected on the basis of group dynamics. In this way we were able to encourage women to identify their own learning needs while providing a framework based on knowledge gained from earlier classes, and to offer a range of teaching methods that were appropriate to the group in question.

This method of developing health education is based on a health promotion model[14] and facilitates a client-centred approach both to content and format. We saw it as important that women worked together with midwives to develop content, and that they regarded us as responsive to their particular needs. Crafter[15] advocates this approach in antenatal education whereby the midwife leads the woman into interaction and builds on this to meet women's learning needs.

Evaluation of the service

Since the early antenatal classes were a new service, it was important not only to include women in their development, but also to access their views of the classes in relation to their needs. To do this we constructed an evaluation form comprising open questions to capture their views of their experience.

On the basis of the feedback given to us about each class, we developed action plans, which included practical ways of making improvements to subsequent classes. Evaluation therefore becomes cyclical and the data obtained were included at regular team midwives' meetings when ideas to improve the classes grew out of reflecting on the process of delivering them. In this way the views of women and of the midwives were synthesised to enhance the content of future classes.

Findings

Since the classes began in 1998 we have now provided sessions every second or third month offered to all caseload women and their partners. A third of caseload women have consistently attended these and these are primarily

COMMENTS MADE BY MOTHERS

'It was very good to be able to spend so much time early in pregnancy with the midwives.'

'Useful to meet other parents and share their views and experiences.'

'I feel this class will be very beneficial to newly pregnant women.'

primigravid women. The main points to come out of the evaluation questionnaires have focused on how women are helped to manage their pregnancy and their felt need for information on topics such as diet, exercise, minor ailments, and fetal growth. Without exception, women attending the classes have found them useful. While the formal elements of teaching and learning are valued, women also feel they gain from the support of meeting other pregnant women, and from meeting the midwives who will be responsible for their subsequent care.

Discussion

Evaluation of antenatal classes has rested primarily on the views of the women who have attended them. The flexible nature of our classes has enabled us to respond effectively to individual women's needs, while providing a broad structure within which to operate.

Enkin et al[16] suggest that because antenatal education is not a clinical intervention, it should be evaluated by educational criteria. Our project has been very much at the formative stage of evaluation – that is, modifying the nature and content of the classes in line with the needs of our users. We have not attempted to do an outcome evaluation to establish whether attendance at these classes changes women's behaviour through pregnancy and so has a knock-on effect in terms of the health of mothers or their babies.

Clearly women who attend these classes are among the most motivated and aware of their health and it is likely to be non-attenders who require additional help. Even so, the high attendance rate and the popularity of the classes indicate that they are fulfilling a need.

The classes now form an integral part of the workload of the team and are provided at regular intervals in accordance with the number of referrals into the caseload. In order to meet the needs of women who do not choose to attend the classes, a one-to-one session is offered to them in order to identify their specific needs and they are encouraged to attend the later preparation for parenthood classes.

In the future we will continue to collect information from the women who attend our classes in order to continue to develop them and integrate them with later antenatal provision. The midwives providing the classes are themselves improving their teaching and facilitation skills to enhance women-focused care.

The provision of this additional class does not make a heavy demand on the team midwives. The benefits to mothers themselves and to improving the relationship between mothers and their midwives are in themselves thought to be adequate benefits. We would like to see more midwives offering this facility and we would be delighted to share our experience with others who may be interested.

REFERENCES

1 Greig F, Bell M. Evaluation of team midwifery project in Newcastle. The Directorate of Women's Services. Newcastle: RVI; 1997.
2 Page L. Effective group practice in midwifery: Working with women. Oxford: Blackwell Science; 1995.
3 Audit Commission. First class delivery: Improving maternity services in England and Wales. Abingdon: Audit Commission Publications; 1997.
4 Redman S, Oak S, Booth P, et al. Evaluation of an antenatal education programme: Characteristics of attenders, changes in knowledge and satisfaction of participants. Australian and New Zealand Journal of Obstetrics and Gynaecology 1991; 31(4):310–316.
5 Murphy-Black T. Antenatal education. In: Alexander J, Levy V, Roch S (eds). Antenatal care: A research-based approach. 2nd edn. Basingstoke: Macmillan Press; 1992.
6 Perkins E. What do women want? Asking consumers' views. Midwives Chronicle 1991; 104(1247):350.
7 Jackson MS, Schmierer CL, Schneider Z. Development, refinement and future usage of the scale: 'Attitudes toward learning in pregnancy'. International Journal of Nursing Studies 1996; 3(1):37–46.
8 Rees C. Antenatal education, health promotion and the midwife. In: Alexander J, Levy V, Roch S (eds). Midwifery practice: Core topics 1. Basingstoke: Macmillan Press; 1996.

9 Nolan ML. Antenatal education: Failing to educate for parenthood. British Journal of Midwifery 1997; 5(2):21–26.
10 Cranston CS. The important first trimester: An educational approach. Journal of Nurse-Midwifery 1980; 25(4):40–42.
11 Ciliska DK. Early pregnancy classes as a vehicle for lifestyle education and modification. Canadian Journal of Public Health 1983; 74(3):215–217.
12 Maybruck P. Early pregnancy classes. International Journal of Childbirth Education 1988; 3(2):17.
13 Lane B. Promoting a great start: Teaching an early pregnancy class. International Journal of Childbirth Education 1997; 12(2):24–26.
14 Ewles E, Simnett I. Promoting health: A practical guide. In: Crafter H (ed). Health promotion in midwifery. London: Arnold Publishing; 1997.
15 Crafter H. Health promotion in midwifery. London: Arnold Publishing; 1997.
16 Enkin M, Keirse MJN, Renfrew M, et al. A guide to effective care in pregnancy and childbirth. 2nd edn. Oxford: Oxford University Press; 1995.

Antenatal education: past and future agendas

Education not indoctrination

Mary Nolan

The recent Report of the Royal College of Midwives, *New Perspectives in Parenting Education*[1] embodies a popular misconception of the nature of health education with its repeated suggestion that midwives in antenatal classes need to advise parents about 'the psychological, emotional and relationship changes they will experience' (p.23). Education is not the same thing as advice giving:

'In education the teacher helps the learner to become free ... we seek to bring the student participants into contact with the primary material and leave them free to use it for themselves.'[2] (p.48)

Paulo Freire, a South American Catholic Priest, who has played a critical part in shaping late twentieth century educational theory, explains how a prescriptive approach to education, that is, telling people what they should do, reinforces a status quo in which the powerless remain subservient and the powerful, dominant:

'Every prescription represents the imposition of one man's choice upon another, transforming the consciousness of the man prescribed to into one that conforms with the prescriber's consciousness. Thus, the behaviour of the oppressed is a prescribed behavior, following as it does the guidelines of the oppressor.'[3] (p.31)

Freire is committed to education because he sees it as a powerful, perhaps the most powerful, means of liberating people from oppression. If midwives want to be 'with women', their role is not to prescribe what women should do but rather to help them understand their options and stand by them when they make their choices, whatever those choices may be. The midwife's first duty is to the woman, not herself, her colleagues or the baby, and her role is to act as the woman's advocate, not advisor.[4] Judith Schott, one of the foremost antenatal teachers in the UK, suggests:

'How would it be if, instead of giving advice, which is often conflicting and sometimes inappropriate, we listened to the woman and encouraged her to talk about what is important to her?... The woman may quite spontaneously find her own

solutions, but, if not, by understanding her situation more fully, we are in a better position to offer the information (not advice) she needs in order to make her own decisions.'[5] (p.3)

The RCM Report, however, considers that:

'In order to provide a realistic preparation for early parenthood... midwives need to be able to offer advice to parents from different social and economic backgrounds, from career women, to single mothers and the ethnic communities in their locality.'[1] (p.21)

Impossible and very unwise, midwives might reasonably retort! Nobody could have sufficient insight into the lives and needs of such divergent groups of women to make it at all realistic to consider offering advice to them all (or indeed to any of them). A concept of education which embraces the aim of assisting people towards greater adulthood does not incorporate advice-giving. Rather, such a concept supports educators' efforts to help women and men decide for themselves how they can best make the transition to satisfying parenthood.[2]

An overview of the literature

In mitigation of the RCM Report's confounding of education and prescription, it can be argued that antenatal education has historically been seen as an adjunct of a medical model of maternity care, and has generally reflected the paternalistic values of obstetrics. GPs, health visitors and midwives have perceived the dominant theme in antenatal education to be medical,[6] for example, one author describes the aim of antenatal education being to:

'ensure that the mother and baby remain healthy throughout pregnancy and that the mother gives birth to a healthy baby.'[7] (p.8)

A considerable proportion of the research that has been carried out into the effectiveness of antenatal education has focused on its impact on the uptake of analgesia by women in labour.[8-14] This reflects both the influence of obstetricians and of anaesthetists in determining the nature of women's experience of childbirth,[15] and the thrust, both perceived and actual, of the work of the early childbirth education pioneers, Dick-Read and Lamaze.

The seminal works of Dick-Read[16] and Lamaze[17] were critical in determining the antenatal education research agenda. For at least the next four decades, that agenda was in remorseless pursuit of an answer to the question of whether women who attend childbirth preparation classes use less pharmacological analgesia in labour than their sisters who do not attend classes. Such research continues until the present day, for example a paper was published in 1996 which concluded that parentcraft education has little influence in determining the type of pain relief used by women in labour.[14]

Other researchers have reached the same conclusion.[8,12,13] One looked at the efficacy of 'breathing and postural techniques' taught at antenatal classes and found that the overwhelming majority of women did not make use of such techniques during labour.[18] However, an American study which investigated 10 women, 5 of whom had attended Lamaze classes and the other 5 no classes, found that the prepared women managed pain more effectively.[10] These researchers tested women's response to a finger prick of increasing intensity applied during labour and concluded that the effectiveness of childbirth preparation was undeniable in the prepared group:

'In the women with childbirth preparation, an analgesic process is activated during labor. While the degree of analgesia is not sufficient to eliminate the pain of labor, the present findings imply that the pain of labor would be more severe if this mechanism did not exist ... It may be that this analgesia during labor is ... a consequence of the activities used during prepared childbirth.' (p.219)

The limitations of the study are self-evident. The sample was extremely small. It is questionable whether testing women's response to a finger prick bears any relation to their ability to cope with late first stage contractions. Nor do the researchers record what pharmacological pain relief the two groups of women used during labour. However, an overview of research from the 1970s and early 1980s, whilst being generally critical of the methodologies employed and aware of the very different teaching approaches deployed in the classes attended by subjects, agrees with the findings of the American study:

'One consistent finding is that women trained in childbirth education use less analgesia and anaesthesia than untrained women.' [19] (p,1:4)

A study of women attending classes at an inner-city hospital in Baltimore bears out the same conclusion.[20] This is a particularly interesting study because more than half the subjects (54%) were black and the vast majority (90%) were clinic patients, i.e. poor women who did not have private medical insurance. Women who chose to attend classes were matched with a control group who chose not to attend classes, for the variables of race, patient status (clinic or private), parity, marital status and age. Far less analgesia was used by the study group, who also achieved more spontaneous deliveries. However, the author clearly acknowledges the many factors which may have influenced her results, such as the degree of self-esteem enjoyed by individuals in each of the study groups, and differences in their stress levels.

All the studies which have been carried out into antenatal education suffer from important flaws. They do not describe the content of the classes that subjects attended, nor the philosophy of the childbirth educators who were leading them. They rarely mention the amount of contact time between parents and educators. Only a few studies comment on the educational aspects of classes such as the size of the group and the teaching approaches employed. In addition to these factors:

'Variables such as parents' goals and expectations, physician attitudes and practice patterns, and hospital labor management routines affect both outcomes and parent satisfaction at least as much as, if not more than, whatever happens in a few hours of childbirth classes.' [21] (p.206)

Such serious limitations make it very difficult to compare with any degree of security the results achieved by different studies.

Clients' agendas for antenatal classes

When evaluating prenatal classes researchers should focus on outcomes which reflect educational rather than obstetric objectives.[22] It is by no means certain that women's only (or primary) goal in coming to classes is to learn how to cope with pain in labour. Remarkably little work has been carried out to discover what it is that women do want from their antenatal education, and even less to ascertain the goals of the men and other support people who increasingly attend classes alongside pregnant women.

Some insights into women's agenda for classes can be gleaned from the literature, most notably from an Australian study which concluded that parents sought confidence and skills (a) to use the healthcare system effectively, (b) to care for their babies, and (c) to make decisions about their family's health and care.[23] Another author noted that her subjects considered classes least useful as a source of parentcraft instruction,[24] a conclusion with which another researcher concurred when reporting that class attenders felt that they had been inadequately prepared for 'coping with the new baby'. [25] (p.276). The desire of class attenders to focus on postnatal issues and not to focus exclusively on labour is borne out by attenders' responses to an open-ended question on the content of antenatal classes conducted in 1997:

- Anything relevant to bringing up a baby: healthcare, clothing i.e. amount of clothing, bathing, temperature for bedrooms etc.
- Recommended ointments, lotions, nappies etc.
- Parentcraft, how to bathe the baby, safety in the home etc.
- Care of the baby and not so much emphasis on pregnancy.[26]

The women interviewed in another study also stated that antenatal classes focused too much on birth and not sufficiently on parenting and breastfeeding.[27] A very recent study reported that women wanted classes to include 'information about local services' and very importantly, to cover the role of the partner both in labour and postnatally.[28]

A lack of realism in antenatal education has been repeatedly identified in the literature as a source of dissatisfaction for class attenders, with some women feeling that they had been inadequately prepared for deviations from the normal course of labour[25] and others criticising classes for their lack of honesty.[29] For example, the women in this last study expressed surprise at the difference between what they had been told about the bearing down stage of labour and what they actually experienced. The study concludes with some advice for childbirth educators that they should 'prepare women more realistically' (p.197).

One study of men in antenatal classes addressed the clients' agenda directly by asking National Childbirth Trust fathers what they wanted to learn about.[30] This small study of a non-representative sample of fathers identified that the fathers wanted to know how they could help their partners during labour and in the early days of their babies' lives; to learn essential babycare tasks; and to meet other men in a similar situation.

Future directions

Five years ago, optimism was expressed that antenatal classes were moving from:

'*Practitioner convenience to consumer needs, power-broking to power-sharing, and from directive practice to negotiated practice.*'[31](p.120)

However, it is clear that it is only possible to put women and their families in the centre of antenatal education if the agenda is theirs and if practitioners are able to recognise that what clients want to learn might be how to challenge the system's priorities (p.120). There is scope for further review of the needs of people who attend antenatal classes (and even more so, of those who do not attend).

A recent study, of NHS and NCT antenatal education, highlighted the role of classes in creating support networks and peer group empowerment for parents.[32] Parents did not originally choose to attend classes principally as a way of accessing parent-to-parent support, but by the end of classes, they rated this as one of the most important things they had gained. Empowerment through support is a vital aspect of adult education[33] and can be realised in antenatal classes when groups are kept small and when teachers provide opportunities for parents to learn from each other's experiences and ideas.[34]

Antenatal classes have a central role to play in creating 'a critical mass of mothers' who will drive forward changes in obstetrical practice once they become aware of the fact that options are available to them.[35] Empowering people to make their own health choices and to structure health service delivery to meet their needs calls for education for change, not for conformity.

Arguably, there is no such thing as a neutral education process; either it facilitates the integration of clients into the logic of the present system or it becomes the means:

'*by which men and women deal critically and creatively with reality and discover how to participate in the transformation of their world*'[36] (p.15).

Such an ideal begs the question of who should be delivering antenatal education. Should parenting education take place in hospitals and clinics, or should it take place in non healthcare settings? Is it possible to educate people for independence as healthcare consumers and as parents within a system that fosters reliance on health professionals? These are some of the fundamental questions that need addressing before antenatal education can move into the next millennium.

REFERENCES

1 Royal College of Midwives. New perspectives in parenting education: Report from the Royal College of Midwives Trust parenting education consensus conference held in London on 29th January 1998. London: Royal College of Midwives; 1998.
2 Rogers A. Teaching adults, 2nd edn. Buckingham: Open University Press; 1996.
3 Freire P. Pedagogy of the Oppressed. Trans Bergman Ramos M. New York: Herder and Herder; 1972.
4 Lee G. Worst case scenario: supporting women who refuse a caesarean section. The Practising Midwife 1998; 1(7):28–9.
5 Schott J. The importance of encouraging women to think for themselves. British Journal of Midwifery 1994; 2(1):3–4.

6 McCabe F, Rocheron Y, Dickinson R, et al. Antenatal care: a lost opportunity. Health Education Journal 1985; 44(1):36–38.

7 Hyde B. Curriculum planning for antenatal health education. Nurse Education Today 1981; 1(6):8–10.

8 Gunn TR, Fisher A, Lloyd P, et al. Antenatal education: does it improve the quality of labour and delivery? New Zealand Medical Journal 1983; 96:51–53.

9 Melzack R. The myth of painless childbirth. Pain 1984; 19:321–337.

10 Whipple B, Josimovich J, Komisaruk B. Sensory thresholds during the antepartum, intrapartum and postpartum periods. International Journal of Nursing Studies 1990; 27(3):213–221.

11 Wuitchik M, Hesson K, Bakal DA. Perinatal predictors of pain and distress during labor. Birth 1990; 17(4):186–191.

12 Redman S, Oak S, Booth P, et al. Evaluation of an antenatal education programme: Characteristics of attenders, changes in knowledge and satisfaction of participants. Australia and New Zealand Journal of Obstetrics and Gynaecology 1991; 31(4):310–316.

13 Lumley J, Brown S. Attenders and nonattenders at childbirth education classes in Australia: How do they and their births differ? Birth 1993; 20(3):123–130.

14 Qureshi NS, Schofield G, Papaioannou S, et al. Parentcraft classes: do they affect outcome in childbirth? Journal of Obstetrics and Gynaecology 1996; 1(6):358–361.

15 Mander R. A reappraisal of Simpson's introduction of chloroform. Midwifery 1998; 14:181–189.

16 Dick-Read G. Childbirth without fear. Oxford: Heinemann; 1951.

17 Lamaze F. Painless childbirth: psychoprophylactic method. London: Burke; 1958.

18 Copstick S, Hayes RW, Taylor KE, et al. A test of a common assumption regarding the use of antenatal training during labour. Journal of Psychosomatic Research 1985; 29(2):215–218.

19 Green JM, Coupland VA, Kitzinger JV. Great expectations: a prospective study of women's expectations and experiences of childbirth, vol 1. Cambridge: Child Care and Development Group, University of Cambridge; 1988.

20 Hetherington SE. A controlled study of the effect of prepared childbirth classes on obstetric outcomes. Birth 1990; 17(2):86–90.

21 Shearer S. Commentary: Randomized trials needed to settle question of impact of childbirth classes. Birth 1996; 23(4):206–208.

22 Perry M. Prenatal Education: how effective is it? Australian College of Midwives Incorporated Journal 1992:15–20.

23 O'Meara C. An evaluation of consumer perspectives of childbirth and parenting education. Midwifery 1993; 9(4):210–219.

24 Gould D. Locally organised antenatal classes and their effectiveness. Nursing Times 1986; 82(45):59–61.

25 Hillan E. Issues in the delivery of midwifery care. Journal of Advanced Nursing 1992; 17:274–278.

26 Nolan M. Antenatal education: failing to educate for parenthood. British Journal of Midwifery 1997; 5(1):21–26.

27 Britton C. The influence of antenatal information on breastfeeding experiences. British Journal of Midwifery 1998; 6(3):12–15.

28 Proctor S. What determines quality in maternity care? Comparing the perceptions of childbearing women and midwives. Birth 1998; 25(2):85–93.

29 McKay S, Barrows T, Roberts J. Women's views of second-stage labor as assessed by interviews and videotapes. Birth 1990; 17(4):192–198.

30 Nolan M. Caring for fathers in antenatal classes. Modern Midwife 1994; 4(2):25–28.

31 Walsh D. Parenthood education and the politics of education. British Journal of Midwifery 1993; 1(3):119–123.

32 Nolan M. Empowerment and antenatal education. Unpublished PhD thesis. Birmingham: University of Birmingham; 1998.

33 Tones K, Tilford S. Health education: effectiveness, efficiency and equity, 2nd edn. London: Chapman & Hall; 1994.

34 Nolan M. Antenatal education: a dynamic approach. Edinburgh: Baillière Tindall; 1988.

35 Enkin M, Keirse MJNC, Renfrew M, et al. A guide to effective care in pregnancy and childbirth, 2nd edn. Oxford: Oxford University Press; 1995: 17–21.

36 Shaull R. Introduction. In: Freire P. Pedagogy of the oppressed. Trans Bergman Ramos M. New York: Herder and Herder; 1972.

Serving up nutrition in your antenatal classes

Andrea Robertson

Everyone loves to eat, and pregnant women have a particularly keen interest in food. So why is nutrition often served up as an indigestible lump of information as though it was the most boring topic on earth? Instead of a smorgasbord of delectable tidbits, the menu often consists of stodgy servings of predigested facts and figures, presented through bland lectures and boring charts. Let's look at how you can get some spice into your nutrition menu and serve up a delicious mix of exciting morsels designed to boost consumption of vital information.

Linking in

Nutrition is one of those topics that can easily be linked to other themes: fetal growth and development, pregnancy discomforts, exercise in pregnancy, 'eating for two', maternal weight gain, nourishment in labour, snacks for support people, celebrations after the birth (birthday cake and champagne!), nutrition during breastfeeding, weaning foods for babies, dieting after birth... the possibilities are almost endless.

Since everyone eats, everyone has a working knowledge of the importance of food. In pregnancy, the nutritional needs of the baby must also be considered, especially if optimal fetal growth and development are the goal. Introducing nutrition by linking it to the baby's needs is often a good place to start, since every woman wants to give her baby the best possible start.

Ideas for action

- Collect a series of photographs of the developing baby (the book *A Child is Born* by Lennart Nilsson is a good source of pictures). Expectant parents are fascinated by the intricacies of fetal growth, and this can easily lead into a discussion starter for small group work: 'What does a baby in the womb need to grow well?'
- The answers generated by the feedback from this discussion can then be channeled into further questions (perhaps one topic per group): 'How can we tell what is in the food we eat?'; 'How much of the five basic food groups does a pregnant woman need?' (you will need reference material for this activity); 'What are good sources of the essential nutrients?' (again, provide reference materials); 'Make a list of quick and nutritious snack foods'.
- Invite women and their partners to review their individual daily food intake. Then, in pairs, compare what they eat to a given list of foods required each day by a pregnant woman. This can then form the basis for negotiation between each couple for making dietary changes to benefit the baby. Working women need to be particularly careful to eat well as long gaps without food can lead to fatigue and periodic inability to cope at work.
- Meal planning can be fun, especially for younger people with little experience. Pictures of various foods can be mounted on cardboard, or plastic imitations (try the pet toys section of your local supermarket) and actual boxes and cans used to form the basis of many activities: combining ingredients for exciting meals, cheap alternatives and substitutes, new flavour sensations.
- Have a loose-leaf resource book with each page dedicated to an effect of pregnancy. Under each heading (e.g. cramps, constipation, swollen ankles, etc.) list as many self-help remedies as you can, including dietary measures.
- Samples of interesting or unusual foods could be introduced. If you have people from different ethnic backgrounds in the group invite them to contribute foods that form the basis of their diets. Pregnancy might be the time to experiment with, for example: tofu, couscous, chickpea spreads, stuffed aubergines, sun-dried tomatoes, muesli, flat breads, tropical fruits and a host of new spices.

- Carry your theme through to the refreshment break. Invite people to bring healthy snacks to share or at least make sure there is something other than tea, coffee and sweet biscuits to eat.
- Jigsaw puzzles made from a 'Healthy Diet Pyramid' chart could be used as the basis for discussing the five food groups. Have a complementary chart showing the nutritional requirements for pregnant woman and use this as a reference for adjusting the diet, discussing substitutes and special dietary needs for those with allergies and strong dislikes of some foods.
- An exercise in reading the labels of packets and cans for nutritional contents can prove interesting, especially when the lists of ingredients are compared to the ideal diet in pregnancy.
- A card game on nutritional facts and fallacies could be prepared. This could take the form of 'Trivial Pursuit' or 'True/False' for a simple team game with a suitable prize (not a bar of chocolate!).
- A large cut-out cardboard female figure could form the basis for 'add-ons' – with overlays of large breasts, bigger thighs and hips, the uterus and the baby, amniotic fluid and the placenta being added to demonstrate the various components of weight gain in pregnancy.
- Ask couples to prepare a list of snack foods for their labour ward 'goody bag', including nutritious drinks.
- Selecting weaning foods for babies leads naturally into a discussion of family foods in general. Since babies tend to help themselves from their parent's plate, what is on that plate is important.

Don't forget that associated issues such as smoking, alcohol, ingesting chemicals (household cleaning materials, etc.) and medications all need to be raised appropriately. The needs of people with food allergies will also have to be covered, and some of the above ideas can be adapted to include their special needs.

Having a variety of teaching ingredients will make your presentation attractive, interesting and relevant. The only thing you need to watch for is overindulging; too many 'helpings' may lead to listlessness and fatigue and encourage everyone to take a post-prandial nap! Regular snacks rather than one, large helping may be the solution to this common problem.

Watch your language!

Andrea Robertson

Pregnant women are some of the most sensitive people you will ever meet. At a time when they are actively seeking information and support from a wide range of contacts, they are highly vulnerable and very suggestible. They listen to everyone and everything, read copiously, ask a myriad of questions and are the recipients of mountains of advice.

Impact

As caregivers, we often fail to appreciate the impact our words are having. We need to think carefully about the language of birth. The words that are used and the manner in which they are spoken can be uplifting and inspiring or devastating and undermining.

When we talk about topics that are familiar and comfortable to us, we need to be very aware that they may seem threatening and scary to others. Sometimes it is not the words themselves, but the impression the words create that does the damage, perhaps leaving the woman feeling anxious and even afraid when the intention was to leave her feeling reassured and comforted.

In working with pregnant women, our main aim must surely be to help them feel competent, capable and powerful as they journey through the most creative work they will ever do. All our actions and words must support the realisation of this outcome, even when we have to convey bad news.

Developing a sensitivity to the impact of what we are saying is an important skill that every midwife, educator and doctor must develop as part of their professionalism. Remember that what you say may have a profound impact on the pregnant woman. This is a very powerful position to be in and we must be careful not to use it accidentally to coerce her, undermine her rights or sap her confidence.

Self-awareness

The skill of 'watching what you are saying' is essential. Practical ways of developing this skill include tape recording your teaching session for self-appraisal later, asking a colleague to sit in as an observer to offer feedback, or even videotaping a session. Watch for the pregnant woman's reactions as you are speaking – note her body language, facial expression and verbal feedback. It is often rather sobering to see yourself as others see you, but it can be a very effective learning experience!

Whenever you are talking to a pregnant woman, try to develop the ability to 'split yourself up' into three parts: the person speaking, the person you are talking to, and an observer noticing the interaction between both of you. Putting yourself in another person's shoes is an important first step in developing effective communication skills and is integral to the processes of negotiation and conflict resolution. Analyse what you observe from these three standpoints and use this to formulate changes to your approach. Notice, for example, what you were saying when she narrowed her eyes – this probably indicated she didn't understand what you were saying. You may need to repeat the information and either paraphrase it or use different terminology.

People are very sensitive to the congruence between what is being said and the accompanying body language of the speaker. Just raising an eyebrow as you are taking a blood pressure can create alarm in a client, even if you are saying 'This seems to be just fine'. Be wary of creating bias through the use of emotionally laden expressions and personal opinion. 'If I were you I would...' and 'In my professional opinion you should...' are messages designed to influence rather than empower.

Masculine and medical

Think carefully about your vocabulary. Most of the terminology used in maternity care is masculine, negative and medical, probably the result of the early textbooks being written by the doctors of the time rather than midwives. One of the worst examples is the word 'delivery'. This has become so commonplace that we hardly notice we are saying it, yet in the wider sense it describes a service that is performed for you, rather than something you do for yourself. This is hardly the impression we want to be giving pregnant women. There is not one occasion when you use the word 'delivery' that you could not neatly excise it and replace it with the word 'birth'. Try saying 'I was at a wonderful birth last night' rather than 'I had a wonderful delivery last night' and see how it alters your perceptions of the whole event, while maintaining the woman in her central role.

In prenatal education, as in all interactions you have with pregnant women, pay careful attention to avoid the use of jargon. Abbreviations (e.g. V.E.) and acronyms (e.g. APGAR) are appropriate for quick communications with colleagues but unsuitable for helping understanding amongst pregnant women. You may need to find whole new ways of describing certain conditions to avoid creating negative impressions with women; think of the impact of being told you are 'failing to progress', have an 'incompetent cervix', or are being given a 'trial of scar'. Even apparently safe words such as 'coping', 'adequate' and being 'in control' need to be reassessed for the impressions they are conveying. It has also been popular to talk about uterine contractions as 'pains', e.g. 'How often are the pains coming now?' What messages are being embedded in this false description? Yes, contractions are usually painful, but to call all contractions 'pains' is inaccurate and potentially damaging to women's perceptions.

Sometimes even apparently innocuous words can have profound effects. 'Still' and 'only' are two examples.

How would you feel about being told, after hours of dealing with contractions 'you're only in early labour', or some hours later 'you've still got a long way to go' or for the full double whammy, 'You're still only 5cms'?

Take responsibility

Many caregivers tend to blame women when communication fails: it is the woman's fault if she doesn't understand. In any educational setting (and these are many and varied in maternity care) if the message is not received then it is the responsibility of the message sender to make amends and find a better mode of communication. A completely different approach may be needed, such as drawing a picture, acting out a situation or using a prop for clarification. Selecting different words will also be important and using vernacular or slang words may work well. Ask yourself, 'How would this woman describe the situation herself?'

During labour, women are particularly alert to what is being said by caregivers. Even though she may look as though she is lost in concentration during contractions, the labouring woman will hear, often acutely, what is being said around her. She looks to the midwife for confirmation that she is doing well, particularly with handling the pain. A few well chosen words of encouragement and support can be more effective than pethidine in achieving relaxation and confidence in the labouring woman.

The midwife at a birth has great influence on the woman's reactions and impressions, so be careful not to introduce your own feelings and biases into the room. This woman is not a 'poor thing' who won't cope without you – she is a strong, innately capable woman uniquely designed for giving birth easily, safely and enjoyably. If you truly believe this then you won't need to watch your language – you will already be feeding this information back to her through your language and responses.

Asian women's maternity language course

Karen Ramsey

'A course to teach you the English you need to know when you are having a baby in England, so you will understand the doctors and nurses and feel confident that you can cope.'

Reading the publicity handout, I wished I could share the optimism that this could be achieved in 11 two-hour classes. It did not take long before my excitement at being offered the chance to teach these classes to Asian expectant mothers gave way to a feeling of overwhelming responsibility.

As a National Childbirth Trust antenatal teacher, I was used to running discussion-based courses in which people pooled their knowledge and analysed advantages and disadvantages. But 'informed choice' seems a distant dream when you don't even know how to make an appointment.

If most women are nervous about hospitals and birth, what must it be like for someone who cannot understand the language? Many of the women who came to classes were very young, having only recently arrived in this country. They had left their own families behind in Pakistan to marry men who lived in England. It was therefore the husbands who did all of the English speaking and communicating with the outside world.

The training

My involvement with teaching Pakistani women had begun 18 months before, when I had responded to a request in the local newspaper for volunteer tutors to teach English to women in their own homes. Training consisted of a term of evening classes, leading to a City & Guilds Certificate in Teaching Basic Skills. I also had to observe classes and, because of my background, I was allocated to the Maternity Language course, which I had not known existed.

The classes were held in Wycombe General Hospital in High Wycombe, Buckinghamshire. They were organised by the English for Speakers of Other Languages (ESOL) section of Adult and Continuing Education, and funded by Buckinghamshire County Council. The tutor for this course was Roma, who taught together with a community midwife or, on a few occasions, a health visitor and a dental health educator.

Roma's gentle manner and effortless switching from English to Urdu made the classes look quite easy. There was also a hospital interpreter translating into Punjabi, the women's first language (although they could also understand Urdu). For some classes, a student midwife accompanied the community midwife, so there were times when we outnumbered the pregnant women!

Having finished my training, I stood in for Roma a couple of times, but never imagined that I would take her place when she retired. I could not speak Urdu and to make matters worse, the hospital interpreter had left. Funding had been cut, resulting in the number of sessions in the course being halved, and there was no money in ESOL's budget for an interpreter.

A joint adventure

The solution was a stroke of genius. Skilled at juggling her dwindling resources, the ESOL manager approached Fareedah, a woman who had attended classes herself, years before. She offered her a place on an interpreters' training course in exchange for translating the hospital classes. This opportunity was as new and exciting for Fareedah as the teaching was for me, so we started together, sharing a feeling of adventure and trepidation.

Neither of us realised how much work the course involved. It was up to us to find the women. Referrals came in patchily from midwives and sometimes health visitors, and it was our job to knock on each woman's door to explain what was on offer. I did the driving, Fareedah did the talking. Surprised that I could often follow the gist of the conversation, I would sit smiling, a little embarrassed and feeling rather like a visual aid: the

English teacher. I was struck by the way we were always invited in; I am not sure we would have been given such a generous hearing – turning up unannounced – at many English households.

Most of the women were living in their husband's family home, so we often found ourselves aiming our pitch at their mothers-in-law, who needed to be assured that this was a suitable class. We were helped by the fact that Roma's classes had been going for 17 years, which meant she had actually taught some of these older women. In fact, it was remarkable that most of them had attended, or at least knew about, the literacy classes run by ESOL.

During these visits, I learned not to assume that a woman had no English, despite what she said. Often the young women understood more than they admitted to, but lack of confidence, especially in front of their family, made them reluctant to speak. Sometimes I would feel quite foolish and patronising if I had spoken in a simplistic way, before realising that a woman could understand quite easily. Seeing the women start to overcome this shyness during the course was one of the rewards of teaching.

No transport

Getting to the classes was a major hurdle for the students. Even if she lived within walking distance of the hospital, it would not be thought appropriate for a woman to walk on her own, or to take a bus. Most of the women relied on their husbands for transport, but the men were generally at work at this time of day.

We therefore had to organise lifts – but we only had two cars and this limited the number of students. One of the plans for future courses was to obtain grant funding for a minibus, to be driven by a woman driver – a welcome improvement from my point of view. Driving around town, picking up the women immediately before a class could be quite hectic. I missed having the time to prepare the teaching room and to talk to students or colleagues after the class, because we would be in a hurry to deliver the women with older children back in time before school finished. Co-ordinating the lifts was as time-consuming as the actual driving, and I found it wise to telephone each woman the night before a class to check whether she planned to come. On the other hand, I did enjoy the opportunity to get to know students better. I found they were quite curious about my family life, and chatted more easily in the car than they would in the classroom.

Different needs

One of the main challenges was meeting the needs of women with different levels of English. Some had had little or no schooling, others had been to secondary school and enjoyed written work. This was made easier after a couple of classes, when the women with more English began to help those who were having difficulty. One student was even able to stand in for the interpreter when she was away for a session. I like to think that this woman might find that the classes help to open doors for her in the future, in the same way as they had done for Fareedah.

Most of the students were first-timers, but one woman was expecting her fifth child. They were all at different stages of pregnancy, joining the rolling programme at any point, and able to continue coming for as long as they wanted.

For a couple of the students, the class was clearly a highlight of their week, and they dressed up for the occasion. Others were not so committed. Attendance was variable: we had eight students registered, but sometimes only a couple of women came. This was a worry because the course would be cancelled if numbers dropped. I had to mark names off on a register and give the office details of attendance for each class. There were also various forms for the students to fill in. Although necessary for funding, I resented the time they took up and felt they were intimidating, particularly for the women who found writing difficult.

The responsibility of preparing these women for birth in England seemed less awesome as I came to realise that simply getting to know the hospital and becoming comfortable with the staff was as important as anything I could teach them. Students often took the opportunity to speak individually to the midwife about any worries and the midwife would occasionally take a woman down the hall to be monitored if there was particular concern. From the hospital's point of view, the classes made communication easier, and the women learned some of the dos and don'ts such as how to fill in a menu card and which bin to use for nappies.

A class joke

We could not take it for granted that everyone knew the full facts about conception, so we started with the midwife's chart showing sperms meeting the egg. There was a lot of embarrassed giggling, as there was about anything to do the bladder or bowels. It became a class joke that so much of the course was taken up with these functions: we had cards and pictures explaining constipation, diarrhoea and cystitis, not to mention a sequencing exercise on midstream urine samples. I wondered whether they might think all this was a British obsession!

I was curious to see what was on the chart that the midwife had been keeping carefully covered up during her talk about conception. This turned out to be a diagram showing a penis and sexual intercourse, which the students would have found offensive. I know that a woman had dropped out of a previous course 'because of the pictures'. Even the usual anatomy and birth charts were not always appreciated. I remember the women being quite shocked by a full-frontal view of a baby's head being born.

The name game

Some of the women were very shy and embarrassed about their pronunciation, so I felt rather a bully making them practise giving their name, address and due date at the beginning of each class. But even the apparently simple question 'What is your name?' which they would be asked every time they went to an antenatal appointment, was not that easy to answer. It is not their tradition to take the husband's name, so misunderstandings about family – or surnames – were common. This could lead to inconsistencies and confusion if the same name was not used on all medical records. I was pleased that, following the class, one woman went back to her doctor to change the name on her notes, having previously thought that she could not say anything.

Some of the students did not know where their husbands worked, so homework after the first class was to find this out in case he needed to be contacted. As their confidence grew, we practised making and cancelling appointments and then role-played telephoning for an ambulance and calling the labour ward.

Sitting comfortably

I did introduce a couple of NCT teaching ideas, with mixed success. We began the course sitting on the floor on mats, leaning against wedges, as was usual for parentcraft classes in the hospital. However, I could see that a few of the women were not happy sitting so casually. It also made writing difficult and meant that not everyone could see the visual aids. We ended up sitting around a table which made life easier, especially when there were forms to fill in! The students were reluctant to try positions or exercises, mainly due to shyness, but I think the formal seating arrangement was a factor.

They did, however, respond well to open questions such as 'What do you like (or dislike) about being pregnant?' I was very aware that, otherwise, most of my questions required answers that were right or wrong, which could discourage less confident students. For example, 'What is the word for this?' or 'Where is the uterus?'

Although I hesitate to generalise, it seemed to me that compared to women in an NCT class, the students were less ambivalent about having a baby, and certainly had more experience of babies in their households. No one said 'it won't change my life'. There was real fear about the pain of labour, but great excitement about becoming a mother. Living with their husband's family created pressures such as the worry that a mother-in-law might expect to be at the birth (not many partners would be attending), or might try to impose her traditional ideas about babycare. But there was also a confidence that there would be several women around to help them with the new baby. A general reaction against the 'old ways' of Pakistan, which they associated with high mortality rates, made this class suspicious of homebirth and unenthusiastic about breastfeeding.

Words and pictures

I had inherited teaching materials from Roma. Most of these were based on 'The HELP Maternity Language Course'[1] (produced in 1980 but, sadly, no longer available). Although this was a little dated, it did have useful line drawings featuring Asian women. As well as helping with explanations, these could be used for checking understanding, for example by asking 'What is happening here?' They could also be cut up to be used for activities such as matching words to illustrations or putting pictures in chronological order. These exercises could be geared to suit different levels of English. For example, some women could pick out a picture when I said the word 'epidural', while others could point to the word on a flashcard. More advanced students could write the word.

I had found a few leaflets with Urdu text in the Trust's store, but resisted the temptation to use all of them just for the sake of having something to give out. In some cases there was no English translation, so I did not know what information they were giving; in others, there was too much product advertising in the illustrations, which is all the more effective when a person has difficulty reading.

The real thing

The most striking visual aid was, of course, the real thing. I was most envious of the way the midwives could lay their hands on anything from forceps to femidoms. Not to mention their free access to the labour and postnatal wards and a plentiful supply of newborn babies.

One of the most moving classes I observed was on ultrasound. During this session, the specialist midwife actually scanned each woman's baby while the rest of us watched. (It was a measure of her dedication that she would come in to do this on her day off.) I felt a little unsure about the extra exposure to ultrasound, but the students found it very exciting and it gave them a unique opportunity to ask all the questions they wanted through the interpreter. It was a disappointment that by the time I became tutor, there was a new midwife who was not happy to do this in case any of the scans showed a problem. Instead, she produced photographs which the women enjoyed puzzling over, but the session did not have the same magic.

Unexpected items caught the students' interest. When I brought in packets of dried fruit for a session on healthy eating, one woman was really excited to hear that these could be bought in England, and the whole class earnestly copied down the word 'apricots'. Another time, there was an enthusiastic response when we looked through a bag of baby clothes – this made motherhood seem more real. It also provoked quite a lot of whispering between the interpreter and the youngest student who finally asked: 'Could we go shopping next week?' This woman had been to the town centre only twice since coming to England and she very much wanted to buy something new for her baby. So we added another class to the course. I can still see her beaming smile as she carried her new baby bath home. It was worth doing the course just for that moment.

The team

We were very fortunate to have Fareedah, who clearly enjoyed coming to the classes, and who had happy memories of her own children's births. (I think it would always be worth debriefing any interpreter's birth experiences.) It took a while to get used to having my explanations translated. It seemed to give my words an added weight of authority which could surely go to one's head! The pace was slower, because I had to pause for Fareedah to translate. Short sentences sometimes took a surprisingly long time to be interpreted, but as Fareedah explained, sensitive topics had to be expressed in a way that would be acceptable – and there were times when she giggled with embarrassment. It was important that

we could trust her to convey what had been said, as too much delicacy could mean the women were not getting the full story. She also needed to translate back what the students said, even if this was just a humorous comment.

I enjoyed the opportunity to teach with midwives, although I was a little nervous at first. My main function as tutor was to make sure that the women were learning the necessary language, whether it was 'contraction', 'push' or 'my address is…', while the midwives dealt with the obstetric information. I was worried about overstepping the mark in my enthusiasm for the subject, although there had been no clear boundary between Roma and her midwife colleague, Maggie, in the classes I had observed. I recognised, from co-teaching at other times, the worry about inadvertently jumping in with information that a colleague was about to give – or missing the chance to mention it if we had in fact been thinking along different lines. I was also conscious that the midwives were initially wary of what my NCT views might be, particularly regarding breastfeeding.

Moving on

Maggie retired shortly after the course began, after which there was less continuity when she was replaced by two midwives. The fact that we were all new to the course made it easier in some ways, although we did sometimes feel we were flying by the seat of our pants. The classes got better as we became familiar with each other's ways, and it is a real regret that because I moved away from High Wycombe, we did not get the chance to perfect our double-act.

Although it feels like an unfinished story, because I do not know how their births went, I relished this chance to support women who would not normally be reached by NCT classes. I do not know whether the 11 weeks were enough to teach them 'all the English you need to know when you are having a baby in England', but I am confident that many of the skills they learned will be useful long after the birth of their babies.

REFERENCE

1 Lewycka M, Mares P, Whitaker N. The H.E.L.P. Maternity Language Course. Leeds: Leeds City Council Department of Education; 1980.

Labour and birth

The area of labour and birth is one which has consistently received the attention of writers; just as this time is often the main focus for pregnant women, midwives and researchers also find it fascinating! Although in theory and discussion we separate labour and birth into the arbitrary first, second, third and fourth stages, in reality midwives know that labour and birth are an inseparable part of the same journey. In many cases, the transition from 'first' to 'second' stage is gradual, and it is often inappropriate to put an exact time on exactly when this transition occurs. For this reason, articles concerning any aspect of labour and birth have been kept together, although, for this edition only, evidence concerning the third stage has been put in a separate section as it was felt that this would reflect the current focus on this aspect of women's experience.

In this section, Maureen Boyle looks at the historical evidence surrounding birthing positions, and the attitudes that surround this. Jilly Rosser's review of the evidence on birth reveals a continued need for research and reflection in this area. A recent publication for childbearing women invites readers to consider whether they would like their babies placed immediately onto their tummies; a common question which at first glance seems relatively empowering. Yet this statement assumes that a woman will be giving birth in a recumbent or semi-recumbent position; it is simply not possible to 'deliver' a baby onto the stomach of a woman who is on all-fours, and not always the easiest option if the woman is upright. A woman who is sitting upright, perhaps in a pool of water, may be catching her own baby, so this statement becomes irrelevant. A seemingly innocuous question shows just how pervasive the assumption that women will be on their backs can be.

Increasingly, midwives are questioning the need to assess the progress of labour by invasive means, particularly in an age where some women experience ten or more vaginal examinations during the course of their labour. Chris Warren, Lesley Hobbs and Ci Ci Stuart all consider this question, and offer some alternatives to vaginal examination. How can we make these alternatives more of an option for women whilst surrounded by systems which place a higher value on technology and the close monitoring of progress in labour by more concrete means?

Another current issue is the rediscovery and development of midwifery skills in supporting women through physiological labour. As we increasingly turn (or return) to 'other ways of knowing', the wisdom of experienced midwives becomes more valuable than ever in reclaiming the kinds of knowledge, skills and tricks which can help facilitate physiological birth, even in the face of technology. Here, Kate Walmsley considers the role of the midwife in helping women through early labour, Deborah Hughes offers some practical ways of helping women cope without pain relief, and Jo Hartley collates the experience of several midwives in helping women to cope with crises in their labour. Two articles by Jean Sutton discuss her description of physiological birth – acting as a reminder of how often we need to revisit the fundamentals of birth physiology – and her suggestions for helping women who have a baby in an occipito-posterior position.

While it is important to enable women to enjoy the entire journey of childbirth, there is little doubt that, for most women, their experience during labour and birth will be remembered more closely than any other aspect of their time with midwives. There is also little doubt that, for most women, the kind of birth they will experience today will differ dramatically from those experienced by their grandmothers and the women who came before them. How can we enable women in the twenty-first century to have birth experiences which are positive rites of passage, rather than episodes of disempowerment and trauma? Do we have time left to recapture more of the traditional knowledge and power surrounding birth before the Caesarean section rate overtakes the number of vaginal births?

Childbirth in bed
The historical perspective

Maureen Boyle

Historically, and in much of the world today, women give birth in an upright position. It is only in Western countries, and over the past one to two centuries that women have 'gone to bed' to give birth.

From the limited data available, it is certainly true that in the United Kingdom most women give birth in a semi-recumbent position in bed. By the end of the 1980s, although most maternity units (87%) said delivery position was the woman's own choice, the same survey showed that 75% of women delivered in the semi-recumbent position.[1] Research at around the same time, this time asking women, showed that 55% of women said they were given no choice in delivery position.[2] However, before attempting to determine what influences the position the woman adopts to give birth, it is useful to look at how women, and their midwives, have arrived at this point in childbirth history.

Early midwives

Throughout history women have always assisted other women in giving birth, and indeed the very earliest writing in all countries details the role of 'midwife'. However, although there was no doubt often a supportive and mutually beneficial relationship, there is also evidence of midwives being directive and perhaps even dictatorial.[3] There are reports from the eighteenth century of midwives tying women to birthing chairs for hours on end,[4] and not only have early midwives in England been described as 'rigid and authoritarian' but these attitudes have also been attributed to their forerunners, the 'handywomen'.[5]

Nevertheless, it is probably true that in the past, and in much of the world today, women who labour in their own homes (and who probably received little labour care, although they are attended during the birth), are more likely to be able to follow their own physiological and emotional feelings in the way they labour and give birth.[6] It is accepted that in most present-day traditional societies the woman giving birth is free to move about and change position as and when she wishes.[7]

'Natural' positions

It is also true that historically 'in almost all depictions of delivery, the woman is squatting and, if any delivery position is "natural" it is this one'.[8] Certainly for many cultures it is the position of choice for resting as well as a position of comfort for many forms of work.

It is also the natural position for excretion in many cultures and even today on a modern Western delivery suite, imminent arrival of the infant is often signalled by the woman wanting to defecate, and therefore move herself from a reclining position.

In the Western world, much medical interest in studies of birthing positions stemmed from an 1882 treatise, *Labor among primitive* people by George Engelmann,[9] at the time the definitive anthropological work. His conclusion, that in no culture other than that in the West do women lie on a bed to give birth, has held true during other observations through the 20th century. A contemporary review of birthing positions around the world describes women in the majority of non-Western cultures giving birth with an upright trunk.[10]

The movement from freedom of movement and upright birth positions, to giving birth (and labouring) in bed, has taken place in the West over the past two centuries. Mauquet de la Motte, an 18th century obstetrician, said

'I have never brought any woman to birth in her bed, unless I was absolutely forced to do so by some urgent need'.[11]

In the 1930s, there was extensive research demonstrating greater efficiency in the birth process with an upright position; however by then the tradition of giving birth in bed passively was already well established, and this research was largely ignored.[12]

However, interestingly, in the USA during the 1950s upright birth positions were reported to have been used for women who 'could not afford the expense of anaesthesia or analgesia' to achieve more comfort in labour and at delivery.[13]

The move to bed

This move 'to bed' was largely inspired by the birth attendants' influence, who felt 'working nearly on ground level, crouching or on his knees... most disagreeable'.[11] These birth attendants were frequently doctors, and as the dominant authority figures, gave their lead to midwives. They not only found a recumbent woman in bed easier to care for at delivery, but also the position was necessary for the newly developed anaesthesia – from the late 1840s ether and then chloroform necessitated a recumbent position and was used not only for pain relief, but also, again, for the doctor's convenience:

'the natural process goes on with more regularity when not under the influence of the will of the patient' [14]

The development of forceps in the mid-18th century and the increase in instrumental deliveries also contributed to the necessity for a recumbent woman.

Although it was doctors who initially began the movement towards the recumbent position for delivery, their ideas were taken up by midwives – there are reports from women giving birth at home with pre-NHS midwives, stating 'they made you lie down on the old iron bed'.[5] In 19th century America, where poor women were often delivered by lay midwives, reports exist of the attendants 'putting a sharp object under the mattress to cut the pain'[15] demonstrating the labouring woman was in bed.

It is not surprising that women and their midwives adopted the medical ideas of birth readily, when doctors so clearly defined the use of any alternative birthing positions as 'low-class if not barbaric'.[4] From the 19th century, obstetricians in France condemned a hands and knees delivery, previously used for difficult births, as 'indecent' and 'too reminiscent of animals'.[11]

By the 1970s in the Western world 'custom, convenience and social attitudes'[16] had all come together to ensure a compliant women who laboured in bed and was delivered of her infant, and a midwifery profession largely acquiescent with the medical model of care of the pregnant patient. There was also evidence that in some formerly traditional societies, women were now lying down for birth, following Western trends.[15]

The medical model

This is probably not surprising considering the history of midwifery in the UK, which began its legal life under medical domination. The Central Midwives' Board, established by the 1902 legislation, was predominantly, and under legal obligation to be, made up of doctors, and indeed the Chairperson of the Central Midwives' Board was not a midwife until 1973.

From 1902 doctors were also responsible for the education of midwives, and presided over their final examination for qualification. The involvement of doctors in midwifery education continued until the late 1980s, with obstetricians still part of the viva for the student midwives' final examination, and consultants' lectures a mandatory part of the curriculum.

It can therefore be of no surprise that 'midwifery knowledge' is deeply influenced by medical research and that the values of the medical profession have been ingrained into midwifery.

The textbooks

The earliest midwifery textbooks were written by doctors, in an authoritative and greatly detailed manner. For example, in a 1924 text[17] attention to such subjects as ventilation of the bedroom

'the lying in room should be thoroughly flushed with pure air at least twice a day by first carefully covering up the patient and then opening wide the window and door for a few minutes'

ensures the doctor is seen as an authority on even those subjects that could be considered to be dependent on common sense, including the personal hygiene of the midwife:

'the midwife will naturally have had a daily bath followed by the thorough brushing and combing of her hair.'

In the same way, clear instruction is given on the position to be adopted for delivery of the baby:

'when in second stage, the patient should lie in the left lateral with legs drawn up.'

Even a doctor with a reputation of considering the physiology, as well as the comfort, of the woman, Grantly Dick-Read[18] gave detailed instructions:

'as soon as second stage is underway, and the mother is helping to push her baby through the birth canal, she should be placed in a semi-sitting position with her knees wide apart. When pushing she pulls her knees upward and outward and supports her feet on her attendants.'

One of the first modern midwifery texts written by a midwife, for widespread distribution in the UK, was *Myles Textbook for Midwives*, the first edition being published in 1953. She suggests that for delivery

'alternative positions can be tried if progress is slow, but the dorsal position is advisable, and exaggerated lithotomy is recommended to facilitate advance of the head.'

The advantages of the dorsal position followed, and these instructions continued unchanged through until the

8th edition in 1975, except that the number of advantages of the dorsal position increased.

De-skilling the midwife

In 1975 the general de-skilling of the midwife is clearly represented:

'midwives are supplementary to and not substitutes for the doctor. They are an extension of his eyes, ears and hands and a helpful assistant in abnormal and operative obstetrics.'

This attitude was clearly demonstrated in the removal of even the small amount of variation of maternal positions left to the midwife's discretion described in earlier editions. In 1975 the position for delivery was 'flat but may prefer patients to be propped up on 3 pillows' with now no mention of alternative positions, although the advantages of the dorsal position continued to be listed. By removing the suggestion of an alternative position to progress birth if necessary, there was no longer any option at all to 'calling the doctor' if there was delay.

By the 11th and 12th editions of *Myles Textbook for Midwives* (1989/1993), now edited by VR Bennett and L Brown, the semi-recumbent position is noted as 'most commonly encouraged in Western cultures' but other positions, including vertical ones are discussed. Other current midwifery textbooks deliver the same message, although Louise Silverton in *The Art and Science of Midwifery* claims: 'most women prefer to remain semi-recumbent upon the delivery bed'[19] with no suggestion that perhaps the popularity of the semi-recumbent position may have little to do with the woman's physiological and emotional choice.

Over the past few decades women have become less ready to accept dictatorial attitudes from doctors and midwives, even during the vulnerable time around childbirth. Many midwives have also become eager to encourage alternative positions, seeing this as a way to empower women and enhance their childbirth experience, as well as for any physiological advantages. But still most women give birth to their babies in a semi-recumbent position on a bed.

The Active Birth movement was founded in April 1982 and by 1985 the World Health Organisation had adopted recommendations for improved practice world-wide: 'each woman must freely decide which position to adopt during delivery'.[20]

'Scientific' birth

As women succeeded in opening the debate and established their right to give birth in an alternative position, the medical establishment moved in to re-assert its dominance by undertaking to define by 'scientific' research what was the 'best' position.

It can be argued that allocating women to a delivery position will influence the outcome by removing the element of choice from the women, as well as removing the chance of her being influenced by her body and how the labour feels to her. This seems particularly true in studies such as the one done by Chan in the 1960s, allocating women to erect or recumbent labour, where women appeared not even to have the choice of withdrawing from the research:

'8 patients in group A complained bitterly of the discomfort of remaining upright and the medical and nursing staff found it no easy task to ensure that the patients were maintained in the erect position.' [21]

Although it is to be hoped that research undertaken more recently would be conducted with an approach more sensitive to women's needs, this may not be so. A study in India in 1992 talks about 200 randomised women being 'kept ambulatory', 'kept in the supine position' during labour, and 'made to squat on the usual delivery cots'.[22] But asking (or forcing) a woman to 'perform' during labour according to preset criteria seems doomed to produce redundant data.

Studying the literature brings forward confusing conclusions relating to women's choices. There are some studies in which women are asked their opinion as to their preference of positions and these report an overwhelming majority choosing upright positions for the second stage.[23] There are likewise some studies that state women choose to 'return to bed' during late first stage.[24] From comprehensive observation, Michel Odent[25] believes the physiology of labour is such that the first stage is optimally spent 'at rest', with the women only receiving the physical urge to become upright and active in the second stage.

Freedom of movement

In considering various positions for birth, it may be that the ability to change positions during the second stage may be more important than a single 'best' position anyway.[16] Most research that has looked at comparing two fixed positions has had ambiguous results. The interest in alternative positions was initially based on positions adopted by other cultures, but the freedom of movement between the postures has been largely ignored by researchers.[7]

Given all the variables influencing the second stage, it is difficult to see how a direct relationship can be made between positions for giving birth (and/or freedom of movement) and outcome. It is not clear whether it is of physiological benefit if a woman can move to a position (or positions) of choice, or if it is of psychological benefit – or, which is more likely, a combination of meeting both aspects are necessary for the best outcome. Lesley Page[26] states:

'in labour our skill also lies in creating an environment where women might follow their instinct to move and find the most comfortable position.'

This then may be the challenge for the midwife – to try and ensure the woman has the freedom to behave during labour as she feels best, to meet her own needs, despite the various constraints of a modern British delivery suite.

REFERENCES

1 Garcia J, Garforth S. Labour and delivery routines in English Consultant Maternity Units. Midwifery 1989; 5(4):155–62.
2 Kitzinger S. Walking through labour [correspondence]. British Medical Journal 1987; 295(6612):1568.
3 Davies ML. Maternity: Letters from working women collected by the Women's Co-operative Guild. London: Virago; 1978.
4 Donnison J. Midwives and medical men: A history of the struggle for the control of childbirth. London: Historical Publications; 1988.
5 Leap N, Hunter B. The midwife's tale: An oral history from handywoman to professional midwife. London: Scarlet Press; 1993.
6 Bryar R. Theory for midwifery practice. London: Macmillan; 1995.
7 Kitzinger S. Childbirth and society. In: Chalmers I, Enkin M, Keirse M (eds). Effective care in pregnancy and childbirth. Oxford: Oxford University Press; 1989.
8 Gebbie D. Reproductive anthropology: Descent through woman. Chichester: John Wiley & Sons; 1981.
9 Hillan E. Posture for labour and delivery. Midwifery 1985; 1:19–23.
10 Russell J. The rationale of primitive delivery positions. British Journal of Obstetrics & Gynaecology 1982; 29: 712–715.
11 Gelis J. History of childbirth: Fertility, pregnancy and birth in early modern Europe. Cambridge: Polity Press; 1991.
12 Rossi M, Lindell S. Maternal positions and pushing technique in a nonprescriptive environment. Journal of Obstetric, Gynecologic & Neonatal Nursing 1986; May/June:203–298.
13 Howard F. Delivery in the physiologic position. Obstetrics & Gynecology 1958; 11(3):318–322.
14 Simpson J. Remarks on the superinduction of anaesthesia in natural and morbid parturition. Lancet 1848; 1:254–256.
15 Priya JV. Birth traditions and modern pregnancy care. Shaftesbury: Element Books; 1992.
16 Roberts J. Alternative positions for childbirth. Part II: Second stage of labor. Journal of Nurse-Midwifery 1980; 25:11–19.
17 Berkeley C. A handbook of midwifery: For midwives, maternity nurses and obstetric dressers. London: Cassell & Co; 1924.
18 Dick-Read G. Childbirth without fear. 5th edn. New York: Harper & Row; 1985.
19 Silverton L. The art and science of midwifery. London: Prentice Hall; 1993.
20 World Health Organization Recommendations. Lancet 1985; August 24th: 436–437.
21 Chan D. Positions during labour. British Medical Journal 1963; 12th January: 100.
22 Allahbadia G, Vaidya P. Why deliver in the supine position? Australian & New Zealand Journal of Obstetrics & Gynaecology 1992; 32(2):104–106.
23 Sleep J, Roberts, Chalmers I. Care during the second stage of labour. In: Chalmers I, Enkin M, Keirse M. Effective care in pregnancy and childbirth. Oxford: Oxford University Press; 1989.
24 Melzack R, et al. Labor pain: Effect of maternal position on front and back pain. Journal of Pain and Symptom Management 1991; 6(8 November):476–80.
25 Odent M. Laboring women are not marathon runners. Midwifery Today 1994; 31(Autumn):23–4, 43, 51.
26 Page L. Putting principles into practice. In: Page L (ed). Effective group practice in midwifery: Working with women. Oxford: Blackwell Science; 1995.

Why should I do vaginal examinations?

Chris Warren

A conversation I had recently with a supervisor of midwives made me think again about vaginal examinations (VEs) in labour. Looking over my practice, there were two or more occasions when she would have undertaken a VE and I had not done so. Our areas of clinical practice and expertise differ greatly and her opinion was different to mine. Time for reflection – was it a matter of right and wrong, or just different clinical judgements?

I only examine a woman vaginally if I am looking for specific information in order to make a decision. This was the case with Georgina, who wanted to give birth in hospital but was making little grunting noises when I arrived at her home. Her membranes were intact but as her cervix had dilated to 9cm, I judged it best to stay home.

The problem is that the birth process is so individual, with such a wide range of normality that, while a lot of information can be gained from VEs (see Table 4.2.1), it is not always easy to interpret.

'Please examine me, now!' was how Sarah, expecting her third, greeted me when I arrived at her house in response to her call. I usually have a cup of tea and give time for my presence to be absorbed but Sarah was insistent. Her cervix had partially effaced and dilated to 3cm. She was reluctant to get into the waiting pool as she had read that it was better to wait until her cervix was 5cm dilated. But she wanted something to help with the pain. I recommended trying the water. Less than $1\frac{1}{2}$ hours later, Sarah delivered Ellory and I guided him up through the water to her arms. The rate, power and consuming energy of her contractions had indicated a well advanced labour, progressing rapidly.

It was very different with Susan, who called me out on three consecutive Friday evenings, with runs of contractions that faded away soon after my arrival.

The first time, when I examined her vaginally I was excited to discover that her cervix was 4cm dilated and I unpacked my bag, ready for the birth. In the morning I repacked my bag and went home. The following week, I did not examine her until the Saturday morning. Her cervix was fully effaced and 5cm dilated but the contractions had stopped completely. 'Don't worry!' I said. 'It will be soon.' Off I went, clutching my bleep, fearing a baby born before the midwife's return. On the third Friday, at 10pm, her cervix was again 5cm dilated. Each time, the baby's head felt well engaged by palpation and its station was 1cm above the spines. I stayed overnight again; some of the contractions had, prior to my arrival, been 'pretty fierce'. This time, we both dozed until 6am when I woke to grunts from Susan. Baby Natalie arrived in time for breakfast.

Sarah and Susan were birthing their third babies but it was the first time they had given birth at home.

In retrospect, I sometimes realise that a vaginal examination might have been helpful. Alison, 35 weeks pregnant, was having occasional tightenings. She had been up in the night with diarrhoea and vomiting; her two-year-old was just recovering from a similar bug. I drank tea and chatted, listened to her baby's heartbeat and reassured her that while bowel activity can trigger uterine action, things would probably settle down. Seven hours and lots more uterine 'irritability' later, she bleeped me, and within an hour was sitting up in bed suckling baby Iolanthe.

An abdominal palpation should precede a vaginal examination, and the information gained considered in the context of this woman, this labour and this time. I find it useful to ask: 'How can I justify this invasive interference?' In response to a wonderful study which I recommend every midwife to read[1] Murray Enkin says that we need to 'recognise that repeated vaginal examinations are an invasive intervention of as yet unproven value.' Like others[3] I have found no research-based recommendations on the timing or frequency of vaginal examinations in labour. Have VEs become so routine that they are no longer seen as an intervention? The RCOG do consider vaginal examinations to be medical interventions and stress that such intimate

Table 4.2.1 Information which can be obtained from a vaginal examination

The condition of the vulva, perineum and vagina: old scars, warts, cysts and prominent veins
The position, length, consistency and dilation of the cervix
The presentation, attitude and position of the baby
The presence of caput, degree of moulding
The relationship of the presenting part to the cervix
The presence of the membranes and their reaction to a contraction
The colour and amount of the liquor

examinations should be undertaken only when necessary. They do not comment on the need for vaginal examinations in labour.[4] The fact that midwives or doctors check on the progress of most labours implies a lack of confidence in a woman's ability to birth naturally. '…the role of the midwife… is to support the woman… not to manage the woman's labour…'

Most women do not like vaginal examinations. They bring up issues of sexual intimacy, invasion of privacy, and vulnerability. For some, they are very traumatic, mentally and/or physically, and may lead to infection.[6] Sometimes, women who have had a difficult birth ask me how often I do vaginal examinations. They tell me that the examinations were the worst part of the birth – others may feel the same. Devane's study found that 'Vaginal examinations are often a source of anxiety, both for midwives and the clients they care for. Many women find them distressing, uncomfortable and embarrassing.' [3]

Vaginal examinations can even be life threatening. Severe reactions to latex are rare, occurring in less than 1% of the general population but rising to 5-17% among healthcare workers,[7] so all midwives should be aware of the possibility. One woman's reaction following a vaginal examination in labour before her allergy to latex was suspected included 'anxiety, hypotension, dyspnoea, congestion of her face and hands and oedema, generalised pruritus and arthralgias.'[7]

Last year, at eight consecutive births I attended, I judged that no vaginal examinations were needed, but at the next two births I did four each time. Both women laboured over three days; one gave birth at home and the other had a Caesarean for fetal distress after we transferred her to hospital in the second stage of labour.

Frequent vaginal examinations in the second stage of labour may well 'reinforce cultural messages about women's powerlessness and imply that the woman's body cannot be trusted to work right.'[1] Any examination, if done primarily for the professional's need, implies a distrust of the woman's ability to birth her baby. This is not to deny that 'vaginal examination to assess the dilation of the cervix is the most accurate method of measuring progress in labour',[8] and there are occasions when the information gained could be critical.

Both the woman and her carer should be involved in the decision to perform a vaginal examination. It is likely that: 'Most women will accept vaginal examination if the necessity for the procedure is explained and the examination is performed by a doctor [sic] who is skilled, sympathetic and gentle'.[4]

It is difficult to find research to direct practice. With such a lack of evidence, it is impossible to know whether routine vaginal examinations constitute effective care. How, then, can we justify routine vaginal examinations? All we can say is that they are useful in certain circumstances. Currently, too many are done and as a result women are unnecessarily discomforted or traumatised. I am worried that they are seen as routine, and that 'necessity' is interpreted differently by different midwives. One particular supervisor and I certainly had different interpretations of necessity.

On reflection, I think I may do too many.

REFERENCES

1 Bergstrom L, Roberts J, Skiliman L, et al. "You'll feel me touching you, sweetie": Vaginal examinations during the second stage of labour. Birth 1992; 19(l):10–18.

2 Enkin M. Commentary: Do I do that? Do I really do that? Like that? Birth 1992; 19(l):19–20.

3 Devane D. Sexuality and midwifery. British Journal of Midwifery 1996; 4(8):413–416.

4 The Royal College of Obstetricians and Gynaecologists. Intimate examinations: Report of a Working Party. London: RCOG Press, 1997.

5 Banks M. Breech birth, woman-wise. Hamilton, New Zealand: Birthspirit Books; 1995.

6 Seaward P, Hannah M, et al. International multicentre term prelabor rupture of membranes study: Evaluation of predictors of clinical chorioamnionitis and post partum fever in patients with prelabor rupture of membranes at term. American Journal of Obstetrics and Gynaecology 1997; 177(5):1024–1029.

7 Santos R, et al. Severe latex allergy after a vaginal examination during labor: A case report. American Journal of Obstetrics and Gynecology 1997; 177(6):1543–1544.

8 Crowther C, et al. Monitoring the progress of labour. In: Enkin M, Keirse M, Chalmers I (eds). A guide to effective care in childbirth. Oxford: Oxford University Press; 1997:199–204.

9 Menage J. Post-traumatic stress disorder following obstetric/gynaecological procedures. British Journal of Midwifery 1996; 4(l):532–533.

Assessing cervical dilatation without VEs

Watching the purple line

Lesley Hobbs

For some time, it has been my ambition to find a reliable way of assessing progress in labour which, as far as possible, does away with the need for internal examinations. Yes, I know, you can assess progress without them, but it makes sense to have some formal mechanism both for the benefit of the client who wants to know how far she's got, as well as the more pragmatic reason that if you have to transfer, it's more credible if there's an established measurement.

A few years ago, I heard about a research study which put the hypothesis that the purple line which creeps up the so-called 'natal cleft' (or bum cleavage for the less scientific amongst us) can be used as a measure of cervical dilatation.[1] The purplish-red line begins at the anal margin at the start of labour and gradually creeps up, like mercury in a thermometer. When it reaches the nape of the buttocks (see diagram), the woman is fully dilated. Allegedly.

I found this intriguing. So I sent off for the article, but also started in a minor way to see if the digital measurements (that's fingers, nothing to do with analogue) corresponded. So far, it has been uncannily accurate. The line starts to appear just above the anal margin at between 0 and 2cm cervical dilatation. It does not seem to rise in strict proportion; there is a longer gap between 4 and 7cm dilatation than there is both before and after.

The nape of the buttocks is the point just below the sacrococcygeal joint, where the coccyx begins to curve inwards (in most people).

A woman for whom I was recently caring was giving some signs of being in late first stage. (She was a primip and the baby was OP.) The contractions were coming thick and fast, she was grunting and deeply under the influence of endorphins and had been 4cm three hours earlier. Bearing in mind the baby's position, however, I was suspicious. I didn't want to do another VE even though she kept asking how she was doing, so I asked her to move from her position straddled backwards on a chair on to all-fours. I also explained why. When I had a look, the line indicated that her cervix was, at most, 6cm dilated. I told her this and she decided to stay on all-fours for a while. To my amazement, as I watched, the line crept up. At the same time, she stopped grunting with the contractions and told me that the 'awful pressure' in her bottom had gone away. Half an hour later, the line suggested that she was about 8cm. An hour after that, the line reached the top of the cleft and she began pushing. In this case, it seems that observing the line told

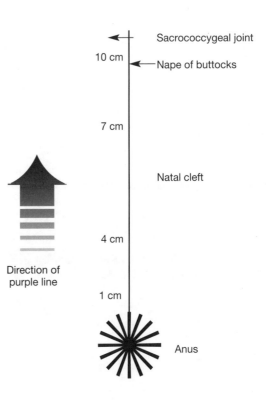

Sacrococcygeal joint

10 cm — Nape of buttocks

7 cm

Natal cleft

4 cm

Direction of purple line

1 cm

Anus

me much more than just an approximation of cervical dilatation; I could tell that the baby had turned and that the rate of dilatation had altered.

Accurate reading would seem to be the key to this practice. I sometimes notice in myself a wish to see the line progressing more quickly than it actually does; when I do this – and then check with a VE, only to find the line is right – I get annoyed with myself and wish I'd trusted my observations. As a clinician, I ought to have got over wishful thinking when women are tired and dispirited, and concentrate on giving them strength and perseverance, but I'm only human.

I'm not quite ready to abandon my training yet – so far it's a very small sample. It does seem, however, that once allowances are made for anatomical diversity (e.g. bad piles make the initial dilatation difficult to assess), the hypothesis is rapidly becoming a demonstrable reality. I have to resist the temptation to make pencil marks (sometimes there are helpful distinguishing features which serve as landmarks) and peering intently at some poor soul's buttocks can, I suspect, have an inhibiting effect on the sensitive. You certainly have to be more intrusive on women with large buttocks in order to be able to observe the line.

As I work in an area with very little ethnic diversity, I have only made these observations on white women. I would love to hear from midwives working with black, Asian or Chinese women, for example, who are interested in exploring the possibilities of this new practice, and who could tell me whether all the above holds true across ethnic and racial groups. For instance, what is the colour of the line on women with black skin?

I can now envisage a time when I shall feel confident enough to use this as my formal measurement mechanism and abandon intrusive and superfluous vaginal exams.

REFERENCE

1   Byrne DL, Edmonds DK. Clinical method for evaluating progress in the first stage of labour. Lancet 1997; 335(8681):122.

Invasive actions in labour

Where have the 'old tricks' gone?

Ci Ci Stuart

In her article, 'Why should I do vaginal examinations?', Chris Warren[1] posed some challenging questions regarding the necessity for performing frequent vaginal examinations during labour. She raised a particularly salient question: Have vaginal examinations become so routine in labour that they are no longer seen as an intervention? The issue of whether it is necessary to perform routine and frequent vaginal examinations during normal labour will be explored in this paper.

History?

Warren's article reminded me vividly of the days when I used to assess the progress of labours without having to resort to the performance of vaginal examinations. This happened in the early 1970s when I was training and working in Scotland – in this particular maternity unit, midwives did not perform vaginal examinations on women during labour unless instructed to do so by medical staff. Student midwives then were required to perform only six vaginal examinations during their training. Margaret Myles' *Textbook for Midwives*[2] was our bible and her writings on midwifery practice were treated as doctrines! On the performance of vaginal examinations during the management of normal labour, Myles had this to say:

'*A vaginal examination should not be necessary during every labour and should always be preceded by abdominal examination. The presentation, position and descent of the fetus can be ascertained by abdominal palpation during the first stage of labour ...*' (Original emphases)

Margaret Myles' wisdom as a midwife was apparent, as she continued thus: '... but there are occasions when it is imperative that a vaginal examination be made'. This advice could account for the inclusion of the honour of performing six vaginal examinations during my training! At the completion of my training, I was confident in my ability to assess progress of labour abdominally but obviously did not possess the same degree of competence about assessing progress vaginally!

The two main criteria I then used to monitor the progress of labours are the patterns of uterine contractions and the descent and flexion of the fetal head, determined by abdominal palpation. Our chant in relationship to contractions was that if labour was progressing normally, contractions should become stronger and longer and more frequent. Abdominal palpations were performed two to three hourly to assess the rate of descent and the degree of flexion of the fetal head. Descent, then, was described in terms of the head being 'engaged' or 'deeply engaged'.[2] Landmarks used to assess descent and flexion were the pelvic brim and the sinciput and occiput of the fetal head.

The midwives possessed a high level of competence and confidence in their abilities to monitor whether labour was progressing normally with information obtained from the measures described above and with the information obtained from the 'usual observations' made of maternal and fetal wellbeing. Their skills and confidence were 'passed on'. I became quite adept at ascertaining the amount of fetal head palpable abdominally, and in many instances, the degree of flexion. I learnt to develop a 'feel' for the sinciput and the occiput as these landmarks feel different abdominally, and also their 'whereabouts' in relationship to the pelvic brim. Therefore, when descent and flexion were taking place, I learnt to ascertain how the positions of the sinciput and occiput would change in relationship to each other and in relationship to the pelvic brim. When the head is deflexed, the occiput and sinciput can be felt to be at the same level to each other. As flexion starts to occur, the occiput can be felt to be lower than the sinciput. Conversely, when the head is extended, the sinciput is lower than the occiput in which case a brow presentation is suspected. Using the pelvic brim as the landmark, I developed a feel for the 'high' head, the 'engaged' head and the head which is flexed and descending and therefore labour was progressing normally. If uterine contractions had developed into the expected pattern and both the maternal and fetal conditions were satisfactory, then all was well. And when 'little' or 'no head' was palpable, it frequently coincided with increasing 'distress' in the woman and soon after, she developed the urge to push, heralding the onset of the second stage of labour, confirmed by the visibility of the presenting part. Frequently, over the many hours of a normal labour, no vaginal examinations had been done, certainly not by a midwife!

Assessing fetal descent abdominally

The practice ethos that had been instilled in me did not include the necessity for performing vaginal examinations in order to assess the progress of normal labour. Vaginal examinations were reserved for labours which fell outside the parameters of normality, such as breech presentations and labours which had been induced or augmented. I had strongly internalised that what are paramount in determining progress are an establishment of longer, stronger and more frequent contractions and fetal head descent and flexion determined by abdominal palpation.

Through radiological examinations, Stewart (cited in Philpott)[3] showed how abdominal palpation of head descent can be made with accuracy. The head that is five-fifths palpable is entirely above the brim; one that is four-fifths palpable is just entering the brim. When three-fifths palpable, the hands can still go partially round the head. When two-fifths palpable, more than half the head has entered the brim. The hands splay outwards. Studd et al[4] equate this abdominal level with the 'engaged' head. In most women, once the head is engaged the bony presenting part is at or nearly at the level of the ischial spines which is equated to station zero as determined by vaginal examination.[16] With one-fifth palpable, only the sinciput can be tipped abdominally and nought-fifths represents a head entirely in the pelvis with no sinciput or occiput palpable abdominally. A pictorial representation of the above discussion is shown in Figure 4.4.1.

Studd et al[4] recommend that fetal head level should be assessed and recorded by bi-manual abdominal palpation and described as the number of 'fifths' of head palpable. This is preferable to the use of the descriptor 'station' of the head with reference to the ischial spines assessed at vaginal examination. Determination of fetal head level by abdominal palpation excludes the variability due to caput and moulding and that produced by a different depth of pelvis. Assessment in fifths is quantitative and easily reproducible. They go on to say that:

'The most important part of the head is that part which still has to enter the pelvis and it is this which should be assessed.'

Internalising new values

With the start of practising midwifery in England, came the requirement for me to perform regular and frequent vaginal examinations as part of the strategy of 'active management' and the partographic control of labour.[5,6,7] Although I had knowledge of the theoretical underpinnings for the necessity for performing vaginal examinations and the information which can be obtained from a vaginal examination, I had only vague recollections of the six momentous occasions when I performed vaginal examinations with the doctors. I rapidly had to learn to perform vaginal examinations. I was very conscious and concerned that noting descent vaginally is much more invasive than noting descent abdominally, even though the latter procedure may cause many women to experience discomfort and some even feel pain. I was, however, alone with my concerns about vaginal examinations; I had no voice: my voice was muted in the presence of more powerful others.[8] In my case, the more powerful others were everyone else who considered regular and frequent vaginal examinations necessary to assess progress of labour. In the presence of such oppression as espoused by Freire,[9] it was easier not to question the frequency with which I performed vaginal examinations. Like the nurses in Roberts' study,[10] as 'the oppressed', I rapidly internalised the values of others who were dominant – I spoke of, and believed in, the value of regular and frequent vaginal examinations. Warren[1] has outlined some psychological side effects for both the woman and midwife, and the potential physical complications for the woman of vaginal examinations. In her haunting and poignant account of having been cruelly sexually assaulted and thus abused, Jo Desborough[11] reminds us that a large percentage of women in our care will have suffered similar abuse. Intimate procedures such as vaginal examinations for these women are likely to induce painful and distressing flashbacks. Desborough pleads for heightened sensitivity for women in our care, particularly when we are performing intimate procedures such as vaginal examinations and assisting with breastfeeding. I examine instances of less than sensitive practice with much soul-searching.

The science of midwifery?

Amongst others, the work of Studd[5,6] and Philpott and Castle[7] became influential in 'diagnosing labours that were not progressing' because the patterns of cervical dilatation of these women did not fit the patterns of cervical dilatation of the normogram and the latent and active phases of labour. I can remember the sense of excitement amongst obstetricians and midwives as we could see how the labour was progressing graphically,

Figure 4.4.1 Head in fifths above the pelvic brim

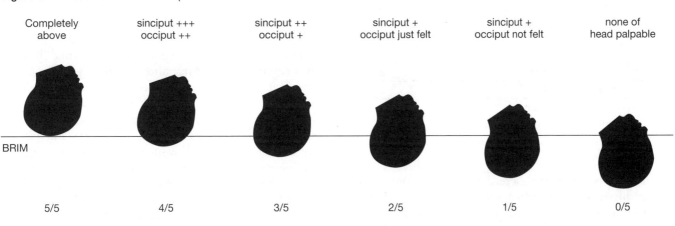

| Completely above | sinciput +++ occiput ++ | sinciput ++ occiput + | sinciput + occiput just felt | sinciput + occiput not felt | none of head palpable |

BRIM

| 5/5 | 4/5 | 3/5 | 2/5 | 1/5 | 0/5 |

and we knew (or so we thought), the action to take if nature's powers were letting the woman down. There was a sense of objectivity as we went about our business of managing the labours. Great emphasis is placed on the rate of cervical dilatation as a measure of the progress of labour. Studd[6] stated that cervical dilatation is the most critical indicator of progress. The usual question asked of progress is: 'What is the cervix on VE?' Rarely, 'What is the station?' And even more rarely, 'Where is the fetal head on abdominal palpation?' The performance of vaginal examinations is accepted as part of the strategy of the management of labours today. However, there is no research-based evidence recommending the frequency of vaginal examinations in labour. In her search to find empirical evidence to support her practice of performing vaginal examinations, Warren[1] concluded:

'It is difficult to find research to direct practice. With such a lack of evidence, it is impossible to know whether routine vaginal examinations constitute effective care. How, then, can we justify routine vaginal examinations?'

Stuart[12] makes the point that aspects of care which are routine become taken for granted, which in turn may lead to unhelpful and even unthinking care-giving. Kirkham[13] stresses that in order to improve care we need to 'see through and beyond the accepted ways of seeing and thinking'. Midwives need to ask whether they need to perform vaginal examinations with the frequency and regularity, as is the custom and practice, in order to assess progress of labour. We need to challenge the taken for granted and consider alternatives. The following question is posed: With what degree of confidence can midwives assess progress of labour using abdominal palpation to ascertain fetal head descent and flexion, and the pattern of uterine contractions, without having to resort to the performance of vaginal examinations as frequently as many are now doing?

Friedman's work in 1967[14] showed that labour consists of a latent phase, associated with cervical effacement and dilatation of up to 3cm, and an active phase, associated with cervical dilatation. Later work by Pearson[15] indicates that the curve of cervical dilatation is mirrored by the curve of descent. During the latent and early active phase of cervical dilatation, fetal descent may be minimal. Once the phase of rapid cervical dilatation has begun, steady fetal descent usually begins, with the most rapid descent taking place when the cervix is nearly fully dilated, and in the second stage of labour.[16] Extrapolating from work done during the last three decades, Bowes concluded that the rate of descent during the active phase can be quantified at 1cm per hour in the primigravida and 2cm per hour in the multigravida.[17] There are exceptions, for example, in the African primigravida, the head does not start to descend until the late first stage of labour.[7]

In their work to determine the mathematical relationships between uterine contractions, descent and rotation of the fetal head determined by vaginal examinations and the degree of cervical dilatation in 50 multiparous women with spontaneous vaginal deliveries, Sallam et al[18] found a good correlation between the amount of descent of the fetal vertex and the degree of cervical dilatation. From the normogram constructed, they concluded that the amount of cervical dilatation can be determined given the descent of the fetal head, the rotation of the presenting part in degrees and the frequency of uterine contractions. Some of their findings are shown in Table 4.4.1.

When no direct evidence is available to support practice, we may be able to extrapolate from indirect sources. The above discussion indicates the correlation between fetal head descent, uterine contractions and cervical dilatation. Midwives can therefore infer cervical dilatation from assessments of the fetal head level abdominally. When labour is progressing normally, there is progressive descent of the fetal head and the establishment of a pattern of uterine contractions. Having the confidence to make such clinical judgement and

Table 4.4.1 Cervical dilatation, fetal head station, zero degree internal rotation and uterine contactions[18]

Cervical dilatation (cm)	Head station	Internal rotation (degrees)	Contractions per 10 minutes
3	-1 cm	0	2
4	+1 cm	0	2
5	+2 cm	0	2
7	+3 cm	0	3
10	+4.5 cm	0	4/5

decision is also important here. This perhaps comes with the acquisition of practice knowledge and wisdom through critical reflection on midwifery practice.[20] Kirkham[21] says that in order to acquire such clinical wisdom, we need to acknowledge the importance of our midwifery experiences and what we can learn from them. Kirkham relates how she made connections between personal feelings of nausea, and even vomiting on occasions, with the onset of the second stage of labour in women who had long labours. Sadly, a midwife's ways of gaining knowledge through practice are frequently discounted as this source of knowledge is not the taught authoritative knowledge – that knowledge which counts and therefore motivates decisions and actions.[22]

Conclusion

The technocratic world of obstetrics and midwifery practice makes it difficult to exercise midwifery wisdom acquired through alternative ways of 'knowing'. But we can exercise the caring and sensitivity that many vulnerable women during childbirth deserve and need. A vaginal examination is an invasive procedure. Performed with regularity and frequency in obstetric units, it has come to be accepted as a routine procedure by many. This may desensitise us to the intrusive nature of vaginal examinations which could result in untoward emotional and psychological consequences. Physical complications, although uncommon today, cannot be excluded. There are alternative ways of assessing progress in labour without having to resort to regular frequent vaginal examinations. We need to develop the confidence to use these alternatives. Such confidence will develop when we start to analyse and interpret our clinical experiences so that patterns which indicate that labour is progressing normally can be recognised.

Every woman is an individual. Every labour is different. Midwifery is also an art. As such, we perhaps need to remind ourselves that the application of a set of rules and policies such as the set timing, regularity and frequency of vaginal examinations for every labour is simply illogical.

REFERENCES

1 Warren C. Why should I do vaginal examinations? The Practising Midwife 1999; 2(6):12–14.
2 Myles MF. Textbook for midwives, 7th edn. London: Churchill Livingstone; 1972.
3 Philpott RH. The management of labour. In: Stallworthy J, Bourne G (eds). Recent advances in obstetrics and gynaecology, no. 13. London: Churchill Livingstone; 1979:137–153.
4 Studd JW, Cardozo LD, Gibb DMF. The management of spontaneous labour. In: Studd JW (ed). Progress in obstetrics and gynaecology, vol. 2. London: Churchill Livingstone; 1982.
5 Studd JW. The partographic control of labour. Clinics in Obstetrics and Gynaecology 1975; 2(1):127–151.
6 Studd JW. Partograms and normograms of cervical dilatation in the management of primigravid labour. British Medical Journal 1973; 4:451–455.
7 Philpott RH, Castle WM. Cervicographs in the management of labour in the primigravidae. I. The alert line for detecting abnormal labour. II. The action line and treatment of abnormal labour. Journal of Obstetrics and Gynaecology of the British Commonwealth 1972; 79:592–602.
8 Johns C. Reflection as empowerment? Nursing Inquiry 1999; 6:241–249.
9 Freire P. Pedagogy of the oppressed. London: Penguin Books; 1972.
10 Roberts SJ. Oppressed group behaviour: Implications for nursing. Advances in Nursing Science 1983; 5:21–30.
11 Desborough J. Sexual assault and flashbacks on the labour ward. The Practising Midwife 2000; 3(4):18–20.

12 Stuart CC. Concepts of reflection and reflective practice. British Journal of Midwifery 1998; 6(10):640–647.
13 Kirkham M. Reflection in midwifery: Professional narcissism or seeing with women? British Journal of Midwifery 1997; 5(5):259–262.
14 Friedman EA. Labor: Clinical evaluation and management. New York: Meredith; 1967.
15 Pearson J. Clinical Forum 7: Midwifery 1 – Partography. Nursing Mirror 1981; July 8: xxv–xxix.
16 Oxorn H. Human labour and birth, 5th edn. Norwalk, CO: Appleton-Century-Crofts; 1986.
17 Bowes WA. Clinical aspects of normal and abnormal labour. In: Creasy RK, Resnik R (eds). Maternal-fetal medicine, 4th edn. Philadelphia: WB Saunders 1999; 541–568.
18 Sallam HN, Abdel-Dayem A, Sakr RA, et al. Mathematical relationships between uterine contractions, cervical dilatation, descent and rotation in spontaneous vertex deliveries. International Journal of Gynecology and Obstetrics 1999; 64:135–139.
19 Reed J, Proctor S. Nursing knowledge: A critical examination. In: Reed J, Proctor S (eds). Nurse education: A reflective approach. London: Edward Arnold; 1993: 14–29.
20 Benner P, Tanner C, Chesla C. Expertise in nursing practice: Caring, clinical judgement and ethics. New York: Springer; 1996.
21 Kirkham M. Bodily knowledge: The wisdom of nausea. Midwifery Today 1999; Winter(52):15.
22 Jordan B. Authoritative knowledge and its construction. In: Davis-Floyd R, Sargent CF (eds). Childbirth and authoritative knowledge. London: University of California Press; 1997: 55–79.

Midwives and women

Coping with pain together

Deborah Hughes

Midwives spend a lot of time with people in pain. Learning how to support a woman with her labour pains without feeling tension, inappropriate sympathy or anxiety is one of the biggest lessons a midwife has to learn and it is something that we have to go on learning throughout our professional lives.

Whilst many midwives may take the analgesia/anaesthesia approach, this has many well-documented, physical and psychological disadvantages for mother and baby.[1] Moreover, satisfaction with the experience of childbirth is not related to the absence or lessening of pain.[2] Many women wish to minimise the use of analgesics and anaesthetics; and many midwives, aware of the problems that analgesia can bring, strive to help women avoid analgesic medications and epidurals. How can we maximise a woman's chance of achieving this? The following suggestions can help.

- Once the woman is in labour, refer to 'contractions', (or whatever name the woman uses) rather than 'pains'. This does not prevent the midwife from acknowledging the woman's pain when appropriate, but it does help remind everyone present of the underlying processes taking place.
- Minimise all activity that worsens the woman's experience of pain. For example, do you really need to do this VE? Do you require the information it will give you in order to make a clinical decision or have you already got a fairly full picture of what is happening from your other observations and examinations? If a VE is not essential to you or the woman, you will cause discomfort for no obvious benefit. The increased discomfort the woman experiences, either from the procedure itself or the position she is asked to adopt for it, may be enough to make her feel she can no longer cope.
- Make sure she has constant support or, if she is being left alone, that she feels this suits her well. Try to do

stage management chores like checking equipment and communicating with other personnel quietly between contractions. Even if you have other things to attend to and there is other support (partner, friend, mother), convey to the client that she remains your priority and that you are available to her at any time. This will increase her sense of support and safety and decrease hormone-blocking anxiety.

- Nurture her sense of wellbeing and that of her birth partner(s) with a touch, smile or quiet word between contractions. Stopping what you are doing and attending to the rhythm of her breathing during contractions will help give her non-intrusive support and help build an atmosphere of psychological safety and calm, positive regard and empathy. All of this will allay fear and panic, create a sense of wellbeing and help the woman and her partner(s) cope with her contractions.
- Other aspects of atmosphere need attention. Is the room pleasant, does the woman seem psychologically comfortable with the surroundings, is everyone physically comfortable and relaxed between contractions? Too much light, noise, activity and people can adversely affect the release of labour hormones[2] and inhibit relaxation – not only in the woman but also in her attendants. Don't be afraid to leave the woman alone or with her partner if this seems to suit them. As long as you remain within earshot, this may, at times, be the most helpful midwifery care you can offer.
- Try not to inhibit the woman's free movement by practice or suggestion. Most labouring women will adopt the positions that are most anatomically advantageous to them but they may need some help to maintain that position comfortably. For example, if she seems to prefer to stand leaning forward slightly, is there a piece of furniture of a suitable height that she could use to take her weight? If she seems to

prefer all-fours, can you help prevent her knees becoming sore by putting soft pillows underneath?

- Group your observations around one or two contractions, explaining what you need to do in the next rest phase. This will minimise inhibiting the woman's regression to primitive brain consciousness and its accompanying hormonal activity. Feed back your findings to everyone present so that they know that all is well and do not begin to build up anxiety.

- Some quiet conversation and humour between contractions can help everyone retain a sense of social wellbeing. Positive feedback is essential for everyone – the woman, her partner and the midwife.

- Don't start using pain-relieving techniques too soon. If the woman is 'coping', bide your time unless she asks for specific assistance. Baths, back-rubbing, vocalisation, hot flannels and intensive help with breathing can all be brought into play as the increasing intensity of the contractions begins to distress her. Take each contraction as it comes and concentrate on helping the woman through that one, introducing non-pharmacological forms of pain relief only as she begins to waver on the brink of distress or asks for help. Use each for as long as it helps and only move on to or add another when necessary. As labour becomes increasingly intense, you may end up using many techniques together, e.g. applying hot flannels to the woman's back in a tub whilst everyone in the room breathes or vocalises with her.

- Stay relaxed. You are not the cause of the woman's pain and are not responsible for it. We are socially driven to alleviate pain and distress and the nurses among us have also been professionally trained to do this. As labour intensifies, remember to breathe calmly, i.e. slowly and abdominally, and to keep your brow, mouth and shoulders relaxed. Soothe your own distress by taking a moment to stretch and release tension.

- Beware of suggesting analgesia at this time unless you are sure you are doing so to meet the real needs of the woman rather than to relieve your own pain and anxiety. If you feel the woman is reaching the end of the road with non-pharmacological options, you can always quietly remind her that she does have other choices. Use open rather than closed questions when you do this – 'How do you want us to help you through your contractions?' is more likely to enable her to consider her options than 'Would an epidural help?'

- Have you had a drink? Have you got support, another midwife you can talk things over with? Are you satisfied with the woman's condition, the baby's condition and the way labour is progressing? Any tension, discomfort and uncertainty you feel about any of these must be recognised and may require a change of plan. Are you too tired to carry on? If so, this can have a detrimental effect on the woman's sense of wellbeing and her ability to bear her labour.

It is lack of attention to these fundamentals of midwifery care which can have a cumulative effect in any labour and render it impossible for a woman to cope without pharmacological analgesia or anaesthesia. The minutiae of behaviour, environment and atmosphere should be the foundation for midwifery care, not afterthoughts.

Drug-free birth has many benefits for mother and baby but is increasingly uncommon in the UK. It is demanding on the midwife because it requires her to attend not only to the woman but also to the environment, the woman's supporters and herself. These skills are under-recognised, undervalued and under-taught. The culture of many labour wards even actively works against them. We should talk about them much more.

REFERENCES

1 Tew M. Safer childbirth? A critical history of maternity care. London: Free Association Press; 1998.

2 Jowitt M. Childbirth unmasked: The science, art and humanity of childbirth. Craven Arms: Peter Wooller; 1993.

Helping women through crises in their labour

Jo Hartley

Midwives interviewed

Mary Cronk
Independent midwife, West Sussex

Becky Reed
Group practice midwife, London

Christine Hone
Hospital midwife, Dorchester

Lesley Hobbs
Independent midwife, Southampton

Chris Warren
Independent midwife, York

Julia Guy
Midwife, Wessex Maternity Centre

Carole Lord
Hospital midwife, Dorchester

Corinne Sims
Midwife, Wessex Maternity Centre

Ros Weston
Independent midwife, Shropshire and integrated midwife, Powys

For the majority of labouring women, there comes a point when they feel that they can't go on. They find themselves overwhelmed by the pain, the sheer relentlessness of the contractions. The fullness of the baby's head descending can cause great fear and panic, sometimes to the point of the woman saying that she thinks she will die. The midwife must draw on all her skills, her strength and experience to support the woman, to provide the reassurance and encouragement that will see her through to a normal, triumphant birth – so the question is, how do we do this? Several experienced midwives share their ideas.

Focusing

Mary Cronk emphasises the need to acknowledge that this is indeed a terrible time. It is not for the midwife to detract from the experience, the woman needs reassurance that it will not last forever, that she is nearly there. Women need to be praised and they need to feel that their fears are accepted. Becky Reed tries to impart to the women in her care how positive she is feeling about their progress: 'If the midwife is smiling it's because we know you are getting there; soon you'll be pushing your baby out'. Becky recommends trying to direct the woman to focus on what her body is doing – describe the cervix opening, emphasise the importance of strong contractions to fully dilate the cervix and push the baby into the birth canal. In a similar vein, Corinne Sims gently directs the focus of the woman back to the labour and birth, possibly asking her to close her eyes, or alternatively asking the woman to look into her (Corinne's) eyes. She encourages the woman to draw strength from visualising the 'contractions pulling the cervix open, the baby's head slowly coming down'. Lesley Hobbs also asks women to look into her eyes while telling them how strong and brave they are. However, she is also cautious of downplaying the woman's distress. 'Pay her the courtesy of acknowledging that she knows what she wants – it is an honour to do something to help if that is what is required and no woman should look back on her labour and birth and be horrified by the experience.'

Several midwives suggested encouraging a woman to try something different when they become distressed. Chris Warren referred to this as 'distraction techniques – for instance a bath, shower, sitting on the loo, something to drink or eat, preparing the room for the baby's arrival'. Julia Guy recommends the woman changes position – if she's in a birthing pool, then she might want to get out, maybe go for a walk outside. Mary Cronk uses massage, hot pads, encourages movement and a trip to the toilet – in fact, recently Mary administered an enema to a woman who was very distressed mid-labour which provided excellent relief and allowed the woman to refocus and take control again. Christine Hone will suggest a woman moves around and uses pelvic rocking. Changing the dynamic in the room can provide temporary distraction. Julia Guy might ask for another (familiar) midwife to come in and Chris Warren sometimes leaves the woman and her birth partner together while she goes and makes a cup of tea or a phone call.

If there are several people at the birth Ros Weston might ask them to leave the woman and her partner alone for a while, or send the partner out of the room to do something useful like make a drink.

Establishing rapport

Carole Lord made the point that establishing a rapport with the woman is the most important goal because without it, however skilled the midwife, she will not be able to support the woman when the pain and tiredness overwhelm her. Ideally, the midwife will have developed a strong relationship with the woman during the pregnancy. However, as is often the case, the initial meeting between woman and midwife will be when the woman arrives at the hospital in labour and this puts considerable pressure on the midwife to assess correctly the woman's emotional and physical requirements.

Lesley Hobbs advises her women to 'go with the moment. Don't be too definitive about what you want in advance'. She often relies upon the 'tell me three times rule'. In other words, judging when a woman genuinely wants to transfer into hospital or have an epidural, she waits until the woman mentions it three times. The midwife may think that persuading the woman she can cope without further pain relief is a laudable achievement whereas in actual fact, the woman does need a greater level of analgesia than the midwife can provide. Again, we return to the guiding principle of tuning into and listening carefully to the labouring woman – a point that was repeated by the midwives again and again.

Chris Warren highlighted the difficulty of letting the woman know that there is further pain relief available without giving in to the natural desire to 'make things better'. Ros Weston also mentioned the need to be vigilant and to ensure that all options are discussed with the woman. The midwife should always have a plan of care constructed within the bounds of normal labour and birth, taking into account her own strengths, and never be ashamed to organise an epidural if that seems appropriate. However, a couple of the midwives felt confident in refusing a woman an epidural if during her pregnancy she had expressed very strong views against their use and she was progressing well in her labour.

Clear explanations

Before the first vaginal examination, Corinne Sims always takes great care to explain what she might find if the woman is in the latent phase of labour. Chris Warren also commented that if the woman thinks she is fully dilated and her cervix has only opened 2-3cm then one has to be 'brutally honest, telling the woman it is time to calm things down, that her body will get used to this if given a chance. The endorphins will start to build up and once the woman is calmer the whole experience will become easier to handle'.

If the woman is in transition then Ros Weston emphasises that this is very encouraging and will only last a relatively short length of time.

One of the most exhausting, disheartening times for women can be when they have a cervical lip, particularly if it is their first baby. Becky Reed will try to push the lip out of the way, usually with the woman on all-fours as it's easier to bend one's fingers the right way rather than negotiate the pubic bone with the woman in a semi-prone position. She warns that the midwife must be confident that it is only a lip of cervix before she attempts this manoeuvre.

Being in tune

Ros Weston has noticed how some women need their midwife to be very physically close during difficult periods in the labour, whereas other women want their midwife to remain present, but not too close – understanding these needs requires the midwife to be constantly alert to changes in the woman's behaviour and reactions. As Carole Lord says, 'The most important thing is the relationship – without trust, empathy and sympathy there is nothing. This can be almost instinctive – you don't necessarily need years of midwifery experience to help a woman deal with her fear and pain'.

Ros Weston said that the midwife should always be aware of the link between the emotional and physical body. 'Although labour is not a counselling session, it can bring back experiences of abuse that can be deeply traumatic and can effectively prevent labour progressing.' This may not be an issue the midwife feels confident to tackle but she should be aware that such fears need to be dealt with using the utmost sensitivity.

Carole Lord recently cared for a woman having her third baby. The woman had previously had epidurals but this time she had no analgesia and became very distraught, repeating over and over again that she couldn't do it, that the pain was too awful. Carole acknowledged her pain and fear and kept telling her how well she was progressing. She was a constant presence, retaining physical contact with the woman. Afterwards, the woman said 'The pain was awful and I doubted my ability to cope but all the time I was aware of the nice, even steady tone of your voice. I can't remember what you were saying but your steady presence made it bearable'.

No magic formula

There is no magic formula that can be used to help women through difficult periods of labour. The midwife must provide sensitive, sympathetic, reassuring care and acknowledge that the woman's experience is of paramount importance. She must establish a rapport with the woman, be ready to help her refocus on the labour, on her body and how well she is doing. At the same time, the midwife must be aware if labour is not progressing well, if the woman really is reaching the end of her resolve and requires extra help in the form of hospital transfer or an epidural.

As is always the case in midwifery, the demands are great and often very draining, but to know that you have accompanied a woman through an experience that she would not have coped with had you not been there, is a privilege and a reward in itself.

Caring for women during the latent phase of labour

Kate Walmsley

Wessex Maternity Centre is a private, 'stand-alone' birth centre offering a range of midwifery-led services. The midwives who work at the Centre carry a defined caseload of women for whom they are responsible. 60% of our clients are expecting their first baby, enabling our midwives to gain considerable experience about the preparation and midwifery care of these women. This article is about their care during the latent phase of labour.

Defining the latent phase

The latent phase of labour is poorly defined and poorly understood. While the active phase of labour has been described as 'pain with progress', by contrast the latent phase is loosely defined as 'a preliminary to true labour'.[1] Others have defined the latent phase as that portion of labour between the onset of regular contractions and the beginning of the active phase.[2] There is little agreement about its normal length; some suggest 20 hours for primigravidae women and 16 hours for multigravidae woman as the maximum duration[3] with others suggesting that six hours is the upper limit of normal for the latent phase.[4] It is difficult to define when active labour begins; it may be at five centimetres' dilatation of the cervix, and it may be as little as three centimetres' dilatation.[3]

It is important to understand the nature of this stage, as ignorance of its normal course can lead to unnecessary Caesarean section for what is erroneously described as 'failure to progress'.

Our early experience of caring for women expecting their first baby at the Wessex Maternity Centre was coloured by our previous hospital experiences; when an effaced cervix was dilated to three centimetres the woman was considered to be in active labour and the partogram was started. It was then expected that a vaginal examination four hours later would reveal significant progress, otherwise there was a very disappointed woman and midwife, the contractions were labelled 'ineffective' and the labour was augmented.

When the Centre first opened, the midwives would encourage each woman to phone in and talk to her midwife as soon as she felt her labour was starting. The midwife would encourage the woman and her partner to stay at home as long as possible, unless her membranes ruptured or she was unduly worried.

That is all fine in principle, but the early phase of labour can be very difficult for a woman to cope with. She may experience short, sharp, painful contractions, which although irregular can be frequent. They tend to start at night and she spends the rest of the night pacing the floor, either because she's trying to keep it going or because she's too uncomfortable to lie down anyway.

Her partner keeps her company, because he would feel guilty if he slept whilst she is 'in labour'. She forgets to eat, or chooses not to eat, doesn't drink enough and as the night wears on they both become increasingly anxious. Today's baby books and magazines rarely mention a latent phase of labour, so by the morning they both believe she has been in labour all night, with little or no progress, and are beginning to think something must be wrong.

When the midwife next sees this woman she is hot, very tired and anxious, her pulse rate is raised, her urinalysis shows ketones present and the baby is tachycardic. Her partner is restless and demanding to know what is wrong and why nothing is happening.

Emotional support

When the couple who have experienced the latent phase of labour at home arrive at the Centre they are exhausted. She will have lost a lot of her determination and resolve to cope with the labour. They will both voice doubts about her ability to cope. One or other of them will suggest transfer to hospital. They feel 'something should be done' to sort the labour out.

Practising in an independent stand-alone unit we offer continuity of midwifery care. However, experience has taught us that, when the foregoing scenario is played out, despite the relationship we have built up, psychologically we have lost this couple. It is very hard to get them back on track. They want to see some action, either an epidural (which will meet his needs), or rupture of the membranes to speed labour up for her, both of which will set in motion that well-known 'cascade of intervention'.

The first thing to do, as a midwife, is to acknowledge that there is a latent phase of labour, and that this stage is painful. Experience suggests that it is important to prepare the woman and her partner for the latent phase of labour. This is best done during antenatal classes and reinforced during the last month of pregnancy. When labour starts we still encourage the woman to stay at home, advising her to rest as much as possible and to eat and drink frequently and we keep in regular contact by phone. But if she or her partner voices any concerns we invite them into the Centre. Often the reassurance that their midwife is at hand if needed is enough. They are made comfortable in a bedroom with beanbags and pillows. The midwife encourages relaxation and gives back and leg massage. If her partner has arrived tired and anxious he is sent home to sleep and ordered not to come back until we call or until he feels rested.

It is important this woman is given constant support at this time. Pain and anxiety in early labour increase catecholamines and cortisol, which may have an adverse effect on uterine activity.[5] Our work at the Centre with primigravidae in the latent phase has shown us that if we give psychological support and physical care at this time, we reduce the need for transfer to hospital for delay in labour. This can create some difficulty for the midwife, because this phase can last for 20-24 hours. The woman and her partner will then require intensive support from a tired midwife during the late first stage and birth of the baby. There is an advantage to working in paired caseloads; the couple know both midwives, so the midwives can take turns to rest at regular intervals.

There is a great temptation for the midwife to undertake a vaginal examination on a woman in any stage of labour 'just to see what's happening'. Yet there is nothing more demoralising for a woman who has been contracting for many hours to be told that her cervix is barely two centimetres dilated. If the midwife is sure of her abdominal palpation and descent of the head per abdomen, then she will not perform a vaginal examination.

There is a big difference between the behaviour and appearance of a woman in the early or latent phase of labour and the woman in active advanced labour. In active labour the contractions are more regular as well as longer and stronger. The woman has a concentration about her that you do not see in early labour. I believe that if you have to do a vaginal examination to diagnose labour then the woman is probably not in labour.

The diagnosis of active labour is difficult and somewhat arbitrary. Whether the woman's cervix is closed or five centimetres dilated is not going to make any difference to her management if she is anxious and in pain in a birth centre environment. The midwife will suggest non-pharmacological ways to cope with the pain, as well as giving constant psychological support. Regular abdominal palpation will give an indication of the descent of the head and the rotation of the baby's position.

The midwife can interpret the sounds and movements the woman makes and the changes in breathing pattern as well as the state of her concentration. Once the woman's endorphins start to work she can appear sedated by drugs with a far away look and dilated pupils. These signs are all suggestive of a move from the latent to the active, progressive phase of labour. In a technocratic birth culture these 'watching' skills have been trivialised or forgotten.[6] They are skills the midwives at the Centre have spent the last four years relearning, and they have enabled us to bring down our rate of transfer to hospital significantly.

Over the years we have come to realise that, to help women achieve an active natural birth, we have to spend the last months of pregnancy preparing them for the latent phase of labour. As midwives we have had to learn that using very basic midwifery skills – watching, supporting and caring for women patiently through this difficult period – is essential to achieving a good outcome.

REFERENCES

1 Crawford JS. The stages and phases of labour: an outworn nomenclature that invites hazard. The Lancet 1983; 30(7):271–272.
2 Freidman EA. Labour: Clinical evaluation and management, 2nd edn. New York: Appleton-Century-Croft; 1978.
3 Cohen WR, Brennan J. Using and archiving the labour curves. Complicated labour and delivery 1. Clinics in Perinatology 1995; 22(4).
4 Cardoza LD, Gibb DMJ, Studd JW, et al. Predictive values of cervimetric labour patterns in primigravidae. British Journal of Obstetrics and Gynaecology 1982; 89:33–38.

5 Wuitchik M, Bakal D, Lipshitz J. The clinical significance of pain and cognitive activity in latent labour. Obstetrics and Gynaecology 1989; 73(1):35–42.
6 Kitzinger S. Communication of pain [MIDIRS abstract]. MIDIRS Midwifery Digest 1994; 4(6):181.

Birth without active pushing

A physiological second stage of labour

Jean Sutton

Since long before recorded history, female mammals have given birth to live offspring. All those species which have been successful have followed the same, involuntary process to survive. Breathing, digestion, elimination, all go on without any need for conscious help – unless the process is disturbed.

Pregnancy and birth too belong to those bodily processes that are controlled by the autonomic system. Each month, the human female's uterus expels its contents unaided. Once, it was perfectly capable of expelling a full-term fetus without help. What has happened to change this? Has the uterus really lost its powers, or are we failing to understand the process properly? As we have gained more and more knowledge of the details, have we lost the main map?

This article aims to look at the broad canvas of birth, and to see if any helpful clues can be found in the almost-lost 'women's wisdom' relating to birth. Before I begin, I should tell you where I am, in today's jargon, 'coming from'.

The loss of normality

I began in the birth world at the age of seven, as a farm child in New Zealand. At 17, I joined the staff of a small country hospital during the baby boom. Later, I worked in several private maternity hospitals, until having my own four children. Thus, from 1951 to 1970, I saw hundreds of babies born. I had observed that mothers having a normal birth always said, breathlessly: 'It's coming' – never: 'I want to push'. I never once saw a mother deliberately push her baby into the world – their uteri were quite capable of managing by themselves.

Was it because they had to suffer more? No, the amount of sedative drugs used was substantial. Most mothers were given either trilene or, if a doctor was present, chloroform, at the end of second stage, so they really couldn't have pushed deliberately if they had wanted to!

When I returned to work in 1977, I was amazed to find almost all women vigorously pushing their offspring out. All that effort, all that instruction in how to push! So many episiotomies, so many haemorrhoids, so many forceps births. What on earth was going on, what had changed since the 1960s? The big difference was that previously women had given birth in the left lateral position. This position allows the pelvis to open as it should, and neither helps nor hinders the baby's descent. Now they were all reclining on their backs and trying to force these babies down and round the corner. How had this happened when, as far back as 1932, Corkill (a New Zealand obstetrician) was stating as given, in a midwifery textbook, that there are 16cms of space at the outlet of the pelvis at the end of second stage[1] (see Table 4.8.1). Where had that extra space come from? More recently, Michel Odent has drawn our attention to the 'fetal ejection reflex'[2] and Sheila Kitzinger has reported the Jamaican midwives' advice that 'The baby will not be born until the mother opens her back'.[3] If birth is to regain its normality, we need to understand the anatomy and physiology behind these observations.

Another major difference between the 1960s and the 1970s was that, in the 1960s, at least 70% of babies presented in early labour as vertex LOA and a further 15% as vertex ROA. There's the 85% normal we should be able to achieve.

Can we regain such results and still have reduced mortality and morbidity? Of course we can, once we study the broad canvas more carefully. It is quite possible to achieve at least 85% normal births in an area, even when mothers are so-called 'high risk' if antenatal education focuses on teaching expectant parents what really happens when a baby makes its amazing journey. But first midwives need to gain more understanding themselves and create the environment at birth where these natural processes can be encouraged, rather than prevented.

The first stage: The process should take place this way:

- Labour begins with the baby vertex LOA
- Contractions begin short and widely spaced
- Length and intensity increase steadily
- The baby moves down and tucks its face under the top of the sacral curve
- The shoulders move from the oblique to the transverse
- The cervix reaches full dilatation and the membranes rupture.

Now there is a pause, sometimes only seconds, but usually several minutes. During this time, the baby finishes its moves: the head becomes directly anterior/posterior and the shoulders enter the pelvic brim in the transverse. The uterus adapts to the partial loss of contents (the liquor and the baby's head) and prepares to change its action. The baby begins to lift its head.

The second stage: To understand real, physiological second stage labour, we must learn about the 'rhombus of Michaelis'. This is the kite-shaped area of the lower spine that includes the sacrum and three lower lumbar vertebrae. We may learn that it has limited flexibility during pregnancy, but nothing about its role in labour.

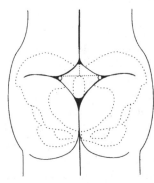

As second stage labour begins, the rhombus of Michaelis moves (this is 'the opening of the back' which the Jamaican midwives spoke to Sheila Kitzinger about). Midwives working with mothers who give birth on all-fours or kneeling without wearing clothes will have seen this as a large 'lump' that suddenly appears on the mother's back. It has been suggested that it is the baby's head pushing the sacral prominence outward, but this is not so. It is the rhombus of Michaelis moving back – up to 2cm. At the same time (but not visible to the observer) the wings of the ilia fan outwards, thus increasing the internal dimensions (see Table 4.8.1).

This movement can only occur if the mother is in a position that puts her weight in front of her ischial tuberosities, with the angle between her spine and her thighs at least 120° (i.e. the distance between her hips and her head is less than the distance between her knees and her head).

What causes the rhombus to move? This explanation is still at the hypothesis stage, but it appears to be something like the following:

The back of the baby's head contacts a nerve plexus at the front of the pelvis, where the bladder and urethra join (this is known in the feminist literature as the G-spot). This triggers the backward movement of the rhombus of

Table 4.8.1 Pelvic measurements

Normal

	Transverse	Oblique	Anteroposterior
Brim	13cm	12cm	11cm
Cavity	12cm	12cm	12cm
Outlet	11cm	12cm	13cm

After rhombus of Michaelis moves

	Transverse	Oblique	Anteroposterior
Brim	15cm	14cm	13cm
Cavity	14cm	14cm	14cm
Outlet	13cm	14cm	16cm (includes 1cm for coccyx straightening)

Michaelis and the fanning open of the wings of the ilia, which makes more space in the pelvic cavity. Then the following actions occur (although these are written as a sequence, they tend to happen simultaneously):

- The mother reaches upward to find a firm object to grasp
- She allows her body to sag forward and knees to roll out
- Her back arches and she begins to wriggle her lower body
- The uterus contracts and forces the baby's body down.

The baby's head (facing directly backwards) passes the spines and is born, followed rapidly by its posterior shoulder. (The anterior shoulder is against the symphisis pubis, leaving plenty of space for the posterior shoulder to be born.)

The similarities between the mother's actions at the end of the second stage labour and the involuntary actions which occur during orgasm (both female and male) are striking.

Compare and contrast

How does this contrast with what we have been taught is normal second stage labour? Very few mothers, even those who remain mobile, seem to give birth unaided. The idea that all babies need to be pushed out is firmly embedded, yet cannot be found in older textbooks. Until the 1960s, women giving birth at home, and in many hospitals, were delivered in the left lateral position. Why was it changed? One midwife can manage perfectly well, as the mother will move her own upper leg if she needs to.

Once mothers were in a reclining position, their babies no longer found the passage from womb to world straightforward, and they ended up far too deep into the back of the pelvic floor. This brought the baby's head into contact with the nerves of defecation, rather than birth.

Then came the need to push, and the idea of 'protecting' the mother's back. Someone decided that a rounded back would be protective – without realising that bringing the knees up brought the spine and the symphisis pubis so close that, unless the baby's shoulders were already in the transverse, they would be stuck at the brim. Then came the ridiculously long second stage labours. If a baby is lined up properly, and his mother keeps her knees down, half an hour is normally plenty for a first baby and ten minutes for a subsequent one.

When things don't go smoothly

Failure to progress in the second stage of labour is so common, but is usually so simple to cure.

If the baby in LOA is not descending in the second stage of labour, then he must have failed to rotate his shoulders. His anterior (right) shoulder will still be sitting on the brim, so his head can't move down. Remember, the shoulders rotate into the anteroposterior position once they are inside the cavity. Only a very small baby can pass through the pelvis without his head turning 90°.

In most cases, all that is needed is to ask the mother to move to a position where her knees are further away from her head than her hips. Left or right lateral, kneeling, in a birth pool, a supported squat with the thighs at least 45cm from the ground – all of these will work, as long as she gets her knees well away from her body.

Any position that brings the knees towards the abdomen reduces the space in which the baby can move. It will also increase the chance of the baby being pushed into the back of the pelvis and into the back of the pelvic floor, instead of pressing against the symphisis. From here a major pushing effort is needed to get the baby out, and the likelihood of tearing the perineum or needing an episiotomy rises.

A few babies manage to get a hand or arm into the pelvis with their head, and these may appear to need pushing. If we are listening carefully, we will have heard the mother complaining about discomfort or pain in odd places. A hand by an ear causes pain on the side of the pelvis; an asynclitic head causes pain deep on the left side of the pelvis behind the spines; an elbow under the chin causes pain in the sacrum during contractions but not between. Getting the mother on her feet and asking her either to visit the toilet (have a wheelchair right behind her) or to lean on the bed and wriggle her hips until the pain goes can be spectacular. If there has been a transverse arrest, once the baby becomes unstuck it will emerge very fast.

Keeping the angle between the spine and thighs at least 120° will also prevent or cure most cases of shoulder dystocia. This is because shoulder dystocia usually occurs when the baby has failed to rotate its shoulders into the transverse at the brim, or into the anteroposterior at the spines. Give it room to move and it will.

The use of epidural anaesthesia during labour, even the walking kind, must have had an effect on the normal movement of the rhombus of Michaelis. If the birth nerves are not stimulated, how can the reflex occur?

Regaining normality

Looking at the normal birth process, shorn of preconceived ideas, would be a useful project for any midwife. Birth is not just a mechanical process, but if the parts are unable to interact as they are designed to do, then the stimulation of hormones and tissues will also fail and the Caesarean section rate will spiral even further, making midwives, who should be protecting the normal, into intensive care nurses.

None of this explains the problems that arise when the baby is right occipito-posterior. These babies may get stuck during first stage and will almost always have problems during second stage. A second article (reprinted as chapter 4.10 in this book) will describe the moves open to OP babies as they try to use all the available space in the maternal pelvis. They have a number of choices, but unless someone is able to help the mothers respond effectively, many will fail, and are destined to become subject to the well-known 'cascade of intervention'.

REFERENCES

1 Corkill TF. Lectures on midwifery and infant care. New Zealand: Whitcombe-Tombs; 1932.

2 Odent M. The fetus ejection reflex. Birth 1987; 14(2):104–5.
3 Kitzinger S. Ourselves as mothers. London: Bantam; 1993.

Women's position in second stage
A Cochrane database review

Jilly Rosser

The suggestion that there are advantages in women adopting certain positions during labour and birth has been around for centuries. This review aims to evaluate the benefits and risks of the use of different birth positions during the second stage of labour on maternal, fetal, neonatal and caregiver outcomes.

Background

The majority of women in Western societies give birth in a dorsal, semi-recumbent or lithotomy position. This is in contrast to women living in societies not influenced by Western conventions, who avoid the dorsal position and change position frequently. In non-Westernised societies, women tend to give birth in an upright position e.g. kneeling, squatting, or hanging from a rope tied to the ceiling.

Theoretically at least, there are a number of physiological advantages in being upright:

- gravity assists the descent of the fetus
- there is less risk of aorta-caval compression, leading to improved acid-base outcomes in the newborn
- uterine contractions are stronger and more efficient
- the fetus is better aligned for passage through the pelvis
- pelvic outlet diameters are increased.

The research on this subject is complicated by the wide variety of possible positions women can adopt, and the fact that no consistent approach has been used by researchers. For the purpose of this review the various positions have been broadly categorised as either neutral or upright. Neutral positions are those in which a line between the centre of a woman's third and fifth vertebrae is more horizontal than vertical, such as:

- lateral
- lithotomy

- Trendelenburg's position (head lower than pelvis)
- knee-elbow.

The upright positions are

- sitting (usually on a birth stool)
- semi-recumbent (with the trunk tilted backwards 30° to the vertical)
- kneeling
- squatting (unaided or using squatting bars)
- squatting with a birth cushion.

Studies included

A total of 18 studies are included. All these studies used a random or quasi-random allocation.

Objectives

To assess the benefits and risks of different positions in the second stage of labour (from full dilatation of the cervix).

Outcome measures

Maternal – pain, use of analgesia/anaesthesia, intensity and frequency of contractions, blood pressure, length of labour, method of delivery, suturing, blood loss >500ml, long-term perineal pain/discomfort, dyspareunia, urinary/fecal incontinence, maternal experience of and satisfaction with the second stage of labour.

Fetal – abnormal fetal heart rate patterns needing intervention, persistent OP position.

Neonatal – neonatal condition, admission to NICU, perinatal death.

Overall, the quality of the studies was poor, and the conclusions must be regarded as tentative.

Results

Because of inconsistencies in the way the included studies were carried out, the comparisons available between different positions were rather limited.

Comparing upright or lateral position with supine or lithotomy position, the outcomes among women allocated to upright or lateral positions were:

- a reduction in the length of second stage (mean 5.4 mins)
- a slight reduction in the rate of assisted deliveries
- fewer episiotomies with a slight increase in second stage tears
- more blood loss >500ml
- less severe pain
- fewer abnormal heart rate patterns.

There were no differences in:

- use of analgesia or anaesthesia
- rate of Caesarean section
- 3rd or 4th degree tears
- need for blood transfusions
- manual removal of the placenta
- unpleasant birth experience
- dissatisfaction with 2nd stage
- feeling out of control
- persistent OP
- admission to NICU
- birth injuries
- perinatal death.

Comparing use of a birth or squatting stool with the supine positions, the outcomes among women allocated to birth or squatting stool were:

- fewer episiotomies
- more second degree tears
- more blood loss >500ml
- less severe pain
- fewer abnormal heart rate patterns.

Comparing use of a birth cushion with supine or lithotomy position, the outcomes among women using the birth cushion were:

- considerable reduction in the length of second stage
- fewer assisted deliveries
- fewer second degree tears
- similar rates of episiotomy and blood loss >500ml.

Comparing use of a birth chair with supine or lithotomy position, the outcomes among women using a birth chair were:

- no difference in length of second stage
- fewer episiotomies
- more second degree tears
- more blood loss >500ml.

Because of the variable quality of the studies, the impossibility of blinding, and the different approaches and definitions used, these results should be interpreted with care.

The considerable reduction in episiotomy was found particularly in women allocated to the birth stool, the birth chair and other upright postures, and was only partly offset by an increase in second degree tears.

Taken together, the reduction in the length of second stage and in the rate of assisted delivery support the suggestion that second stage bearing down is more efficient in upright positions.

The increased diagnosis of blood loss >500ml should be interpreted with caution; this is a notoriously inaccurate measurement, and in the women using the birth chair, blood was collected in a receptacle (so none was absorbed into bedding etc.).

Implications

With the possible exception of increased blood loss, no harmful effects were found from women giving birth in upright positions. Current evidence on the effectiveness of various delivery positions is inconclusive. Therefore, during the second stage women should be helped to use whatever positions they prefer.

Questions

This review provides very little of the information which most midwives would like to have to inform their practice. It tells us nothing about how birthing women will respond to being encouraged (both through their labour environment and through the guidance of their caregiver) to freely choose the positions which are most comfortable for them. It also tells us nothing about how women in different clinical situations – baby in the occipito-posterior position, slow descent etc. – may be helped by the use of specific positions.

Many midwives suspect that the ability to move about and change position during the second stage may be more important than the adoption of any particular position. However, addressing this question would be nearly impossible using a randomised controlled trial.

Policy makers considering how to turn this review into labour ward guidelines will have to work in the context of considerable uncertainty. The suggestion that upright positions reduce the amount of perineal trauma and the instrumental delivery rate is compelling. Other labour ward practices restrict the movement of labouring women. This should be considered by caregivers, and explained fully to women.

Date of the most recent substantive amendment: 23 March 1999

Citation
Gupta JK, Nikodem VC. Women's position during second stage of labour (Cochrane Review). In: The Cochrane Library, Issue 1, 2000. Oxford: Update Software.

STUDIES INCLUDED IN THIS REVIEW

Allahbadia GN, Vaidya PR. Why deliver in the supine position? Aust NZ J Obstet Gynaecol 1992; 32(2):104–106.

Bhardwaj N. Randomised controlled trial on modified squatting position of birthing [abstract – personal communication for rest of information]. Int J Gynaecol Obstet; 46:118.

Chan DPC. Positions during labour. BMJ 1963; 1:100–102.

Crowley P, Elbourne DR, Ashurst H, et al. Delivery in an obstetric birth chair: a randomized controlled trial. Br J Obstet Gynaecol 1991; 98: 667–674.

de Jong P. Randomised trial comparing the upright and supine positions for the second stage of labour [letter]. Br J Obstet Gynaecol 1999; 106:292.

de Jong PR, Johanson RB, Baxen P, et al. Randomised trial comparing the upright and supine positions for the second stage of labour. Br J Obstet Gynaecol 1997; 104:567–571.

Gardosi J, Hutson N, Lynch CB. Randomised controlled trial of squatting in the second stage of labour. Lancet 1989; 2:74–7.

Gardosi J, Sylvester S, Lynch CB. Alternative positions in the second stage of labour: a randomized controlled trial. Br J Obstet Gynaecol 1989; 96:1290–1296.

Gupta JK, Brayshaw EM, Lilford RJ. An experiment of squatting birth. Eur J Obstet Gynecol Reprod Biol 1989; 30:217–20.

Hemminki E, Virkkunen A, Makela A, et al. A trial of delivery in a birth chair. J Obstet Gynaecol 1986; 6:162–165.

Humphrey M, Hounslow D, Morgan S, et al. The influence of maternal posture at birth on the fetus. J Obstet Gynaecol Br Cmmwlth 1973; 80:1075–1080.

Johnstone FD, Aboelmagd MS, Harouny AK. Maternal posture in second stage and fetal acid base status. Br J Obstet Gynaecol 1987; 94:753–757.

Liddell HS, Fisher PR. The birthing chair in the second stage of labour. Aust NZ J Obstet Gynaecol 1985; 25:65–68.

Marttila M, Kajanoja P, Ylikorkala O. Maternal half-sitting position in the second stage of labor. J Perinat Med 1983; 11:286–289.

Radkey AL, Liston RM, Scott KE, et al. Squatting: Preventive medicine in childbirth? In: Proceedings of the annual meeting of the Society of Obstetricians and Gynaecologists of Canada 1991; 76.

Stewart P, Hillan E, Calder A. A randomised trial to evaluate the use of a birth chair for delivery. Lancet 1983; 1:1296–1298.

Stewart P, Spiby H. A randomized study of the sitting position for delivery using a newly designed obstetric chair. Br J Obstet Gynaecol 1989; 96:327–333.

Turner MJ, Romney ML, Webb JB, et al. The birthing chair: an obstetric hazard? J Obstet Gynaecol 1986; 6: 232–235.

Waldenstrom U, Gottvall K. A randomized trial of birthing stool or conventional semi-recumbent position for second-stage labor. Birth 1991; 18(1):5–10.

Occipito-posterior positioning and some ideas about how to change it!

Jean Sutton

This article considers the baby who presents in the OP (occipito-posterior) position at any stage from 36 weeks gestation, and suggests ways to help him and his mother avoid the trauma of a long 'backache' labour. OP babies are the ones who fail to enter the maternal pelvis on time, and become subject to a 'cascade of intervention'. Most can be persuaded to change their position before labour begins, but midwives need ideas to help the birthing pair if the baby remains OP.

It is a mistake to think that if a baby presents in the occipito-posterior position at the start of labour, there will be no problems. In fact, in older textbooks, the OP presentation was always found in the section on abnormal labour.

The space available in the female pelvis for the passage of the baby forms a triangle. The back wall of the triangle is quite long, as is the base, but the front, or symphysis, is shallow. An OA (occipito-anterior) baby can tuck his head in, and slide into the cavity. An OP baby cannot do this because his back is too straight and lying against his mother's. His neck is unable to bend sideways sufficiently to allow him to get into the cavity and under the sacrum.

Detecting the OP baby in pregnancy

The mother whose baby is in the occipito-posterior position walks freely and without a 'duck waddle'. She has a tidy, high abdomen and people comment that she is 'carrying well'. Unfortunately, most mothers are happy to look like this, and feel sorry for the girl carrying the OA baby with her bulky abdomen and generally 'full-blown' look.

The OP baby makes lots of small movements as his limbs are all at the front. The mother's abdomen has a dip around the umbilicus, marking the space between her baby's arms and legs. The baby tends to lie on her right side, with his back more or less between her hip bone and spine. His heartbeat is heard well over on his mother's right hand side.

Preventing OP positioning

The OP baby has difficulty engaging in the pelvis. His head is too straight and, because of its angle, bumps on the top of the symphysis. As this is extremely painful, and may go on for up to twenty minutes without pause, his mother tries to lift him off her pubes, perhaps by lying on her back. This results in her baby's head being high at term, a situation with which midwives are all too familiar.

Because there is insufficient stimulation of the cervix by the baby's head, the maternal tissues fail to become as soft, stretchy and flexible as they should. Very few OP babies arrive on time.

Braxton-Hicks contractions have no effect on the baby's position. If the baby is to be persuaded to move, midwives must show his mother, without frightening her, how to help him turn.

The support given to the baby by the mother's abdominal muscles must be reduced and this can be achieved if the mother adopts any 'tummy down', knees well down, posture. The abdomen then becomes more like a hammock, and the baby makes himself comfortable in the OA position, with his back to his mother's front.

Most first time mothers have puffy feet at the end of pregnancy, and tend to rest with their feet up. This means that the baby is only comfortable in the OP position with his spine against his mother's. To provide the baby with the maximum space in which to turn, the mother must keep her knees down, and rest on her side so that her abdomen is level with or below her spine.

The baby who is ROP often objects to his mother sleeping on her left side, which is the side he should be on. He doesn't like having his support removed, so until he turns, a small pillow can be placed between the mother's bump and the bed.

Most of the positions recommended in active birth literature for the mother to practise during pregnancy are helpful with OP babies, but squatting with the thighs not parallel to the floor must be avoided. In deep squatting, the pubes and spine are too close together, and present an unnecessary obstacle to the OP baby's turning. To prevent their babies settling in the OP position, mothers need to avoid having their knees higher than their hips by not sitting on low furniture, or spending long periods in a car.

Problems during first stage

The OP baby does not fit easily into the pelvic cavity. If he uses the back of the cavity, he becomes a face presentation, putting considerable stress on his cervical spine. He can't bend forward properly, because the symphysis is in the way. Although the OP position is sometimes described as 'flexed' or 'deflexed', flexion is minimal above the spines. If flexion were greater, the baby's shoulders would be trying to enter the brim and this would add up to rather more than 11cms.

The OP baby encounters further difficulties in trying to descend through the pelvis with his head upright. The force of contractions is directed in front of his spine, and through the area of the anterior fontanelle which meets the uterus about 2-3cms in front of the cervix, stretching the lower uterine segment rather than helping dilate the cervix. This results in the familiar situation of the mother who 'fails to progress' at 5-7cms and is given a syntocinon infusion plus an epidural for the pain.

Results are variable. If enough syntocinon is used, the contractions may be strong enough to dilate the cervix, but in many cases, fetal distress occurs, and an emergency Caesarean section is required.

If the mother is mobile and provided with something to lean on and a small stool to raise one leg, her baby will rotate at this stage. The essential thing is to ensure that the mother's weight is above, or better, in front of her ischial tuberosities. This provides relief for her continuous backache, opens her pelvis as wide as possible and helps her baby turn. Because an OP baby has his posterior shoulder on the wrong side of the sacral prominence, he can't rotate his shoulders unless he can get well forward.

Problems during second stage

If the OP baby gets through the cervix, his head must mould sufficiently to enable him to pass between the spines. These are normally about 10.5cms apart, so unless he is directly anterior/posterior and can find enough space behind them, he may well get stuck. If he succeeds,

he will be born 'face to pubes'. In this case, his shoulders enter the pelvis in the transverse position, and rotate to anterior/posterior in the cavity. This is only possible for relatively small babies.

The baby also encounters problems if his head has rotated to the transverse position with his right shoulder sitting on the brim and his left shoulder on the opposite side of his mother's spine. Because his firm spine is towards his mother's back rather than his soft arms, it is difficult for him to move his left shoulder past the sacrum and descend into the cavity. His attempts to do so cause the mother severe pain.

In many of these cases, if the mother can get on her feet or knees (with her weight in front of them) she can flex her pelvis and 'unstick' her baby with dramatic results. This is the situation where a transverse arrest suddenly resolves itself and the baby is born in three contractions with no need for forceps or ventouse.

In general, whether the OP baby has serious problems in second stage depends on the shape of his mother's pelvis, and whether or not she is mobile. Unless he rotates into an OA position, he stimulates the nerves at the back of the pelvis, rather than those at the front. Consequently, the fetal ejection reflex is not triggered and the extra internal space available to the baby when the rhombus moves is denied him.

If the mother is mobile and has an anthropoid pelvis, her baby will usually turn as soon as he reaches the pelvic floor and be delivered easily. Rotation is less common if the mother has a gynaecoid pelvis. If she has an android pelvis which narrows towards the outlet, the baby has no space to turn and will be unable to deliver. The outlet from the platypelloid pelvis is so spacious that, once the baby has managed to engage, he can be born easily.

Labouring on the bed

All the difficulties encountered by OP babies are magnified when the mother is confined to bed. Whether she is sitting upright with her legs outstretched, or reclining with an epidural in situ, she has tipped the triangle of her pelvis upside down. The symphysis should be level with, or lower than the coccyx, but when the mother's legs are raised, the symphysis becomes level with the sacral prominence and the baby has no space to use.

If the baby goes into the sacral curve, he becomes a face presentation. The small amount of usable space can be demonstrated by inserting a straight piece of pipe into a model pelvis. There appears to be plenty of room, but the baby can only use the space that is inside the pipe. At best, considerable maternal effort will be required if the baby is to descend, presuming that he gets his shoulders sorted out at the brim. Often, the baby will fail to descend and will need to be delivered by forceps, ventouse or Caesarean section.

Bed should be a last resort for the birthing pair when the baby is posterior. The rigidity of the mother's pelvis, splinted by the maternal thighs, means that the baby cannot help himself.

Supporting the mother during labour

Considering the difficulties that OP babies and their mothers face during labour, it is easy to see how important it is for as many babies as possible to start labour LOA. This position enables them to slip easily into the pelvic cavity and trigger off the proper sequence of hormone and nerve stimulation.

However, the midwife can do much to support the mother of an OP baby even after labour has commenced. She should advise and assist the mother to keep her knees down, move her hips during contractions, and focus on where the pain is. The mother will thereby find her own ways to minimise the pain and help her baby turn as early as possible. If her membranes have not ruptured, they should be left intact, as the baby needs the fluid to move in to change his position.

Morbidity following OP labour

The mother with an OP baby is likely to have a difficult labour with continuous backache that becomes worse with each contraction. She needs the continuous and wholehearted support of the midwife.

Apart from the long tedious labour that is often caused by an occipito-posterior baby, there is also considerable postnatal morbidity. The mother is exhausted after her efforts, and should have special support as she recovers. The portion of the baby's skull below his ears and his neck have been compressed for many hours at unnatural angles and the resulting pain and discomfort may make him hard to feed, settle and generally 'get along with'. Years ago, the OP baby would have been treated with rest and minimal handling after birth, as if he had been suffering from concussion. Today, he's likely to be sent to Special Care, undergo hypoglycaemia tests, and be over-handled.

Cranial osteopaths have much to offer babies who have birthed as OPs. Their heads are gently lifted away from their shoulders, and their necks are made much more comfortable. The same effect was achieved when babies were held up by their feet at birth to 'drain'. The weight of the head released the compression between head and shoulders. However, this is not a practice to which we would wish to revert!

Midwife versus obstetric nurse

The only babies who need real help at term are the OPs and breeches presenting RSP. The intervention rate is the true measure of how many or how few babies begin the journey through their mother's pelvis in a position that ensures a short, safe, easy birth. If midwives can reduce the number of OP babies by showing mothers antenatally how they can help their babies enter the pelvis in the anterior position, they will be acting as the guardians of normal birth. If they can use their knowledge and skills to support the mother of an OP baby during labour, they will enjoy the wonderful feeling of helping a mother have a good birth under difficult circumstances. Such skills mark the difference between a midwife and an obstetric nurse, and challenge the policies, protocols and training which support a medical model of birth.

Reflecting on labour and birth

- How can we assist women (especially those who choose hospital birth) to move about in labour, to utilise different positions and to avoid sitting on a bed for the length of their labour? In so many places, the bed is the focus of the birth room and women assume that they need to get in to it on arrival. What do we need to do to address this, and enable women to feel that they can move around and get into the positions that feel right at the time?
- How many midwives feel proficient at assessing progress in labour without vaginal examination? How far do we trust our knowledge of the sounds women make at different stages, their (lack of) ability to talk or rationalise, the physical changes that occur during the course of a woman's labour? Even if you have no choice about doing vaginal examinations, do you make your own assessment of progress first, and how often are you surprised by what you find? Does something later 'explain' why the difference may have occurred?
- What information do women need to help them make choices in labour? When do women feel they need it? When are the best times to offer that information? What are the best formats in which to offer it? How do women evaluate the quantity and quality of the information they receive, and the times at which they received it?
- How do you feel about birth plans? How can midwives – especially those who do not have the advantage of getting to know women before their birth – best help women to use birth plans in a positive way, while acknowledging that birth is a dynamic journey, which may not progress as planned! Have you ever written a 'midwifing plan', describing your hopes for your experience in being with a labouring woman?
- One of the challenges to midwives occurs when they meet a woman in labour who has already started on the 'cascade of intervention'. How can we best help these women to positive birth experiences?

Group exercise

Many midwives have a strong sense that we need to recapture the skills and knowledge that comprise the art of midwifery. All midwives have at least a couple (and sometimes hundreds!) of hints, tricks, insights or reflections which they use when helping women in labour.

Gather a group of midwives with differing levels and kinds of experience, and prepare some questions that will act as triggers for discussion and sharing of these hints. Some examples of questions might be:

- How do you help a woman through transition?
- What can you do to support a woman who does not want pain relief but is finding a stage of her labour difficult to cope with?
- How do you help a woman who is having a physiological third stage?
- What can you do to help a woman who is in early labour to relax?
- How can you help a woman who has an epidural but is finding it difficult to push?

Some other resources for developing and discussing midwifery skills are available on the Internet. The following web pages have links to midwifery email lists and sites which collate midwifery discussion:

www.midwifery.org.uk
www.radmid.demon.co.uk/index.htm
www.gentlebirth.com/archives
www.midwiferytoday.com
www.jiscmail.ac.uk/lists/midwifery-research.html

Focus on:

The third stage

Active versus expectant management of the third stage of labour

A Cochrane database review

Tricia Anderson

There has been a great deal of debate over the last decade about the optimum method for the safe expulsion of the placenta after childbirth. The Cochrane review on the subject has just been updated to include the findings from the recent Hinchingbrooke Third Stage Trial. It summarises the best research evidence with which to guide care and offer informed choice.

Background

Postpartum haemorrhage (PPH) is, by far, the commonest cause of maternal mortality in the world, causing approximately half of the 500,000 deaths which occur worldwide. Therefore the optimum management of the third stage is a matter of great concern, and it is perhaps surprising that there is no professional consensus about the best way to prevent haemorrhage. Two quite different approaches are widely practised across the world: expectant management and active management.

Expectant management (also known as physiological or conservative management) involves a 'hands-off' approach, waiting for signs of placental separation and allowing the placenta to deliver spontaneously (possibly aided by gravity and nipple stimulation). This approach is popular in some northern European countries, in some units in the USA and Canada, and in births which take place at home throughout the developing world.

Active management consists of three interdependent interventions:

i the administration of a prophylactic oxytocic drug immediately after delivery of the baby

ii early cord clamping and cutting

iii delivery of the placenta by the birth attendant using controlled traction on the umbilical cord.

This approach is standard practice in the UK, Australia and several other countries.

Studies included

Four studies have been undertaken in the last decade to attempt to find out which approach is best. All met the criteria for inclusion in the review. Three took place in the UK and one in Ireland, and together they studied over 4,600 women.

Objectives

This review aims to compare the effects of active versus expectant management of the third stage of labour on blood loss and other maternal and perinatal complications of the third stage of labour.

The outcomes considered were:
- Moderate PPH (500-1000ml)
- Severe PPH (over 1000mi)
- Haemoglobin concentration 24-48 hours post delivery
- Postnatal blood transfusion
- Iron tablets in the puerperium
- The need for therapeutic oxytocic drugs
- Length of third stage
- Manual removal of placenta
- Subsequent need for surgical evacuation of retained products of conception
- Maternal blood pressure
- Maternal vomiting and nausea
- Maternal headache
- Maternal pain during third stage of labour
- Maternal satisfaction with the management of the third stage of labour
- Secondary PPH
- Maternal fatigue at six weeks postpartum
- Breastfeeding.

In addition, the neonatal outcomes considered were Apgar score, admission to SCBU and jaundice.

Limitations of the studies

- In three of the studies, active management was the standard practice of the units involved. In only one centre (Hinchingbrooke) was expectant management regularly practised prior to the trial.
- The three largest trials are of good methodological quality. In the Brighton trial women were withdrawn from the trial after randomisation had occurred, which may bias the results.
- Three trials included only women who were at low risk of postpartum haemorrhage; only the Bristol trial included high risk women as well.
- The midwives involved in the trials could not be 'blinded' to the method of third stage management, and therefore there exists the possibility that their assessments of blood loss might be biased. However, the researchers tried to minimise this by using objective indices of blood loss where feasible, as well as clinical assessment.

Results

Active management of the third stage resulted in a statistically significant decrease in the incidence of:

- Moderate and severe PPH (as defined above)
- Postpartum maternal haemoglobin less than 9g/dl
- Postnatal blood transfusion
- The need for therapeutic oxytocics
- Third stages lasting more than 20 minutes.

Women were more satisfied with the third stage if they had had active management.

However, active management also resulted in a statistically significant increase in the incidence of:

- Maternal diastolic blood pressure greater than 100 mmHg
- Maternal vomiting, nausea and headache post delivery.

There is inconsistency in the results with regard to the need for manual removal of placenta and secondary PPH. In the Dublin trial these complications were more common following active third stage management, but in the Bristol trial they were more common in the expectant management group. The remaining two trials found no difference between the groups, as does the overall summary: there is a tendency for the active management group to have a higher incidence of manual removal and secondary PPH, but this does not reach statistical significance. The oxytocic drug used in the Dublin trial was intravenous ergometrine, whereas the other three trials used intramuscular syntometrine, which could be the reason for the difference.

There was no statistically significant difference in neonatal outcome or breastfeeding rates, and no difference in longer term maternal outcomes, such as maternal fatigue at six weeks postpartum.

In the Hinchingbrooke study, the mean blood loss in the active management group was 268ml and the mean length of the third stage was 12 minutes. In the expectant group, the mean blood loss was 336ml and the mean length of the third stage was 21 minutes.

Implications for the practising midwife

The policy of routine active management of the third stage of labour offers protection against greater blood loss and results in a shorter third stage. This results in less need for blood transfusion and for iron supplementation postnatally. Women appear to be more satisfied with this method of third stage management.

However, the longer term clinical significance of this reduction in blood loss is less clear, and needs to be balanced against an increase in unpleasant maternal side effects when syntometrine or ergometrine is used. The potentially hazardous increase in maternal blood pressure associated with the use of ergometrine is well documented in a separate Cochrane review, which suggests that Syntocinon 10 IU is nearly as effective in preventing major PPH without the unwanted side effects.

Women should be given unbiased information about the relative benefits and hazards of the different approaches of third stage management, applied to them individually. Relevant clinical information such as risk factors for haemorrhage, blood pressure level and previous third stage experience (if any) should be included in the discussion. Women should then be supported in their choice by midwives skilled in both approaches to third stage care.

Questions still outstanding

- What are the longer term outcomes associated with increased moderate maternal blood loss?
- Are there any risks associated with reducing blood loss below the physiological norm?
- None of the trials looked at long term neonatal outcomes which might be affected by elements of third stage management, particularly the timing of cord clamping and cutting.
- It would be useful to evaluate the three components of active management separately.

- There is a need for further evaluation of third stage management in different situations, such as in the home setting, particularly in the developing world where the risk of maternal mortality from haemorrhage is high.

Date of the most recent amendment to this review: 8th July 1998.

Citation
Prendiville WJ, Elbourne D, McDonald S. Active versus expectant management of the third stage of labour (Cochrane Review). In: The Cochrane library, Issue 4, 1998. Oxford: Update Software.

STUDIES INCLUDED IN THIS REVIEW

Thilaganathan B, Cutner A, Latimer J et al. Management of the third stage of labour in women at low risk of postpartum haemorrhage. Eur J Obstet Gynecol Reprod Biol; 48:19–22.

Prendiville WJ, Harding JE, Elbourne DR, et al. The Bristol third stage trial: active vs physiological management of the third stage of labour Br Med J; 297:1295–1300.

Begley CM. A comparison of 'active' and 'physiological' management of the third stage of labour. Midwifery; 6:3–17.

Rogers J, Wood J, McCandlish R, et al. Active vs expectant management of the third stage of labour: the Hinchingbrooke randomised controlled trial. Lancet; 351:693–699.

The Hinchingbrooke third stage trial

Jane Rogers   Juliet Wood

The results of the Hinchingbrooke randomised controlled trial, comparing active with physiological (expectant) management of the third stage of labour, were published recently in The *Lancet*[1] and have provoked comment from several authors.[2-6]

This article briefly describes the trial and results, and then goes on to discuss the practical implications for midwives in practice.

The background to the trial

The trial aimed to answer questions relating to outcomes of third stage management which had not been answered by previous similar research.[7-9] As well as collecting information immediately after the birth, data were collected up to six weeks postpartum, some relating to subjective information ('soft data') provided by the mothers. We considered it very important to find out from the women what they felt about their experience of third stage and of being involved in research. Likewise, the experiences and views of the participating midwives were also of interest.

Women were only included in the trial if they were thought to be at low risk of postpartum haemorrhage (PPH). There was random allocation of the women (similar to tossing a coin) to either a supine or an upright posture for third stage, and to either expectant or active management, so producing four groups altogether. Prior to the trial, Hinchingbrooke had an explicit philosophy of minimum intervention, so the midwives were already confident and experienced in the practice of physiological and active management, thus ensuring a fair comparison (in terms of midwives' expertise) between the two groups.

The method

The main outcome was the incidence of PPH (defined as a blood loss (≥500 ml), estimated by the midwife. Sixteen other outcomes, which it was thought may be related to third stage management, were also measured; these were both short-term and long-term, included 'hard' and 'soft' data, and related to both mother and baby.

The components of active management were: an intramuscular injection of syntometrine (or syntocinon 10 IU for those with hypertension) within two minutes of the birth, immediate clamping and cutting of the cord, and delivery of the placenta by maternal effort or controlled cord traction. With physiological management no prophylactic drug was given, the cord was left intact until pulsation ceased and the placenta was delivered by maternal effort.

Results

Although 1512 women took part in the study, this was only about a quarter of the total number of deliveries which took place during the recruitment period of two and a half years. Just over half of the women were excluded for medical and obstetric reasons, such as placenta praevia or augmentation of labour. Almost 20%, although eligible, did not want to accept allocation by randomisation, but wished to choose one of the two types of management.

The response rate of questionnaires completed by midwives and mothers was extremely good, which probably reflects the commitment of the mothers to the research, and also the thoroughness in the way the midwives carried out the consent process.

Those who had the full 'package' of allocated management was 93% in the active group and 64% in the physiological group. Although this means that a significant proportion of women allocated to the physiological group did not actually receive physiological management, this was a higher compliance rate than in any of the previous similar trials.[7-9] Where it occurred, deviation from the allocated management appeared to happen for good clinical reasons.

The results showed that the group which received physiological management had a PPH rate two and a half times greater than that of the actively managed group (16.5% vs 6.8%). This means that ten women need to have active management to prevent one PPH. All other measures of blood loss, including a postnatal haemoglobin measurement, supported this finding. Twenty women in the physiological group received a blood transfusion, compared with only four in the active group, so 48 women would need to have active management to prevent one transfusion being given.

The average length of third stage was 15 minutes in the physiological group compared with eight minutes in the active group, but there was no difference in the incidence of manual removal of placenta.

As expected, there was a raised incidence of side effects (attributed to ergometrine) in the active group.

The babies in the physiological group were on average 67g heavier (probably due to the extra blood received via the pulsation of the umbilical cord at birth).

An examination of the 'soft' and long-term data showed that there was no difference between the two groups in terms of feelings of tiredness and depression, or with problems related to bleeding, or the number of days breastfeeding.

Women were on the whole satisfied with whichever management they had, and a great many positive comments were made by them about their involvement in research. We were surprised by the number of women who said how pleased they were to have the opportunity to be involved in clinical research 'in order to improve care for others'.

Interestingly, the mothers who were allocated physiological management were three times more likely than the other group to make either positive or negative comments about their experience of third stage. Positive comments from this group were mostly concerned with a feeling of achievement and satisfaction at having 'done it all' without intervention, while the negative views centred on the length of time it took and the extra effort involved. There were very few comments from women about blood loss, despite the fact that altogether 177 mothers in the trial experienced a PPH.

In the context of these findings, and related research on the choice of oxytocic, we concluded that guidelines for third stage management in similar settings should advocate the use of active management with oxytocin alone, but that decisions about individual care should take into account the weight placed by pregnant women and their caregivers on the risk of PPH and blood transfusion versus the perceived advantages of non-intervention.

Implications for practice

In terms of midwifery practice, several things can be learnt from the results of this trial.

Firstly, it is clear that when physiological management is offered to women as a reasonable option, many will choose it, as did 52% of the 'eligible' women who chose not to take part in the trial.

Secondly, not every woman will interpret the results of the evidence in the same way, as demonstrated by the comments from the participants. An individual woman will view a PPH as being more or less significant, according to her own values, beliefs and priorities.

Unfortunately, we often make wrong assumptions about what is important to women. Midwives' awareness of the influences which might affect a woman's views about third stage management is, of course, crucial, and should be a part of the decision-making process. At Hinchingbrooke we have written a leaflet for parents who wish to know more about third stage than is covered in the average antenatal preparation. It presents the information in an unbiased and simple format and invites the woman to discuss her plans with the midwife. Clearly, this information needs to be consistent with practice guidelines.

If we believe that this research is for women, as well as for midwives and doctors, then it is our responsibility to share the information and discuss it with women as part of the preparation for birth, rather than to use it to create rigid policies for routine management.

It is also our responsibility to be competent and confident in our practice. This is a difficult issue, because many midwives have either never been taught physiological management, or do not practise it regularly, and are therefore 'out of practice'. This is because over the last couple of decades most units have supported a policy of routine active management. We suggest that students are, at the very least, taught the principles of physiological management, with an emphasis on recognising subtle deviations from the norm. Midwives who are experienced in this area of practice should be valued and used as teachers of this method.

Questions still unanswered

This study had limitations and has not answered all the questions there are about third stage management. It was, for example, limited to a hospital setting.

More work needs to be done on the way PPH is defined. Currently this is done by estimated blood loss, but our research showed poor agreement between haemoglobin levels and estimated blood loss when examined on an individual basis (although overall in the trial there appeared to be good agreement). This means that in terms of providing information about individual women, blood loss estimates do not seem to be helpful.

The Hinchingbrooke trial has not shown what it is best to do when physiological management has to be interrupted, for example for infant resuscitation. This group is of interest, because for those women who ended up with a mixture of both managements the PPH rate was 21%, compared with 8% for those who had the full active management package, and 11% for those who had every element of physiological management. Also not clear is which component of active management accounts for the reduction in the incidence of PPH.

Conclusion

It is clear that there are a number of things to consider when discussing third stage management with women.

We need to give unbiased and relevant information at an appropriate time, acknowledging the lack of some information, and respecting the right of the woman to take responsibility for her decision.

What is perhaps of outstanding importance is that when we offer a woman the choice of physiological management, we also offer a competent and confident midwife to provide that form of care.

Acknowledgements
We are grateful for the immense support of our collaborators, Diana Elbourne and Ann Truesdale, now at The London School of Hygiene and Tropical Medicine, and Rona McCandlish and Sarah Ayers at the National Perinatal Epidemiology Unit, Oxford. Our thanks also go to the midwives and mothers at Hinchingbrooke who participated in this study with such energy and enthusiasm. The study was funded by a grant from Anglia and Oxford Regional Health Authority.

REFERENCES

1 Rogers J, Wood J, McCandlish R, Ayers S, et al. Active versus expectant management of third stage of labour: the Hinchingbrooke randomised controlled trial. Lancet 1998; 351(9104):693–699.
2 Keirse M. What does prevent postpartum haemorrhage? Lancet 1998; 351(9104):690–692.
3 Prendiville W. Active versus expectant management of third stage of labour [letter]. Lancet 1998; 351:1659.
4 Cooke P. Abstract: Active versus expectant management of third stage of labour: the Hinchingbrooke randomised controlled trial. MIDIRS Midwifery Digest 1998; 8(3): 337–338.
5 Perez-Escamilia R, Dewey K. Active versus expectant management of third stage of labour [letter]. Lancet 1998; 351:1659.
6 Odent M. Active versus expectant management of third stage of labour [letter]. Lancet 1998; 351:1659.
7 Prendiville W, Harding J, Elbourne D, et al. The Bristol third stage trial: active versus physiological management of the third stage of labour. BMJ 1988; 297:1295–1300.
8 Begley C. A comparison of active and physiological management of the third stage of labour. Midwifery 1990; 6:3–17.
9 Thaliginathan B, Cutner A, Latimer J, Beard R. Management of the third stage of labour in women at low risk of PPH. Eur J Obstet Gynecol Reprod Biol 1993; 48: 19–22.

Don't manage the third stage of labour!

Michel Odent

Medical journals periodically publish prospective randomised controlled trials of the third stage of labour. The 'Bristol trial'[1] and the 'Hinchingbrooke trial'[2] were published in very authoritative journals and they provide the main references.

In these trials, whatever the details of the research protocol, one group is randomly assigned to 'active management' (i.e. injection of a uterotonic within two minutes of birth followed by immediate cord clamping and controlled cord traction). The other group is assigned 'physiological management' (Bristol study) or 'expectant management' (Hinchingbrooke study). The main objective is to evaluate the risks of postpartum haemorrhage.

The point is that in all groups the third stage is 'managed'. Yet there is an obvious incompatibility between the words 'physiological' and 'management'. Furthermore, in all research protocols the definition of 'expectant management' is negative (no use of uterotonic drugs and no clamping of the cord). But those who have a good understanding of birth physiology understand that there are probably factors that can positively facilitate the release of oxytocin by the posterior pituitary gland. These factors are not included in research protocols, whereas the effects of artificial substitutes for the pituitary oxytocins are studied in depth.

What researchers should look at

One of the main factors researchers should look at is a perfectly adjusted thermo-environment, because if the woman is cold, it will increase the levels of catecholamines. The concentration of catecholamines affects the risk of postpartum haemorrhage. This is more than empirical knowledge. A team from Sapporo (Japan) has studied the levels of catecholamines during the different phases of labour extensively by a noninvasive method[3] (recording with a patch and analysing the skin microvibration pattern of the palmar side of the hand)

and confirmed the findings of a previous study in which plasma catecholamines were measured through indwelling catheters.[4] The Japanese team clearly demonstrated that postpartum haemorrhages are associated with high levels of catecholamines.

Some experienced midwives also find it plausible that undisturbed eye-to-eye and skin-to-skin contact between mother and baby during the hour following birth influences the maternal hormonal balance and, in particular, the release of oxytocin.

Learning from decades of practice

Over the years I have gradually come to the conclusion that postpartum haemorrhages are almost always related to inappropriate interferences. Postpartum haemorrhage would be extremely rare if a small number of simple rules were understood and taken into account. I am so convinced of the importance of these simple rules that I have twice accepted to attend a home birth, although I knew that the woman's previous birth was followed by a manual removal of the placenta and a blood transfusion. I use this opportunity to summarise my own attitude during the third stage of labour, in order to stress the differences between this and the 'expectant' or so-called 'physiological' management used in randomised studies.

When the conditions are physiological, at the very moment of birth most women have a tendency to be upright (that is probably the effect of a peak of catecholamines). They may be on their knees, or standing up and leaning on something. After an unmedicated delivery, it only takes me a few seconds to hear and to see that the baby is in good shape. Then, in most cases my first preoccupation is to heat up the room. In the maternity unit in Pithiviers where I used to work, we just had to pull a string to switch on heating lamps. In the case of a planned home birth, I do not give a written list of what to prepare, but focus on the need for a transportable heater that can be plugged in anywhere and at any time (including practical details, such as the need for an extension cord). When the heater is on it is possible, within a few seconds, to warm up blankets or towels and if necessary to cover the mother's and the baby's bodies.

From that time my main concern is that the mother is not distracted at all and does not feel observed. I want to make sure that she feels free to hold her baby and to look into its eyes. It is easier to avoid unhelpful distractions if the light is kept dimmed and if the telephone is off the hook. I often invite the baby's father (or any other person who might be around) into another room to explain that this first interaction between mother and baby will never happen again and should not be disturbed. Many men have a tendency to break the sacredness of the atmosphere that may follow an undisturbed birth.

During the hour following birth, I keep a low profile and most of the time I sit down in a corner behind mother and baby. Minutes after birth many mothers are no longer comfortable in an upright position. This is most likely the time when the level of catecholamines is decreasing and when the mother feels the contractions associated with the separation of the placenta. Then the birth attendant may have to hold the baby for some seconds, in order for the mother to find a comfortable position, almost always lying down on one side. After that there is no excuse to interfere with the interaction between mother and baby.

For an hour I don't try to learn anything about the cord and the placenta. Clamping the cord when it stops pulsating is not necessary and it requires that somebody is touching the cord every so often to detect 'the right time'. The cord can be cut after the delivery of the placenta. Suggesting a position to the mother is another unneeded distraction. The position is the consequence of the level of catecholamines.[5] When the level of catecholamines is low and the mother feels the need to lie down, it would be cruel to suggest an upright position.

It is only an hour after the birth – if the placenta is not yet delivered – that I dare to disturb the mother in order to check that the placenta is separated. With the mother on her back I press the abdominal wall just above the pubic bone with my fingertips: if the cord does not move, it means that the placenta is separated. In practice, the placenta is always either delivered or separated an hour after birth if the third stage has not been 'managed'.

Immersion in water

In the particular case of the use of water during labour, most women feel the need to get out of water for the very last contractions before birth[6] and therefore the third stage occurs entirely on dry land. If the woman has not time to get out of the bath this suggests that there was a powerful 'fetus ejection reflex'[7] and the placenta will probably be separated during the first minutes following birth. This is the right time to clamp the cord and to get out of the pool.[8] Only in the case of an intentional and planned birth underwater is there cause for concern. Water immersion makes the uterine contractions more effective for an hour or two; after that the contractions may become weaker.[9] If a woman has planned a birth underwater and is the prisoner of her project, the baby may be born at a time when the contractions are already less powerful: they will be still weaker at the time of the delivery of the placenta.

Developing and 'developed' countries

These considerations about the physiological processes in the perinatal period are also highly relevant to developing countries, with their high maternal mortality rates. Postpartum haemorrhages represent a major cause of death in third world countries where the first contact between mother and baby is routinely disturbed by cultural beliefs or rituals. For example the belief that 'colostrum is bad' is associated with an early separation of mother and baby.

Bias

Whatever country we consider, the results of the current randomised controlled trials are of limited use to those who have acquired a good understanding of birth physiology. First of all, in these trials the physiological processes are highly disturbed both in the study groups and in the control groups. Also there are important biases. For example, in the Hinchingbrooke trial the number of women who refused to participate in the study (976) was higher than the number assigned the expectant management (764) or the 'active management' (748). Also 243 women were eliminated from the study because their haemoglobin concentrations were below 10g/dl.[10] The results of large studies, however, indicate that haemoglobin concentrations of 9-9.5g/dl are associated with optimum perinatal outcomes (they reflect good plasma volume expansion).

The future

The widespread 'active management of third stage' supports the belief that women are unable to release their own oxytocin. The possible long-term effects on our civilisations of the routine use of substitutes for oxytocin during the third stage should be considered seriously.

It seems that, in medical circles, it is not yet well understood that oxytocin has behavioural effects and has been called 'the hormone of love'. Whatever their perspective, all the scientists who study the development of the capacity to love give great importance to the perinatal period and use the concept of a 'critical' or 'sensitive' period. Where human beings are concerned, one must always think in terms of civilisation.

REFERENCES

1 Prendeville W, Harding J, Elboume D, et al. The Bristol third stage trial: active versus physiological management of the third stage of labour. BMJ 1988; 297:1295–1300.

2 Rogers J, Wood J, McCandish R, et al. Active versus expectant management of third stage of labour – the Hinchingbrooke randomised controlled trial. Lancet 1998; 351:693–699.

3 Saito M, Sano T, Satohisa E. Plasma catecholamines and microvibration as labour progresses. Shinshin-Thaku 1991; 31:381–99. (Also presented at the Ninth International Congress of Psychosomatic Obstetrics and Gynaecology, Amsterdam 28-31 May 1989 (Free communication no.502).

4 Lederman RP, Lederman E, Work B, et al. The relationship of maternal anxiety, plasma catecholamines and plasma cortisol to progress in labour. Am J Obstet Gynaecol 1978; 132:495–500.

5 Odent M. Position in delivery [letter]. Lancet 1990 (May 12); 1166.

6 Odent M. Birth underwater. Lancet 1983 (Dec 24); 1476–1477.

7 Odent M. The fetus ejection reflex. Birth 1987; 14: 104–105.

8 Odent M. Use of water during labour – updated recommendations. MIDIRS Midwifery Digest 1998; 8(1):68–69.

9 Odent M. Can water immersion stop labour? Journal of Nurse-Midwifery 1997; 42(5):414–416.

10 Odent M. Active versus expectant management of third stage of labour [letter]. Lancet 1998; 351:1659.

Further thoughts on the third stage

Sara Wickham

The third stage of labour has, for some time, been one of the hottest clinical topics in midwifery. Although both of the major research studies[1,2] which have been carried out to compare the physiological birth of the placenta with active management suggest that the latter leads to less blood loss and 'better' outcomes, their findings have been challenged by many.

One of those taking issue with the research is Michel Odent, who suggests that it is impossible to compare the two types of management of the third stage without first understanding the positive steps we can take to facilitate physiological third stage.[3] I would like to add another observation to this debate; the amount of blood loss in the hours following birth, which I believe may account for the differences reported in the above studies.

My observations arise from a time when I worked on a hospital postnatal ward, where women were admitted from the labour ward a couple of hours after they had given birth. Most of these women had had their third stages actively managed, and their recorded blood loss after the birth was usually around 100-200 ml.

I would generally help these women to the bathroom the first time they felt they wanted to get up. Invariably, as I waited outside, women would call me in to inspect blood or clots which they had passed into the toilet or bedpan; they were often concerned about how much blood they had lost. Sometimes almost as much lochia was passed at this point as at the birth itself. Although I reassured the women that this was normal and there was no problem, the pattern started me thinking.

I realised that their blood loss was probably more noticeable to me because I had previously been practising in a situation in which the majority of women chose physiological third stage. After a physiological third stage, the women did not have the pattern of heavy bleeding delayed for a few hours after the birth that I was observing in the women who had had active management in the hospital.

It struck me that this might account for the different amounts of blood lost between women who had physiological and managed third stage. Could the use of an oxytocic in any way inhibit the normal blood loss at birth, but cause the blood to be somehow retained by the woman's body and expelled later? This would account both for the difference in recorded blood loss at birth and the later loss of blood in women experiencing active management.

Physiologically, this would make sense. The use of an oxytocic drug causes a strong and sustained contraction of the uterus. The uterus is too well contracted to release a large amount of blood at this stage, which is why the blood loss is small in most cases. This is seen by many as 'a good thing', and cited as one of the advantages of using oxytocics in the third stage.

However, if the woman's body is physiologically adapted to losing more blood, it wouldn't be until the effects of the oxytocic had started to wear off that the uterus would be able to relax sufficiently to achieve this. So it may be that the average amount of blood lost during physiological third stage is 'normal', while the lesser amounts of blood lost during active management are abnormally low. If we recorded the amount of lochia lost in the first few hours after birth together with that lost during the birth itself, would the figures for the two types of third stage correlate more closely? Could it be that the total blood loss in women experiencing active management might actually be higher?

We also know that the administration of exogenous oxytocin inhibits the body's own production of endogenous oxytocin,[4] which may be another factor in explaining this later blood loss. The effects of the oxytocic drug wear off before a woman's body has time to increase its own supplies of oxytocin to compensate. All midwives are aware of the need to consider the continuation of syntocinon for a while after the birth, because the woman's body may not be able to produce enough oxytocin to keep her uterus contracted. Does the same type of process happen when oxytocics are used in the third stage?

When comparing the outcomes of the two types of third stage, we tend to assume that 'less is better'. But could it be that, for some women, the use of an oxytocic somehow inhibits the normal bleeding which is meant to occur at birth? Does this account for the slightly higher blood losses in women having physiological third stage? Why is it that, simply because women choosing physiological third stage may have higher blood loss initially, this is automatically viewed as pathological, when we may be causing the real pathology by our intervention in the process? We know that women's blood volumes increase during pregnancy, and some of this blood clearly needs to be released by the body in the first days and weeks after the birth.

Of course there are other issues; we need to understand more about how the third stage works physiologically and ensure we are employing the positive intercessions which assist this before attempting to compare physiological with active management. We need to be very clear about when the amount of blood loss is normal and when it becomes pathological; we also need to reflect upon what the causes of any truly pathological blood loss might be.

There are myriad aspects of the third stage which midwives need to consider and debate. Perhaps mine is an unusual experience, and others could add to these thoughts. The evidence which relates to this area needs to come from all sources; from midwives' experience and understanding of physiology as well as research trials.

Whatever the answers may be, we do not yet have a complete enough picture for us to be able to fully inform the women in our care. And it is they who need to make the final decision about how their third stage will occur.

REFERENCES

1 Prendeville W, Harding J, Elbourne D, et al. The Bristol third stage trial: active versus physiological management of the third stage of labour. BMJ 1988; 297:1295–1300.
2 Rogers J, Wood J, McCandish R, et al. Active versus expectant management of third stage of labour: the Hinchingbrooke randomised controlled trial. Lancet 1998; 351:693–699.
3 Odent M. Don't manage the third stage of labour! The Practising Midwife 1998; 1(9):31–33.
4 Robertson A. The pain of labor. Midwifery Today 1997; 39: 19–21, 40–42.

The postnatal experience

SECTION CONTENTS

The character of Cinderella has been used many times as an analogy to describe the relative neglect that the postnatal period receives in relation to other aspects of childbearing, and I make no apology for bringing her name up again. For some reason, the postnatal period and the experience of women at this time hasn't received as much attention as other issues, and some aspects of midwifery practice in this area have remained relatively unchallenged for a number of years. Yet, as Judith Ockenden shows, this is a time of immense importance, and there is much that midwives can do to facilitate this time being a positive rite of passage for women and their families.

But one possible Prince Charming may be on the horizon in the form of the research studies which are offering new evidence to inform practice. Fiona MacVane Phipps considered the difference between women's and midwives' perceptions of pain in the postnatal period, while Becky Reed and Sarah Clement evaluated the practice of not suturing perineal tears after birth and the impact of this on women's experience. These are important studies within this aspect of midwifery, not least because they focus on the women's own perceptions and views of their experience.

The physical aspects of the 'postnatal check', often grouped on a checklist in women's notes, are another series of screening tests designed to assess normality and diagnose problems. But how familiar are we with the normal limits of the postnatal period? Sally Marchant and colleagues offer new evidence on the normal range of postnatal blood loss and uterine involution. These midwives also highlight the different – and sometimes difficult to interpret – ways of recording this information, which not only have implications for communication between midwives, but also for the women themselves, who often hold their own notes during this time and who may be confused or worried by what is written.

What do we want women to get out of the contact they have with midwives in the postnatal period? Just as we need to remember that a woman who turns up to book with a midwife brings with her all of her life experience, the time we spend with a woman in the first few days of her baby's life is only the beginning of her experience as a mother. How can we best use midwifery knowledge and skills to help her to feel powerful and strong in this role? And how do we meet the postnatal needs of women who do not have happy births, or happy endings, or even a live baby?

Midwives have often noted that many women find it difficult to think about the postnatal period until they have actually given birth, finding it hard to 'see beyond' their labour and birth. Yet women may need a vast amount of information and support at this time. How can we provide a service which takes these issues into account, particularly in the light of increasing time constraints on practice?

The longest postnatal visit I ever carried out took three hours. I had been the second midwife for the woman, who had a beautiful vaginal birth at home, albeit after a very long labour. My first visit after the birth was on the seventh day, my midwife colleague having seen her almost every day prior to that. She had no physical problems. She said that she would not change one thing about her labour and birth experience. She just needed to tell me her birth story again. She needed me to know what the experience was like for her, and how the first week with her new baby had been. She had spent a week telling my colleague all about it, and now she needed to tell me too. It was an important part of ending her 'babymoon' and it took over two hours. She breastfed throughout most of the telling, and illustrated parts of her story by showing me her legs and inviting me to feel her uterus.

We took some photos, cuddled and checked the baby and went downstairs for a cup of tea. Just before I left, I picked up her notes and we filled them out. It was my (mis)perception that, after such a long discussion, she had probably told me everything that was important to her that day. But I discovered, when asking about bowel function, that she was experiencing a reduction of sensation, which we would need to monitor. It was an important reminder to me of the need to combine a woman-centred approach with a midwife's knowledge of the postnatal period, and of the kinds of issues which, for whatever reason, women may not tell us about spontaneously. We do need to listen for as long as we can, enabling women to direct the time they spend with us and put their experiences into their own words. But we still need to ask our questions!

After the birth is over...

Rest and support for new mothers

Judith Ockenden

New motherhood is a rite of passage marked by rituals in all societies.[1-3] Special food and clothing may be prescribed, and prolonged rest is a particular favourite, sometimes in seclusion. In the lying-in hospitals of the eighteenth century, a woman had to stay in bed for 28 days after birth.[4]

Now it is nearer 28 minutes, after which time the new mother is encouraged to get up and shower if she has had a straightforward delivery, so as to reduce the risk of thromboembolism. In the UK, the subsequent stay on the postnatal ward will be 1-3 days.

Length of hospital stay

'...*appears to be determined more by fashion and the availability of beds than by any systematic assessment of the needs of recently delivered women and their new babies.*'[4]

An illustration of this is a fascinating turn of affairs that occurred in America during the Second World War.[5] For decades before 1940, obstetricians had insisted that prolonged bed rest was crucial for

'...*physical recuperation as well as mental respite from the demands of home and family life.*'

In the war years, however, these opinions were suddenly revised. Scientific evidence was rapidly produced to show that morbidity was less, and uterine involution quicker, in active women than in those having a couple of weeks in bed.

Market-driven maternity services

By the early 1990s, insurance companies in the US were paying out only enough for women to have 'drive-through deliveries', and, in response to public outcry, President Clinton legislated for a minimum two-day hospital stay, saying:

'*Parents may rush to the hospital, but they shouldn't be rushed out.*'

I came across similar drive-through sentiments recently, on a steering group reviewing maternity services. Two of those involved – an accountant and a local GP – expostulated that hospitals were not hotels and it was the responsibility of the women's families to support them after childbirth. I voiced my shock at their attitude, wondering whether lack of early support might lead to greater use of the NHS in later months.

Was I right to be concerned? After all, several studies have found that early postnatal discharge does not increase maternal and newborn morbidity.[4,6] Does this indicate that all is well in postnatal life?

What do women experience?

For three days after childbirth women may feel euphoric.

Because she feels so well... she may do too much, especially when she is transferred home early from hospital.[7,8]

A woman who has had a 'normal' vaginal delivery will certainly be coping with considerable loss of lochia during this time, and be trying to re-establish contact with her bladder and bowels. She may have perineal stitches and bruising that make sitting uncomfortable. Her breasts will be large and tender, and her nipples may already be sore. Her back may ache, and she may experience afterpains as her uterus contracts, especially when she breastfeeds her baby. She will have many visits and telephone calls. The euphoria may end with the baby blues, when she feels unaccountably miserable.

New mothers are expected to continue with life as usual – as well as coping with the baby.[1] But as time goes by, being on 24-hour call to her new baby, combined with the constant process of learning to understand and care for her child, may lead to extreme fatigue.[9] Lack of sleep and disturbance of sleep cycles, preventing deep restorative sleep, affects mental and physical wellbeing. After 2-3 days of sleep deprivation, the ability to perform even simple tasks is impaired.

Depression is related to fatigue, and so the mother's relationship with her baby is impaired. So too is her closeness to her partner. Half of couples report that their relationship is worse in the first three years after they have a baby; frequency of sex falls by 30-40% in the first year.[3,9,10]

On top of all this, around 20% of mothers in Western society are also overcoming the major surgery of a Caesarean section at the same time as adjusting to motherhood.[2]

In time, the new mother may reflect on the contrast between reality and the 'Johnson and Johnson' image of motherhood.[2]

Making motherhood better

A contented transition to motherhood can be facilitated in three ways: good education, supportive attitudes and practical help.

Education

Reducing stress reduces tiredness and unhappiness and concomitant problems.[9] There are many ways in which antenatal education for parenting can help; for example:

- Realistic expectations. Western imagery surrounding motherhood does not match the reality.[2] In antenatal classes, parents can participate in games and activities which help to bring home to them how much time babies take up, and how they can plan and prioritise to help themselves.[11]
- Babyproofing the relationship. Anticipating areas of disagreement and planning postpartum adjustment[3] can begin to address Underdown's 'six domains in the transition to parenthood'.[10] Sexuality and sex help to sustain both the individuals and their relationship. Confronting this issue is vital, as 'it is tragic to lose this form of internal sustenance when it is most needed'.[12]
- Confidence. I often come across parents who are waiting to be told what to do. Knowledge, and tools to help them practice assertiveness can give them confidence to use their own instincts and common sense in looking after their child.[11]
- Support.
  - Men often want to help their partners, but sometimes feel rebuffed, thinking they will never be able to do things to their partner's satisfaction.[1] A complex renegotiation of roles may be needed.[10]
  - Close family members may themselves be working, and unable to provide the traditional support of the past.[10] Parents need to be reassured about accepting offers of help, and to know how to contact local and national self-help organisations. They need to form support groups with their peers: new mothers have symbiotic relationships, 'sharing the same situation, helping one another and learning together'.[13]

- Coping strategies. Parents can be taught ways to relax themselves and their babies.[11] This promotes a feeling of wellbeing and helps compensate for what new parents miss most: sleep. Penelope Leach[14] gives very sensible advice on how to help parents get more rest:
  - drop the term 'sleeping through the night' and give the facts about when babies develop sleep patterns similar to those of their parents
  - discourage thinking in disciplinary terms and promote flexibility (for example, mothers who keep their babies with them get more and better quality sleep[9])
  - think through the implications of common practices, particularly feeding.
- Caring for the baby. Some parents complain that they do not get the help and advice they need.[8] Practice before birth[11] and sensitive guidance afterwards is not difficult to organise.
- Caring for themselves.
  - 'When your reservoir is empty, it is difficult to pay proper attention to others.'[12]
  - The couple can discuss ways of finding time for themselves, individually, and as a couple.

Underdown[10] suggests that midwives and health visitors should work together to prepare parents. I would add that using the skills of qualified antenatal teachers, who are trained in adult education, would complement the practical and theoretical knowledge of health professionals.

Attitudes

In the West, many women are unhappy after birth.[2] Although cultural rituals may not always be in the best interests of mother and baby, care that applies a 'disease and problems perspective' is not helpful either.[13]

- Caring. Health professionals are perceived to attach greater importance to monitoring the return to physiological normality than to information and support.[8] In hospital, the 'task-centred culture' seems to exist primarily for the convenience of the personnel.[13] This begs the question:
  - 'How to become and how to dare to be caring in a rational, biomedically dominated hospital culture.'[13]
  - Women value the 'philosophy of care and beautiful calm environment' of birth centres,[15] and they are happier with community care than with that in hospital for the first 0-3 days.[8] Engendering positive

attitudes to birth at home or in birth centres would begin to address the issues. Leaving hospital early would also seem to be a good idea in this context, but here we get back to my worries about support in the community. This should comprise support from health professionals, and support from the community as a whole.

- Partnership between women and health professionals. The evidence clearly shows that women do want help. This does not mean going back to the 'we know what's best for you' attitude of the past. From the perspective of the new mother, postpartum care is sharing her new life situation.[13] She needs to learn to look after herself and her new baby, but often doesn't get the advice she needs about childcare, breastfeeding and future life.[8,13] Often she doesn't complain, considering her problems normal and therefore to be endured until they resolve.[16] Abandoning prescribed routine care, so allowing more time for empathic listening, would go along way towards individualised caring.[16] If the advice they are given is consistent and evidence-based, and tailored to their own situation, women are much more likely to act on it.
- Making motherhood special. Cultures which practice rituals (seclusion, assistance from relatives and explicit recognition of change of status) associated with the postpartum period seem to promote mothers' mental health. Where the postpartum period is not celebrated as a special time, high incidences of postnatal depression are reported. We need to address the underlying problems of social circumstances in which women begin their mothering. New mothers must be given value and the practical help they need so that they find the experience less exhausting and more enjoyable.[2]

Practicalities

In the early days after birth, a new mother needs peace and quiet to develop a bond with her child and regain strength, but this environment

'can easily turn into a prison-like experience if there is an absence of care.' [13]

What practical measures can promote a restful and caring atmosphere, in hospital and in the community?

- Hospital environment.
  - Noise could be controlled by suitable flooring or carpeting, smaller or individual rooms, and considerate visiting times.
  - Temperature could be moderated, as many women complain that hospitals are too hot.[8]

- Consistent and evidence-based breastfeeding support could be available all the time.[8]
- Adequate pain relief. Ninety-five per cent of new mothers report that they suffer postnatal pain, and 42% say that pain relief is inadequate.[9]
- Staffing levels should be adequate, as women recognise that lack of time is a significant factor in poor care.[8]

- Organisation of care. Here the 'three Cs' of *Changing Childbirth* come into play again: Give clients **choice** by responding to individual needs. The possibility of planning visits on this basis has been explored.[16] If implemented, this would give **control** to women. And the system might be facilitated by **continuity** of care. Few would argue that caring is more important than who is caring,[15] but surely the building of a relationship through continuity of care increases the chance that women will elicit support and express needs.
- Support.
  - Postnatal visits in the UK fell by 20% between 1990/91 (6 million) and 1998/99 (4.6 million).[17] The importance of postnatal visits is shown by studies on women at low risk for postpartum complications that picked up postnatal complications in 14% of women and 11% of babies.[6]
  - Women need more expert counselling and support for breastfeeding, and for longer.[8] Only 25% of mothers in the UK are breastfeeding at 3 months, soreness and tiredness being important factors in giving up.
  - Some women find that having a mother, or mother figure, to take care of them rather than the baby, is helpful.[1] Studies are ongoing of the provision of community support workers,[18] something akin to the current system in The Netherlands.[9,16] The nearest women can get to this at the moment is to employ a Doula.[3]

Aiming for the (baby) moon?

'Caring aims at helping the patient to be and become more human, to exist for others, and to mitigate suffering.' [13]

It is time for postnatal care to be based on individual need rather than fashion, convenience or economics. The balance needs to tip towards support, and away from medical monitoring. I envisage a time when motherhood is celebrated and valued; mother, father and baby will be allowed to rest and recuperate, and to form a family in a period of supported time we could call the babymoon.

REFERENCES

1 Bewley C. Postnatal depression. Mental Health Practice 2000; 3(7):30–35.
2 Barclay L, Kent D. Recent immigration and the misery of motherhood: A discussion of pertinent issues. Midwifery 1998; 14:4–9.
3 England P, Horowitz R. Birthing from within: An extraordinary guide to childbirth preparation. Albuquerque: Partera Press; 1998.
4 Enkin M, Keirse MJNC, Neilson J, Crowther C et al. A guide to effective care in pregnancy and childbirth, 3rd edn. Ch. 45. Oxford: Oxford University Press; 2000.
5 Temkin E. Driving through: Postpartum care during World War II. American Journal of Public Health 1999; 89(4):587–595.
6 Trends in length of stay for hospital deliveries – United States, 1970-1992. Morbidity and Mortality Weekly Report 1995; 44(17):335–337.
7 Sweet BR. Postnatal care. In: Sweet BR (ed.) Mayes midwifery, 12th edn. London: Baillière Tindall; 1997: 472-95.
8 Singh D, Newburn M. Women's experiences of postnatal care. London: National Childbirth Trust; 2000.
9 Larkin V, Butler M. The implications of rest and sleep following childbirth. British Journal of Midwifery 2000; 8(7):438–442.
10 Underdown A. The transition to parenthood. British Journal of Midwifery 1998; 6(8):508–511.
11 Nolan M. Antenatal education: A dynamic approach. London: Baillière Tindall; 1998.
12 Leonhardt-Lupa M. A mother is born: Preparing for motherhood during pregnancy. Westport: Bergin and Garvey; 1995.
13 Bondas-Salonen T. New mothers' experiences of postpartum care: A phenomenological follow-up study. Journal of Clinical Nursing 1998; 7:165–174.
14 Leach P. When babies are wakeful, who has the sleeping problem? Professional Care of Mother & Child 1999; 9(5):117–120.
15 Kirkman S, Bale B. Made-to-measure midwives. British Journal of Midwifery 2000; 8(4):196–197.
16 Bick D. The provision of community-based midwifery postnatal care in the UK: Making a difference? MIDIRS Midwifery Digest 2000; 10(2):227–231.
17 NSPCC. Protecting babies from harm: The professional's response. London: National Society for the Prevention of Cruelty to Children; 2000.
18 Morrell J, Stapleton H. Supporting postnatal women: Views from community support workers. MIDIRS Midwifery Digest 2000; 10(3):362–366.

Pain in the early puerperium

Women's experiences following normal vaginal delivery

Fiona MacVane Phipps

'Most women's experiences of becoming a mother are considerably and uncomfortably out of tune with the expectations they have absorbed from professional advisors to mothers about what the process will be like.' [1]

The literature available concerning women's experience of pain following a normal vaginal delivery suggests that this has been a somewhat neglected area of midwifery care. While pain relief in labour assumes a high priority – both in antenatal education and in the consciousness of midwives providing intrapartum care – the very real discomfort that some women suffer in the first days following childbirth may surprise the women themselves, and go unrecognised by the midwives providing postnatal care. This study was carried out in a large, university-affiliated teaching hospital in the north of England. It focused on the early puerperium pain experiences of six women and explored their perceptions of pain. The results highlight the lack of information provided to women on the reality of pain following a normal vaginal delivery (NVD).

Literature review

The literature review was undertaken to gain an overview of the topic, in order to provide a framework for women's post-delivery experience. To gain an increased understanding of pain as a subject itself, and to explore the published information on post-NVD pain, I reviewed the literature on the following areas:

- Current perspectives on the experience of pain
- Interventions used to assess or relieve acute pain
- Common causes of post-NVD pain
- Pharmacological and non-pharmacological methods used to relieve post-NVD pain.

The literature suggests that culture and environment shape the human experience of pain. In western healthcare settings, the predominant model of care is the medical model, which influences health professionals' perceptions about pain and its appropriate treatment. [2] However, recent literature suggests that over-reliance on this model results in the experience of pain only being validated where an underlying pathology provides a link between the cause of pain and its experience. [3] This, in turn, influences the pain management techniques most commonly adopted by healthcare professionals. [4] Where the medical model falls short is in its neglect of the psychological, social and cultural factors which influence an individual's perception of pain. [5]

Regarding the midwife's role in assessing and managing pain, two major questions emerged:

- Do midwives have a comprehensive understanding of the nature of pain?
- Do midwives employ an effective strategy of pain assessment and management?

Although there was little information available within the midwifery literature which answered these important questions, studies from both the British and American nursing literature indicate that pain knowledge and assessment are inadequate in the very professionals who have the greatest responsibility in this area. [6] Much of the research into postnatal pain has focused on perineal pain, e.g. the West Berkshire perineal trial [7] and the 1995 review of perineal care. [8] While this is undoubtedly a significant cause of pain following vaginal delivery, the very fact that perineal pain has been so extensively researched may blind midwives to other possible causes of pain following vaginal delivery. While perineal discomfort fits neatly into the medical model's understanding of pain – as it has a visible and identifiable cause – other types of postnatal pain, such as uterine cramps, breast tenderness and unspecified vaginal discomfort, may be more difficult to classify, and therefore easier to overlook.

The study which most influenced this current research project was one of the few to explore a broad spectrum of post-delivery pain.[9] This confirmed empirical evidence from clinical practice that, although perineal trauma is an important cause of pain, other factors also play a significant role in women's experience of discomfort following vaginal delivery.

Design and methodology

Although a quantitative methodology could have been employed in the investigation of post-delivery pain, qualitative research was chosen in order to provide an insight into the experience of women in the early postnatal period. A qualitative methodology gives a voice to the subjects of the study, offering an insight into the individual nature of each participant's experience, and enabling the researcher to observe the development of common themes.

This research project was developed as a small-scale ethnographic study, which pinpoints a specific or narrow area of inquiry.[10] Ethnography seeks to gain an understanding of the cultural values and beliefs which shape the behaviour and social interactions within a group.[11] Researchers use ethnography in healthcare research in order to become close to their informants and to gain an understanding of how people are affected by their state of health or illness.[12]

Ethics committee approval was obtained and the women considering participation in the study were told exactly who would have access to the research.

Participants were selected using a non-probability or convenience sample. In simple terms, this means that they were readily available at the time that the research was being conducted.[13] All of the women included in the study were booked under the care of one of two consultant obstetricians, both of whom had agreed to collaborate with the research.

The exclusion criteria for the study were as follows:

- Women who did not speak English. Although the experience of women from all ethnic backgrounds is highly relevant, reliability and confidentiality could have been compromised by conducting interviews through an interpreter.
- Women with obstetric complications such as infection or postpartum haemorrhage. Both of these factors could exacerbate a woman's fatigue and discomfort, thereby altering the true picture of 'normal' postnatal experience.
- Women who sustained a third degree perineal tear, as the level of pain associated with this type of laceration usually elicits a high degree of midwifery intervention, with stronger and more frequent analgesia being offered than is the norm following an NVD.

Women were eligible for inclusion in the study if they had delivered vaginally, with no complications, within the three days preceding the interview. All interviews were conducted in the hospital setting.

Data management

The primary method of data collection was through semi-structured, tape-recorded interviews. The interviews were supplemented by careful reading of the obstetric notes, which I undertook to gain an impression of the informant's pregnancy and labour, with special attention to pain. This information was not included in the research data. Although this introduced a potential source of bias, I favoured this approach because, in some instances, it enabled me to approach the informant with a developing picture of her attitudes and reactions to pain.

In addition, I kept a fieldwork journal.[14] This contained brief entries documenting any information which seemed relevant at the time of the interview. These included observations of the informant and information gleaned from reading the case notes. The journal, kept as contemporaneously as possible, provided valuable assistance in 'fleshing out' the interviews when I later transcribed them. In effect, this provided a triangulation of data.[15]

The six interviews were conducted using the patient information sheet to ensure that the same issues were explored with each informant. In addition, the women were encouraged to discuss any aspects of their individual experience which they felt held particular relevance. The interviews lasted approximately 20 minutes and were followed by a period of 'winding down' with the tape recorder switched off. This time was used for an initial reflection, with the informant, of what seemed to be the major points that had come out of the interview. This is a step which is considered helpful in establishing the reliability of qualitative data.[16]

The data were analysed using an adaptation of Burnard's fourteen-stage process.[17] All statements relating to the aims of the research were extracted and numbered. Initially, 18 separate categories were identified, e.g. parity, feeding methods, attitudes toward pain relief and perceptions of the ability to provide infant care while experiencing pain. Data which fell outside the established research criteria were set aside, but were returned to frequently, in order to maintain a clear picture of the informants as individuals. In this way I was able to place their 'pain statements' within a framework.

The four final themes which emerged once categories had been trimmed and combined were:

- Perineal pain is not the only discomfort. (Physical focuses of post-delivery pain)

- It really puts you off. You can't concentrate because it hurts so much. (Attitudes to post-delivery pain)
- I'm waiting for the time to run out so I can have my next tablet. (Attitudes to analgesia)
- Nobody talks about afterward, just about labour pain. (Education and advice).

Results

All six women experienced some pain, which included perineal pain, uterine pain, vaginal pain, pain on micturition, back pain, leg pain and breast pain. This finding is congruent with an earlier study examining the 'neglected' area of postnatal pain.[18] Although these were all significant focuses for pain, the most frequently mentioned, as well as the most debilitating, was uterine pain. Comments on uterine pain ranged from 'Like short little blasts', through 'Like contractions. Mild contractions. I wouldn't say it was agony but it's like mild contractions and cramps in the tops of my legs', to 'Like going into labour all over again'. One informant described uterine pain as 'Like a dull backache that starts in my hips and around my back, then becomes like a strong period pain'. Another woman spoke of vaginal pain that occurred with uterine pain: 'I had these sharp pains in my vagina. They made me want to curl up and cry'.

Various attitudes towards pain were observed. One new mother denied that she had any pain and was rather proud of her refusal of analgesia. She later described how she resorted to crawling about the floor on all-fours, or pacing up and down the ward to cope with the uterine 'discomfort' she was experiencing! Other women found that their ability to cope lay in the transient nature of pain: 'I wanted to phone my mum but I couldn't stand talking as it hurt so much. It puts you off doing things but you can go back to them because the pains don't last long.' 'They don't last long. A few minutes while I am feeding, or walking, but then they go.'

Equally, attitudes toward pain relief varied, but the overall impression was of under-medication rather than over-use of analgesia. One informant described paracetamol (the only form of pain relief she had been offered) as totally inadequate, but declined stronger medication because of the transient nature of her pain. Another woman described her refusal to take analgesia as 'being a martyr'. She went on to say:

'I'm not a pill popper. It doesn't help. At the end of it, the pain is still there and I think it makes it worse.'

Some informants were unsure as to when pain relief should be taken, and women tended to wait until they experienced quite strong pain before requesting analgesia. One informant, whose fear of pain had prompted her to accept analgesia while still only

experiencing discomfort, seemed relieved when she was reassured that this was in fact the optimum time to take medication:

'So it was OK to have those tablets? I thought I should have waited but I didn't want to feel too uncomfortable. I had some discomfort and I was afraid that if it got worse I wouldn't feel like taking care of her [the baby].'

One informant described her experience of analgesia as:

'I don't know what they are called. That strong tablet. It's just taken the edge off so I can bear it but I can still feel the pain. I'm waiting for the time to run out so I can have another tablet. I don't think I could stand any more pain.'

When asked about the education and advice they had received in pregnancy, the women did not remember having been prepared for post-delivery pain and felt that in the immediate postpartum period, they were given little help in coping with the pain. Typical comments were:

'All about labour and breathing exercises. I don't think anyone said much about after the birth at all.'

'Everyone talks about labour pain. Then it's supposed to be all over. I knew because I'd had after pains last time and I was dreading it.'

'I don't think anyone warned me. But, I sort of knew, you know, common sense. I went to parentcraft classes but I think the emphasis was all on labour. No one really talked much about what it would be like afterwards. You just think about the labour. How will I cope with that pain?'

Other women reported advice from friends or family:

'Well I was forewarned by a couple of friends. They said beware afterwards! They made out like I'd be in full-blown labour for another couple of days.'

Discussion and conclusion

As the aim of this small, mini-ethnographic research study was to explore individual women's personal perceptions of, and responses to, postnatal pain, it would be inappropriate to formulate any broad hypotheses from the data collected.

While these results may not provide midwives with any radically new knowledge about the puerperium, they should remind us that post-delivery pain has a significant impact on the women who experience it. Several major themes emerged from the research which warrant consideration, both from the practising midwife and from the midwifery researcher.

The women in this study:

- Experienced uterine pain as the primary focus of post-NVD discomfort.
- Tended to delay requesting analgesia until 'discomfort' escalated into a more severe physical

sensation, thereby inhibiting the effectiveness of pharmacological pain relief.

- Felt that traditional antenatal education focused too heavily on pregnancy and labour, resulting in ignorance about both the physical processes of the puerperium and the pain that these processes could engender.
- Identified a lack of information concerning non-pharmacological forms of pain relief.
- Demonstrated the need to talk about their experience of birth and the puerperium, and to feel that problems were taken seriously.

The overall aim of this study was to explore the perceptions of women during this important, but often ignored portion of the childbirth experience, and to assist midwives' understanding of post-delivery pain. If this article helps midwives to reflect on their own practice, as it has stimulated me to reflect on mine, then I have fulfilled my objectives in undertaking the research.

Midwives have some way to go in understanding the normal puerperium from the viewpoint of the new mother, to whom the experience may feel anything but 'normal'. Ensuring that education for childbirth does not stop with the birth itself, and taking the time to really listen to women following NVD, are important first steps in making the early puerperium a positive experience for women.

Further research into women's early experiences following NVD could use a quantitative methodology. This would allow some of the issues highlighted in this small study to be explored using a much larger population and would provide an interesting addition to studies of long-term morbidity following childbirth, such as Bick and MacArthur's research into the extent and severity of post-delivery health problems.[18]

The real value of this study is its insistence that women are the focus of the research, not an abstract idea of pain, or the bodily parts where pain occurs. This philosophy should be the cornerstone of any other project that may lead on from this piece of work.

REFERENCES

1 Oakley A. In: Beattie A, Gott M, Jones L, et al (eds). Health and wellbeing. Basingstoke: Macmillan; 1993:119–28.
2 Achteburg J. Woman as healer. London: Rider; 1990.
3 Wilkinson R. A non-pharmacological approach to pain relief. Professional Nurse 1996; 2(4):222–224.
4 Wakefield A. Pain: an account of nurses' talk. J Adv Nurs 1994; 21:905–910.
5 Waddie N. Language and pain expression. J Adv Nurs 1996; 23:868–872.
6 Kubecka K, Simon J, Boettcher J. Pain management knowledge of hospital based nurses in a rural Appalachia area. J Adv Nurs 1996; 23:861–867.
7 Sleep J, Grant A, Garcia J, et al. West Berkshire Perineal Management Trial. BMJ 1984; 289:587–590.
8 Sleep J. Postnatal perineal care revisited. In: Alexander J, Levy V, Roche S (eds). Aspects of midwifery practice. London: Macmillan Press; 1995.
9 Dewan G, Glazener C, Tunstall M. Postnatal pain: a neglected area. British Journal of Midwifery 1993; 1(2):63–6.
10 Leininger M. Ethnography and ethnonursing: models and modes of qualitative data analysis. In: Leininger M (ed). Qualitative research methods in nursing. Orlando: Grune & Stratton; 1985.
11 Helman CG. Culture, health and illness. Oxford: Butterworth-Heinemann; 1994.
12 Davies R. Introduction to ethnographic research in midwifery. BJM 1995; 3(4):223–227.
13 Polit D, Hungler B. Essentials of nursing research: Methods, appraisal and utilization. Philadelphia: JB Lipincott Company; 1993.
14 Phillips R, Davies R. Using diaries in qualitative research. BJM 1995; 3(9):473–476.
15 Redfern S, Norman I. Validity through triangulation. Nurse Researcher 1994; 2(2):40–55.
16 Woods C, Catanzaro M (eds). Nursing research, theory and practice. St Louis: Mosby; 1988.
17 Burnard P. A method of analysing interview transcripts in qualitative research. Nurse Education Today 1991; 2(6):461–466.
18 Bick DE, MacArthur C. The extent, severity and effect of health problems following childbirth. BJM 1995; 3(1):27–31.

To stitch or not to stitch

A long-term follow-up study of women with unsutured perineal tears

Sarah Clement Becky Reed

The question of whether or not to suture perineal tears is an important issue facing midwives. One of us is a member of a group of midwives who have been practising non-suturing of some perineal tears for several years. Having observed good outcomes at 28 days postnatally we were interested to find out whether these outcomes are maintained in the longer term. We felt it was important to examine not only long-term physical wellbeing, but also psychosocial aspects of women's experiences following an unsutured perineal tear. Here we report the findings of our follow-up of 107 women who had unsutured perineal tears between six months and seven years previously.

Until recently the majority of women with perineal tears were sutured. For example, one survey carried out in 1993 found that just 4% of women reported that their tears were unsutured.[1] However, practice is changing, and there have been increasing references to the nonsuturing of perineal tears.[2] Nevertheless there is anecdotal evidence that many midwives and obstetricians are concerned about the consequences of leaving perineal tears to heal naturally.

A literature search revealed that there is very little research on unsutured perineal tears. There appears to be only one published study on the effectiveness of nonsuturing.[3] This study found that no women reported any complications from not having tears stitched, and when women compared their experiences of an unsutured tear with their previous experiences of a sutured tear, pain levels were lower and sexual intercourse was resumed earlier. However, the study was small, involving only 55 women, the questionnaire used was short, and long-term outcomes were not examined. Indeed Head[3] concluded that 'the long-term effects of leaving a perineal tear unsutured are not known'. An on-going audit of nonsuturing of second degree perineal tears found that, to date, the tears have healed well and women appear to experience less pain.[4] A randomised controlled trial has recently been completed comparing suturing versus nonsuturing of the final skin layer,[5] and the non-suturing approach was found to be superior, but this is a different issue from the non-suturing of perineal tears.

Although there are no prospective studies comparing women with sutured and unsutured tears, there is some literature on the effects of suturing. In one study it is reported that 12% of women found the suturing afterwards the worst thing about their birth.[6] In the same study, it was found that 68% of women experienced some pain during suturing, 5% reported that their sutures were too tight, 5% had problems with gaping/undone stitches and 3% had stitches which became infected. In another study, 10-12% of women with sutures experienced long-term perineal pain, 25-39% of women experienced painful intercourse, and 0.4-1.6% of women had to be resutured.[7]

The aim of the study reported here was to examine and describe the views, experiences and long-term perineal health of a sample of women cared for by a group of midwives who have been practising non-suturing of some perineal tears for several years.

Method

A questionnaire was sent to women who had given birth between six months and seven years previously and had been cared for by one or more of five midwives working together in South East London with a socially and ethnically diverse caseload. The questionnaire was sent to all women except those who did not speak English, had a Caesarean section, had a baby who died or had a serious problem and those known to have moved for whom the midwife did not have a new address. Out of 288 questionnaires sent, 240 were returned, giving a response rate of 83%. In addition, data were extracted from the midwifery notes, with women's consent. Half (52%, 125/240) of the respondents had sustained a

Table 6.3.1

TYPE OF DELIVERY	% (proportion)
Spontaneous	97% (104/107)
Ventouse	3% (3/107)

TYPE OF PERINEAL TEAR*	
First degree	17% (17/100)
Second degree	72% (72/100)
Third degree	0% (0/100)
Unspecified	11% (11/100)

DIRECTION OF TEAR*	
Midline	48% (48/100)
Other	25% (25/100)
Unspecified	27% (27/100)

NUMBER OF PREVIOUS VAGINAL BIRTHS	
0	46% (48/105)
1	42% (44/105)
2	11% (12/105)
3	1% (1/105)

TIME BETWEEN DELIVERY AND FOLLOW-UP	
6 - 12 months	20% (20/100)
13 - 24 months	30% (30/100)
25 - 36 months	19% (19/100)
37 - 48 months	9% (9/100)
49 - 60 months	8% (8/100)
61 - 72 months	7% (7/100)
73 - 84 months	7% (7/100)

*as recorded in the women's midwifery records

Where the denominator is not 107, this is due to missing data (i.e. a few women not answering a particular question, or the midwifery notes not being available).

perineal tear, and 86% (107/125) of these tears had not been sutured. The remainder of the women had an intact perineum (44%, 106/240), an episiotomy (3%, 8/240) or an episiotomy and a tear (0.4%, 1/240). For this research we focused solely on the 107 women who had unsutured tears and these women are referred to as the study sample. The majority of the tears were recorded as midline second degree, and were of varying severity. The characteristics of these women are shown in Table 6.3.1.

The questionnaire was developed specifically for this study by the authors (a midwife and a research psychologist). The questionnaire was piloted before use. It was anonymous, but carried a code number to enable reminders to be sent to non-respondents. The questionnaire included the Present Pain Intensity Scale of the McGill Pain Questionnaire,[8] questions used in other research studies and questions designed by us. The questionnaire directed women to answer in relation to a particular birth, that is, the one they had under the care of the midwives in the midwifery group practice (the most recent one if more than one). This is referred to below as the index birth/baby. The questionnaire covered: decision-making, women's views, perceived advantages and disadvantages, satisfaction and worries, perineal problems, pain and discomfort, continence and subsequent births. It contained both closed and open-ended questions. The total number of words written in response to the open-ended questions was over 12,000.

Data from the closed questions were analysed using the Statistical Package for Social Sciences (SPSS v7.0). A thematic analysis was undertaken on the qualitative data from the open-ended questions. In a provisional analysis of the data we each separately identified the main themes in the data, then met together to agree a revised list of key themes. One of us (SC) then undertook and wrote up the main qualitative analysis based on the agreed themes. The other (BR) then read the account of the qualitative findings (below) along with the raw data to verify that the account reflected that data.

Results

Decision-making

The majority of women (70%, 71/102) felt that they were given a choice about whether or not to have stitches. 30% (31/102) of the women reported that they felt they did not have a choice. The questionnaire did not ask for further details about this. The majority of women who felt they had a choice found it very easy to decide not to have stitches when they were offered this option, with only one woman finding it a difficult decision (see Table 6.3.2).

We asked women how much the information or advice given by their midwife influenced their decision about whether or not to have stitches. Most felt that it had a big influence (68%, 47/69) or a small influence (26%, 18/69), with only 4 women (6%) feeling that it had no influence. We then asked women how they felt now about their decision and the vast majority of women felt that they had definitely or probably made the right decision (see Table 6.3.3).

To find out what factors women were weighing up when they made their decision not to be sutured, we asked them to think back to that time and to recall what they saw as the main advantages of having stitches and not having them. The numbers in parentheses are the number of women who gave each type of response or gave a response categorised to a particular theme. Typical verbatim quotes are presented for each theme.

Table 6.3.2 Perceived difficulty of deciding whether or not to have stitches

	% (proportion)
Very easy decision	64% (47/73*)
Quite an easy decision	34% (25/73)
Quite a difficult decision	1% (1/73)
Very difficult decision	0% (0/73)

* The denominator is 73 because women who felt they did not have a choice about whether or not to have sutures were directed to skip this option.

Table 6.3.3 How women feel now about their decision not to have stitches

	% (proportion)
Definitely made the right decision	77% (57/74*)
Probably made the right decision	19% (14/74)
Unsure about whether I made the right decision	1% (1/74)
Probably made the wrong decision	1% (1/74)
Definitely made the wrong decision	1% (1/74)

* The denominator is 74 because women who felt they did not have a choice about whether or not to have sutures were directed to skip this question.

Many women felt that being sutured had no advantages (30). 'I could not see any advantage in having stitches.' Some women wrote that stitches might be necessary to help a very bad tear to heal (4), or to stop bleeding (4). 'Maybe if I had a very deep/big tear or episiotomy I may have felt some stitches were necessary.' Many also speculated that sutures might promote better healing (18). Women mentioned several different aspects of healing that might be better with stitches, but their responses were generally very tentative. These aspects included the appearance of the perineum (6). 'The possibility – by no means certainty – of a marginally tidier undercarriage; the sexual function of the perineum (2) 'Felt to be more likely to be more likely to be good for sex'; the speed of healing (4) 'Possibly quicker healing'; and the size of the vaginal opening (3) 'Possibly tidier/tighter vaginal opening once healed'. Some felt that stitches might give a sense of security or less worry to women during the healing period (4) 'Reassurance – the tear would have to heal if held together', 'Psychological reassurance that wouldn't tear more'. The only other possible advantage of being sutured alluded to was that it was the conventional thing to do (4) 'I think I was also influenced by a lifetime of hearing how stitches were sort of part of the birth', 'There was a feeling that because it is accepted practice with many midwives/doctors that it must have some advantage'.

Women wrote more about the possible advantages of having an unsutured tear. Many felt that having an unsutured perineum would result in better healing (27) in that the perineum might heal more quickly (7) 'I believed the tear, which was very small, would heal more quickly'; with less chance of having an infection (14) 'No stitches to go rotten'; being stronger for future births (2) 'I strongly believed that a natural heal was stronger and less likely to tear again'; being less likely to result in complications (2) 'Avoiding complications about stitch removal or problems with dissolving stitches'; with less scarring (5) 'Stitches I believe can cause uncomfortable scarring'; and would be less changed by childbirth (1) 'Feeling that my perineum would have more chance of being "the same" as before childbirth'. There were some concerns about badly-done sutures, and one perceived advantage of leaving tears to heal naturally was that it would avoid this eventuality (7) 'Sometimes stitches are not done correctly and have to be done again weeks after', 'Avoiding the possibility of a bodged job'.

Women also felt that the healing period would be less painful with an unsutured tear than a sutured one (15). Women's perceptions were not formed in a vacuum, they were often rooted in their own previous experiences (13) 'The healing process would be less painful and quicker than with stitches, which I had after a previous birth and it was very unpleasant', 'Having had stitches with my first child I felt that the healing process was very painful and very unsatisfactory'. First-time mothers sometimes based their perceptions on the accounts they had heard about other women's experiences (4) 'My decision was based on conversations with friends, some of whom seemed to suffer more after having stitches than others who had not'.

As well as mentioning the anticipated pain of a sutured tear in the days or weeks after birth, women also mentioned pain generally (13), or specifically mentioned pain during the suturing procedure itself (16) 'I had stitches with my first baby and the pricking and pulling was a nightmare', 'Stitches are a long, painful process'. However, it was not solely pain that made having stitches a difficult experience for women. Some women described being stitched as an unpleasant experience regardless of any pain involved (11) 'Not having to go through the discomfort and indignity of having it done', 'I did not want to be messed about with further'. In addition three women specifically mentioned a dislike or phobia about needles 'I'd need to be knocked out since I'm needle-phobic and being "needled" in any way was my worst fear'. The words women used to describe the stitching process ('endure', 'awful', 'horrifies', 'barbaric', 'nightmare', 'trauma', 'intrusive' and 'violated') were powerful and emotion-laden reflecting the fact that, for some women, perineal sutures are not perceived as a purely clinical procedure. Some women felt that the pain or unpleasantness of suturing would be particularly hard

Table 6.3.4 Perineal problems experienced since one month after the index birth

Problem	Extent of problem*	Treatment	Still a problem?
Minor spotting after sex	1	None	No
Thrush	3	Dietary treatment	Yes (at 42 months PN)
Tenderness, slight bleeding, thrush	1	None	Yes (at 13 months PN)
Not completely healed	2	None	Yes (at 30 months PN)
Took a couple of months to heal properly	1	None	No
Finding sex painful. It was felt that I had a build-up of scar tissue from first labour when I was massively stitched that was aggravated by next baby's birth	2	None	No
(Problems) from time to time passing stools	1	None	Yes (at 27 months PN)
Painful intercourse	2	None	Yes (at 9 months PN)
Mild pain	1	None	No
Infection because tear took a long time to heal	2	Silver nitrate treatment (x2)	No
Thrush, which was more painful around the tear than elsewhere	1	Caneston	No
Irritation	2	None	Yes (at 16 months PN)
Some tenderness	2	None	No
Pain on penetration during intercourse and on inserting tampon	2	None	No
Very sore and had a lot of problems in sitting on a chair without cushions	3	None	No
Periods leak at the side of the pad and on pant	3	None	Yes (at 11 months PN)
Area was quite sensitive, sort of numb, different to before	1	None	No
Tendency to constipation	1	None	No

*1 = minor problem, 4 = major problem PN = postnatal

Table 6.3.5 Pain levels during various activities currently and after birth

Activity	Any pain now?	Any pain in first few days/first time	Mean (sd) pain level* in first few days/first time
Sitting	0% (0/105)	84% (86/102)	1.8 (1.3)
Walking	1% (1/105)	77% (79/102)	1.3 (1.2)
Passing urine	1% (1/104)	82% (85/104)	2.0 (1.5)
Moving bowels	1% (1/104)	84% (84/100)	1.9 (1.4)
Inserting tampon	4% (3/75)	26% (18/68)	1.1 (1.3)
Sexual intercourse	12% (11/94)	59% (54/91)	1.0 (1.2)
Other sexual activities	3% (2/73)	21% (14/68)	0.4 (0.8)

0 = no pain, 1 = mild, 2 = discomforting, 3 = distressing, 4 = horrible, 5 = excruciating

to bear at the emotionally and physically vulnerable time just after giving birth (6) 'I was so sore after the birth that I really don't think I could have borne anyone touching me down there, plus I was too exhausted to endure anything else', 'That I wouldn't have to cope with the pain of a needle going into my skin, the thought of that was unbearable after giving birth, and that I would be left alone to start recovering from the birth'.

Some women reported opting for non-suturing out of a belief in the natural healing process (11) 'I had faith that my body would heal naturally', 'Natural healing, if possible, seems a better choice'. Others were more matter of fact about it (3) 'If it will heal naturally, why bother?', 'Natural healing happens'. Some women were keen to avoid intervention in childbirth generally, and not having stitches fitted in with this preference (10) 'Not having stitches fitted in with the rest of the birth – the experience of doing the birth myself, rather than having it done to me', 'The less intervention the better'.

The final theme to emerge from the data was not

Table 6.3.6 Comparison of pain levels after sutured and unsutured tears by women who had experience of both

Activity	Mean (sd) pain level after unsutured tear	Mean (sd) pain level after sutured tear	P value*
Sitting in first few days	2.0 (1.4)	3.1 (1.6)	0.007
Walking in first few days	1.5 (1.3)	2.5 (1.6)	0.015
Passing urine in first few days	1.9 (1.6)	2.9 (1.7)	0.016
Moving bowels in first few days	2.2 (1.3)	3.3 (1.3)	0.003
Using tampon for first time	0.3 (0.6)	0.5 (1.3)	0.317
Having sexual intercourse first time	1.1 (1.4)	1.6 (1.6)	0.013
Other sexual activities first time	0.4 (0.8)	0.6 (1.4)	0.180

*Derived from Wilcoxon signed ranks test

Table 6.3.7 Frequency of urinary incontinence

	Percentage (proportion)
Never	33% (35/106)
Very occasionally	42% (44/106)
Less than once in the last week	10% (11/106)
Once or twice in the past week	10% (11/106)
Three or more times in the past week	5% (5/106)

Table 6.3.8 Women's views about whether they would have stitches for a similar tear in a future birth

	Percentage (proportion)
No, definitely not	82% (85/104)
No, probably not	10% (10/104)
Really don't know	7% (7/104)
Yes, probably	0% (0/104)
Yes, definitely	2% (2/104)

wanting the interruption that suturing would bring at a time when women were greeting and welcoming their new baby (5) 'I didn't want anything to disturb me and my new baby', 'I didn't want an optional or unnecessary medical procedure detracting from time with my new baby'.

Perineal problems

We asked women whether they had an infection in their perineum after the birth of their index baby. Two women (2%, 2/106) reported having an infection. We then asked them if they had had any problems with their perineum since their index baby was one month old. Nineteen (17%, 19/105) reported having a problem. Details of these

problems are given in table 6.3.4. It should be noted that some of the problems, e.g. thrush and constipation are unlikely to be related to having an unsutured perineal tear. The majority of the problems were perceived to be minor, i.e. rating one or two on a four-point scale (1 = minor problem, 4 = major problem). Three women reported having treatment for these problems. The majority (61%, 11/18) of the problems had now resolved. None of the women reported having had an operation on their perineum.

Comfort and pain

We presented women with a list of activities that might be painful after a perineal tear, and asked them to rate their pain for each activity using the Present Pain Intensity Scale of the McGill Pain Inventory.[8] Women rated their current pain, and their pain in the first few days/the first time an activity was done after the index birth. These findings are presented in Table 6.3.5. We found that few women were currently experiencing pain, that many women experienced some pain in the first few days after the birth or the first time an activity was undertaken, but the levels of pain reported were relatively low. The 20 women who had had a sutured tear in the birth prior to the index birth were asked to indicate their pain levels after that birth. This enabled us to compare pain levels following sutured and unsutured tears. Women who had experience of both sutured and unsutured tears recalled the sutured tears being significantly more painful for five of the seven activities examined.

Continence

Half (50%, 53/106) the women in our sample reported experiencing stress incontinence ('at the moment, do you ever leak urine when you cough, sneeze or laugh?'), and a third (30%, 32/106) reported experiencing urgency incontinence ('at the moment, do you ever leak urine when you have an urgent desire to pass urine and there is no toilet nearby?'). The frequency of incontinence was low, with the majority reporting that this happened 'very occasionally' (see Table 6.3.7). Eighteen percent (14/77) reported wearing a pad due to leaking urine, either occasionally (12 women), frequently (three women) or every day (two women). Three women (3%, 3/104) reported having a problem controlling their bowels.

Subsequent births

Twenty of the women in the sample had had a vaginal birth since the index birth. In these subsequent births 40% (8/20) had an intact perineum and 60% (12/20) had a perineal tear. There were no episiotomies in subsequent

Table 6.3.9 Number of women reporting worries

	Worry level					
	Not a worry	1	2	3	4	5
Own experience of sex	76% (77/101)	12	3	7	0	2
Partner's experience of sex	78% (76/98)	9	6	5	1	1
Pain in the perineum	88% (90/102)	10	2	0	0	0
Leaking urine	50% (51/103)	28	12	7	3	2
Lack of bowel control	93% (95/102)	6	1	0	0	0
How well perineum has healed	85% (86/101)	9	5	0	0	1
Way perineum looks	74% (76/103)	14	8	0	1	4

0 = not a worry, 5 = major worry

births. Two of the subsequent tears were sutured, ten were not.

Women's views

To assess women's overall levels of satisfaction with having an unsutured tear, we asked women 'if you were to have another baby, and you had a tear similar to the one you had this time, would you choose to have stitches?' Two of the 104 women who answered this question said they would have stitches, and 82% (85/104) said that they definitely would not have stitches (see table 6.3.8). Women's answers to our question about whether they felt they had made the right decision in not having sutures are also an indication of the high level of satisfaction with unsutured tears.

To explore whether women had any worries that might relate to the perineum, we listed some potential worries and asked women to rate these (0 = not a worry and 5 = a major worry). Table 6.3.9 shows the numbers of women reporting each worry. The most common areas of worry were leaking urine, their own and their partner's experience of sex and the appearance of their perineum, but the overall level of worry was low.

When examining the views people hold about the

Table 6.3.10 Comments by women who had negative views about not having stitches
(all relevant comments reproduced verbatim) N = 2

'I was told stitches were painful, so I thought it will be an advantage not to have it and let the tear heal naturally... The tear did not close together as I was told... Periods leak at the side of pad and on pant due to the nature of the tear.'
(reported in questionnaire, 11 months postnatally)

'I feel like the channel tunnel down there... I would like to think that my lower region was not so gaping... The whole area feels gynormous and when I have intercourse, I can't believe it's much fun for my husband. I wish it had been explained to me exactly how it would have felt if I'd chosen stitches or not. I was told that I'd only need one or perhaps two, so it was hardly worth it – so I was told.'
(reported in questionnaire, 52 months postnatally)

healthcare they receive, it is important to consider the context in which views are given. The questionnaires in this study were sent by and returned to a researcher who was, for some of the women, the midwife who cared for them during labour. To ascertain whether this might have made women more reticent about expressing any dissatisfaction with the management of their perineal trauma, we compared the worry ratings given by women cared for by one of us (BR) with those given by women cared for by other midwives in the practice. We found no statistically significant differences for any of the worries, suggesting that women felt relatively free to express their true feelings.

The qualitative data from open-ended questions in the questionnaire can inform us about why the women in the study were generally satisfied with their unsutured tears, and why the small minority who were unhappy felt as they did, giving a richer picture of women's views and experiences than the quantitative data above. Women were categorised as having negative, mixed or positive views about not having had stitches, on the basis of their answers to the two questions about whether they felt they had made the right decision in not having stitches, and about whether they would choose to have sutures for a future similar tear. Two women had negative views, and seven had mixed views. The relevant comments made by women in these two categories are reproduced in Tables 6.3.10 and 6.3.11. Ninety-eight women had positive views. Table 6.3.12 shows what these women saw as the main advantages of not having stitches. Their answers mirror, to a large extent, the advantages they reported perceiving when deciding whether or not to be sutured.

Discussion

The data above provide a detailed descriptive picture of women's experiences of having an unsutured perineal tear from a long-term perspective. We found that women were

Table 6.3.11 Comments by women who had mixed views
about not having stitches

(all relevant comments reproduced verbatim) N = 7*

'It depends on the circumstances. I didn't have stitches because it was assumed that the tear would heal up naturally and it did... Management fine.'

(reported in questionnaire, 68 months postnatally)

'Maybe [with stitches I would have] a neater looking perineum but I'm only talking aesthetically and I do not know if having stitches would have been able to achieve better results... I'm quite happy apart from that so unless I have lots more facts/knowledge I can't judge or tell if there is anything else I should know... If I've missed out a lot of facts or reasons for and against I would rethink but as far as I know I feel I made a good decision at the time and I know nothing since that has made me change my mind.'

(reported in questionnaire, 35 months postnatally)

'The advantage I saw of having stitches was that my perineum would eventually be the same as before giving birth and was frightened that it could open more, if left unstitched... I only had a small tear, and thought that nature would heal it properly... [With stitches there] maybe, less problems in the future... If the tear is small, why interfere with something that nature could take care of... How many tears can you leave to heal naturally – without stitches? One does not matter too much, but for two, I am not sure.'

(reported in questionnaire, 27 months postnatally)

'I don't know much about stitches... A tear is not something that they can stitch... After the birth of my baby I never feel any pain in my perineum. What worries me now was that my baby is a year old now and we are looking forward to have another one. When me and my husband meet, after a month, what I was expecting is to miss my period, but now am still seeing it. So I don't know why this should be may be is because of the perineum tear I don't know. In fact am confused. I don't know what to do. Please can this have any effect on me?'

(reported in questionnaire, 12 months postnatally)

'[With stitches] I might have healed quicker.'

(reported in questionnaire, 9 months postnatally)

'At the time I was very tired and had been in a lot of pain, I did not want to be messed about with further. I had also heard that sometimes the stitches are not done correctly and have to be done again weeks after... [With stitches] I may have healed quicker? – It took 3-4 months before I felt no pain... I was very sore and had a lot of problems in sitting on a chair without cushions. I used to take pain killers for it.'

(reported in questionnaire, 12 months postnatally)

---

*One woman made no comments

---

generally very satisfied with having an unsutured perineal tear. They appeared to view having/not having stitches from a holistic perspective, weighing up perceived short and longer-term psychosocial and physical factors.

Some women reported experiencing perineal problems. Although meaningful comparative data can only be obtained from randomised controlled trials, it may be helpful for the reader to see the level of problems experienced by the women in our sample in the context of previous studies (see Table 6.3.13). These comparisons suggest that the problems reported by women in our sample are broadly similar to those reported by postnatal women generally.

The problems reported in this study were generally perceived as minor and had often been subsequently resolved. Perineal problems are important, but this study cannot tell us whether the problems would have been more or less likely to have occurred with sutures. The women generally experienced some pain in the first few days after birth. This was less than the level of pain after a sutured tear recalled by those who had experience of both sutured and non-sutured tears. Women reported having some worries. We do not know if these worries are unique to women with unsutured tears. Two of the 107 women were clearly unhappy with having an unsutured perineum, which suggests that leaving tears to heal naturally is not necessarily the best option for all women. The experiences of these two women need to be seen alongside the positive views of the majority of the women in this study, and alongside the prevalence of reported problems with sutured tears.[6,7]

The limitations of this study should be borne in mind. Firstly it was a retrospective study, and women may not have accurate recall of past events or feelings. Secondly, although the response rate was high for a study of this type, not all women answered the questionnaire, so we know nothing about the views or experiences of the non-respondents. Thirdly, women may have felt reticent about expressing dissatisfaction in a questionnaire from the midwife who cared for them, although our data does not support this possibility. Lastly, a descriptive study of this type does not provide comparative data, therefore we do not know whether the outcomes experienced are better or worse than the outcomes for women with sutured tears.

Implications for future research

There is clearly a need for a randomised controlled trial of sutured versus non-sutured perineal tears. This study provides reassuring evidence to support the introduction of non-suturing in a trial context. It has also demonstrated the wide range of outcomes that are important to women, and any trial should incorporate such outcomes. The study also raises a note of caution for those planning trials in that when women were offered the opportunity of not having sutures, the vast majority found it easy to decide not to have stitches. The implications of this for recruitment rates and trial design require careful consideration.

Implications for practice

As far as we are aware, no trial comparing sutured and unsutured tears has been done or is under way. In the absence of trial data, women and midwives need some evidence on which to base their decisions and advice. We

Table 6.3.12 Comments by women who had positive views about not having stitches
(response to question about current perceptions of advantages of not having stitches) N = 98

Theme	Frequency	Typical quotes
Less painful healing	28	'Comfort, both in the early days and since then' 'There is no pain experienced when the tear is healing unstitched' 'Much less painful postnatal period' 'I did not realise that a stitchless tear would give me no discomfort at all'
Quicker healing	17	'More rapid healing' 'Faster healing' 'Tear heals up more quickly'
Avoidance of infections	22	'Less problems with infections' 'Less chance of infection' 'Perhaps less risk of wound infection'
Avoidance of scar tissue	12	'No scar tissue' 'No permanent change or scar tissue on my perineum' 'You don't have the same problems of scar tissue build-up' 'No scarring'
Avoidance of possibility of bad suturing	7	'Not having to suffer the discomforts of being badly sewn up' 'Less chance of bad stitching leading to further problems later on'
Less to worry about during healing period	3	'No worries about stitches bursting' 'Stitches are worrying for a lot of people' 'No worry about looking after the stitches'
Less likely to tear in future births	2	'I feel that the area is more resilient to tearing next time around' 'Possibly less problems with future vaginal births'
Better for sex	3	'A quicker recovery and hence able to recommence sexual relations sooner' 'More rapid less painful healing all making a return to a normal sex life easier'
Better for breastfeeding	1	'Ability to sit down and breastfeed more easily'
Avoidance of a painful procedure	9	'Having stitches means extra pain and injections' 'No pain of stitches being done'
Avoidance of an emotionally difficult procedure	11	'Less emotional sense of having been "tampered with"' 'Not being subjected to indignity of having stitches put in' 'Less trauma – physical and psychological – following birth'
Avoidance of a difficult procedure at a vulnerable time	4	'No intrusive intervention at the most vulnerable recovery time that you/your perineum could be at' 'The stitching itself is very painful at a vulnerable time'
Belief in natural healing	21	'To heal naturally must be better' 'I believe the body is quite capable of repairing itself, without intervention'
Avoidance of intervention	10	'I always think minimal interference is a good idea' 'No more intervention than is absolutely necessary'
Increased confidence in body	5	'Increased my confidence in my belief in my body's ability to heal itself' 'Being able to enjoy one's body's ability to heal itself' 'More positive feeling about own body's abilities'
Sense of control over own body	8	'Feel more control over it' 'It was a small way of controlling my own healing process' 'It allows you to stay in charge of your own body'
No interruption in time with new baby	3	'You don't have to undergo the indignity of being stitched up when you want to get on with being "you" and being "a mother" and being "a family"' 'No interruption in the bonding time with the new baby'
Benefits for midwife/NHS	1	'It takes less time and is cheaper'

believe that the findings of our study provide some evidence for the safety and acceptability of leaving some perineal tears unsutured, and make an important contribution to this under-researched area of midwifery practice.

The implications for practice drawn from this study will depend on the perspective taken. On the one hand, it can be argued that non-suturing is a new, relatively untested form of care, and as such, should not be offered outside the context of a randomised controlled trial.[9] On

Table 6.3.13 Comparisons between the morbidity reported in this study and morbidity reported in studies of general postnatal/adult populations

This sample (6-84 months PN)	Studies of general postnatal/adult populations
Perineal pain	12% (12/102) reported having some worry about perineal pain 10% reported perineal pain 2-18 months PN[12]
Intercourse	12% reported some pain on intercourse 20% reported intercourse sore or difficult 2-18 months PN[12]
Urinary incontinence	50% reported stress incontinence '50% of women aged 18+ will have mild stress incontinence'[13]
Anal/fecal incontinence	3% reported having problems controlling their bowels 4.9% reported fecal incontinence at 3 months PN[14] 2.2% of the adult population report anal incontinence[15]

PN = postnatally

the other hand, where there is no evidence from randomised controlled trials to support an intervention (i.e. suturing), we believe, like Sackett and colleagues, that evidence-based practice 'is not restricted to randomised trials... And if no randomised trial has been carried out... we follow the trail to the next best evidence and work from there'.[10] Furthermore, we support the basic principles of Enkin and colleagues that 'the only justification for practices that restrict a woman's autonomy, her freedom of choice and her access to her baby, would be clear evidence that these... practices do more good than harm, and... that any interference with the natural process of pregnancy and childbirth should

also be shown to do more good than harm. We believe that the onus of proof rests on those who advocate any intervention that interferes with either of these principles'.[11] From this perspective, it would be appropriate for women to make their own informed decisions based on the currently available evidence and their own prospective study of women's expectations and experiences of preferences about the management of perineal trauma. We hope that the findings of our study will help women make such decisions.

Key points

- Six months to seven years after childbirth the vast majority (n=98/107) of women with unsutured perineal tears felt positive about not having had stitches. Two women had negative views and seven had mixed views.

- Women in this study viewed non-suturing from a physiological and social point of view, as well as a physical one.

- Evidence from prospective randomised controlled trials is urgently needed in this important, but under-researched, area of midwifery practice.

- In the absence of evidence from randomised trials, we feel that it would be appropriate for women to make their own informed decisions based on the currently available evidence and their own preferences about the management of perineal trauma.

We would like to thank all the women who took part in our study; also Alison Coyle and Julie Dennison for transcribing qualitative data, and Laura Reed and Martha Reed for secretarial help. Becky Reed received an RCM Professional Development Award (Emma Jane Award) to cover some of the costs of undertaking this study. Sarah Clement is supported by South Thames Primary Care Research Network.

REFERENCES

1 Greenshields W, Hulme H, Oliver S. The perineum in childbirth: A survey of women's experiences and midwives' practices. London: National Childbirth Trust; 1993.
2 Lewis L. Tea-time: using herbs to help heal the unsutured perineum. MIDIRS Midwifery Digest 1994; 4(4):455–456.
3 Head M. Dropping stitches. Nursing Times 1993; 89(33):64–65.
4 Anonymous. Unit round-up. The Practising Midwife 1998; 1(10):7.
5 Gordon B, Machrodt C, Fern E, et al. Ipswich Childbirth Study: a randomised evaluation of two stage postpartum perineal repair leaving skin unsutured. British Journal of Obstetrics and Gynaecology 1998; 105(4):435–440.
6 Green JM, Coupland V, Kitzinger JV. Great expectations: A prospective study of women's expectations and experiences of childbirth. Cambridge: Childcare and Development Group, University of Cambridge; 1998.
7 Howard S, McKell D, Mugford M, et al. Cost-effectiveness of different approaches to perineal suturing. British Journal of Midwifery 1995; 3:587–605.
8 Melzak R. The McGill Pain Questionnaire. Pain 1975; 1:277–299.

9 Steen M. The abused perineum. British Journal of Midwifery 1998; 6:428–429.
10 Sackett DL, Richardson WS, Rosenberg W, et al. Evidence-based medicine. Edinburgh: Churchill Livingstone; 1997: 4–5.
11 Enkin M, Keirse MJNC, Renfrew M, et al. A guide to effective care in pregnancy and childbirth, 2nd edn. Oxford: Oxford University Press; 1995: 389.
12 Glazener CM. Sexual function after childbirth: women's experiences, persistent morbidity and lack of professional recognition. British Journal of Obstetrics and Gynaecology 1997; 104:330–335.
13 Dawson C, Whitfield H. ABC of urology: Urinary incontinence and urinary infection. British Medical Journal 1996; 312:961–964.
14 Wilson PD, Herbison RM, Herbison GP. Obstetric practice and the prevalence of urinary incontinence three months after delivery. British Journal of Obstetrics and Gynaecology 1996; 103:154–161.
15 Nelson R, Norton N, Cautley E, et al. Community-based prevalence of anal incontinence. Journal of the American Medical Association 1995; 274: 559–561.

How does it feel to you?

Uterine palpation and lochial loss as guides to postnatal 'recovery'

I – THE BACKGROUND

Sally Marchant   Jo Alexander   Jo Garcia

These three articles are about the postpartum uterus, its involution and how this is recorded by midwives and described by the women themselves.

A two-year research study of routine assessment of postnatal uterine involution by midwives was undertaken in two health districts in the South and West Region during 1995 and 1996. For one aspect of this work, the observations made of uterine fundal height and vaginal fluid loss were collected from the midwifery records of 729 postnatal women. Using this information the methods used by midwives to assess uterine involution are described and discussed in relation to current clinical practice. Standards for record keeping are reviewed, based on the presumption that accurate records of clinical observations are important where continuous assessment of clinical progress is part of the rationale for providing care.

The two districts differed quite substantially in how the observations of uterine fundal height were recorded. In one district, midwives were more likely to use a range of descriptive language to report the position of the uterus and the state of involution. In the second district, it was more common for midwives to give these observations as a form of quantifiable measurement. The final article reports women's own descriptions of their postpartum uterus from the prospective survey of postnatal women and their experiences of vaginal loss.

The findings are discussed within the context of routine assessment of uterine fundal height by midwives and the purpose of record keeping in relation to outcomes.

Purpose of the study

Midwives use an assessment of uterine fundal height in the postnatal period to establish that women in their care are recovering from childbirth and to detect deviations from this normal process. However, the value of this assessment as a screening measure to predict or prevent women from developing subsequent morbidity had not been established. There is also a lack of information about the normal pattern of postnatal uterine involution and vaginal loss. Midwifery practice is changing to reflect the need to involve women in their care at all stages of childbirth[1] and it is important to evaluate both traditional and emerging practices in the clinical field.

We therefore undertook a research study into the routine assessment by midwives of postpartum uterine involution and a survey of women's experiences of vaginal loss from 24 hours to three months after childbirth.[2]

Medical and midwifery textbooks describe involution of the uterus as a complex physiological process through which the uterus gradually reduces in size following delivery until it has returned to its non-pregnant size.

During this process, contraction and retraction of uterine muscles control blood loss from the uterus and the placental site becomes incorporated into the newly forming endometrial lining.[3] The standard textbooks suggest that the return to the non-pregnant position and size of the uterus is normally complete by 6 weeks after childbirth.[4,5,6,7]

Inhibition of the involution of the uterus can lead to serious consequences for the woman. Haemorrhage can occur when the blood vessels are not occluded because the uterine muscle layer fails to contract and retract effectively. This may occur immediately, or in the first few hours after delivery from causes which include trauma, and physiological disorders which lead to uterine atony.

Excessive or prolonged vaginal bleeding can also occur several days or weeks after the birth; this is usually thought to be associated with uterine infection or retained products from the pregnancy.[4] Where uterine infection occurs, it can develop into a life-threatening septicaemia.

At the start of the 20th century, haemorrhage and puerperal fever were the most common reasons for the large numbers of postpartum deaths, with puerperal fever accounting for about 40% of maternal deaths.[8]

The use of antiseptics and antibiotics significantly reduced deaths from uterine sepsis. Changes in obstetric practice, lower parity, better nutrition and emergency life-saving strategies, such as blood transfusion, contributed to the reduction in the number of women who bled to death from primary or secondary haemorrhage after childbirth.[9]

It is not clear when assessment of uterine involution became part of the standard care offered to postpartum women. An obstetrician writing in 1906 considered that it was essential for the practitioner to assess the descent of the postpartum uterus on a daily basis.[10] However, care following childbirth was largely the remit of the 'monthly nurse' who usually required payment, so her attendance was more likely to relate to social circumstances and the ability to pay, rather than medical need.

The duties of the midwife over this period were described in the form of a *Handbook for Midwives* which was issued from time to time by the Central Midwives' Board.

In the 1919 Handbook, the duties for the midwife attending the postpartum mother were initially described very specifically: Midwives were instructed to give attention to the presence of fever, abdominal swelling or tenderness and persistent offensive lochia (along with several other symptoms), but there is no reference to the palpation of the uterus or the assessment of uterine involution.[11]

Other literature from the same era identifies that uterine palpation and observing deviation from a normal daily reduction in uterine size are important observations.[12,13]

One book[12] describes the method of palpation and measurement of the uterine involution:

'this is best done by sinking the hand, palm to pubis, into the abdomen above the navel, and bringing it down until it is checked by the fundus…

…each day the fundus may be measured with a foot rule. The first day it is about 5¹/₂ inches above the pubis and it usually descends about ¹/₂ [an inch] a day.'

In addition, advice is given on the relationship of these observations to normal progress:

'…it is not the level of the fundus which is of so much importance as to whether it is lower on one day than on the previous one. On consecutive days it should not remain at the same height.'

Current practice

The observation and measurement of postpartum fundal height has become incorporated into routine postnatal care, which predominantly consists of an overall physical examination of the postpartum mother. Current midwifery textbooks describe the average size and weight of the postpartum uterus, the physiological process of involution and the role of the midwife in observing the mother's health in the postpartum period.[5,6,7] There is general agreement among the textbooks that there is a progressive reduction in uterine size until it can no longer be palpated above the symphysis pubis by about the 10th to 12th postnatal day, and that this occurs at a rate of between 1 and 2.5cm a day.

Until recently, this routine practice of assessment of postnatal uterine involution had not been questioned or evaluated.[14]

In addition, studies which have reviewed the use of ultrasound scans of the postpartum uterus have produced conflicting information about the use of ultrasound at this time and its diagnostic role in assessing for pathology.[15,16]

The context within which routine postnatal observations are undertaken has also changed. The daily visits and physical examinations of the mother and baby for the first ten days have largely been replaced by a more flexible approach to the number and frequency of postnatal visits to women in their own homes.[17] Possible reasons for this include: pressure on resources resulting in rationalising of midwifery time, a changing approach to maternity care which involved women more in planning their care, and the appreciation of the importance of continuity from those providing the service.[18]

It might also be considered that, for developed countries such as the UK, a fatal outcome from uterine infection or haemorrhage is now comparatively rare and different priorities have arisen in relation to outcomes for postpartum women.

Against this background, midwives are questioning the role of postnatal care[19] and women are reported to be less satisfied with postnatal care than with other aspects of the maternity services.[20] It is only recently that the extent of morbidity in the postnatal period has been identified.[21,22] The usefulness of routine postnatal observations has been questioned, as has the possible impact of such observations on subsequent morbidity for women, and whether the value traditionally ascribed to these assessments could be supported by evidence.[23,24,25]

A fairly recent study addressed one of these issues by evaluating measurement of the symphysis fundal distance (SFD) by the use of a tape measure.[26]

Two groups were compared: multiple measurements obtained by the same midwife on the same woman, and the measurements obtained by different midwives who measured the SFD on the same women. Cluett and colleagues demonstrated that where the same midwife repeated measurements of SFD by tape measure, these could be expected to vary by nearly 3cm (2.94cm). Where two midwives undertook this measurement, the extent of variance increased to over 5cm (5.01cm).

These findings took place in a controlled environment over a period measurable in minutes, so similar observations in clinical practice are likely to demonstrate much larger degrees of disparity. Such imprecision makes them unreliable as an aid to clinical decision making.[26]

In the second part of Cluett and colleagues' work, a prospective survey of the involution patterns of 28 postnatal women revealed considerable variability in uterine descent over a period of up to 23 days postpartum.

This suggests that the uterus does not always descend with the uniformity described in the textbooks: for some women, several days passed where the uterus did not reduce in size with no associated morbidity and the timing when the uterus became no longer palpable varied considerably.[25]

Conclusion

Clearly, history had resulted in midwives performing screening tests that looked for patterns of change in the uterus and lochia, the normal parameters for which had never been established. Furthermore, the predictive value of these 'tests' had never been demonstrated. Research seemed warranted, and this will be described in Part 2.

Note. Some of the material included in this paper was first presented at the 1997 Research and the Midwife conference.

REFERENCES

1 Department of Health. Changing Childbirth: The report of the expert maternity group. London: HMSO; 1993.
2 Marchant S, Alexander J, Garcia J, et al. A survey of women's experiences of vaginal loss from 24 hours to three months after childbirth (the BLiPP study). Midwifery 1999; 15:72–81.
3 Williams JW. Regeneration of uterine mucosa after delivery, with especial reference to the placental site. American Journal of Obstetrics and Gynecology 1931; 22:664–696.
4 Beischer N, Mackay E. Obstetrics and the newborn. The normal puerperium: anatomy and physiology, 2nd edn. London: Baillière Tindall; 1986.
5 Ball, J. Physiology, psychology and management of the puerperium. In: Bennett VR, Brown LK (eds). Myles textbook for midwives. 12th edn. Edinburgh: Churchill Livingstone; 1993.
6 Silverton, L. Postnatal care. In: Silverton L (ed). The art and science of midwifery. New York: Prentice Hall; 1993: 433–462.
7 Abbott H, Bick D, MacArthur C. Health after birth. In: Henderson C, Jones K (eds). Essential midwifery. London: Mosby; 1997.
8 Loudon I. Puerperal fever, the streptococcus, and the sulphonamides, 1911-1945. British Medical Journal 1987; 295:485–490.
9 Loudon I. Obstetric care, social class, and maternal mortality. British Medical Journal 1986; 293:606–608.
10 Longridge CN. The puerperium or management of the lying-in woman and newborn infant. London: Adlard and Sons; 1906.
11 Central Midwives' Board. Handbook incorporating the rules of the central midwives board, 5th edn. London: Central Midwives Board; 1919.
12 Calder AB. Lectures on midwifery. London: Baillière, Tindall and Cox; 1912.
13 Berkeley C. Handbook of midwifery, part IV. London: Cassell and Co; 1924.
14 Montgomery E, Alexander J. Assessing postnatal uterine involution: A review and a challenge. Midwifery 1994; 10(1):1–4.

15 Hertzberg B, Bowie J. Ultrasound of the postpartum uterus. Journal of Ultrasound Medicine 1991; 10:451–456.
16 Tekay A, Jouppila P. A longitudinal Doppler ultrasonographic assessment of alterations in peripheral vascular resistance of the uterine arteries and ultrasonographic findings of the involuting uterus during the puerperium. American Journal of Obstetrics and Gynecology 1993; 168:190–198.
17 Garcia J, Renfrew M, Marchant S. Postnatal home visiting by midwives. Midwifery 1994; 10(1):40–43.
18 Garcia J, Marchant S. The potential of postnatal care. In: Kroll D (ed). Issues in midwifery care for the future. London: Baillière Tindall; 1996.
19 Walsh D. Hospital postnatal care: The end is nigh. British Journal of Midwifery 1997; 5(9):516–518.
20 The Audit Commission for Local Authorities and the National Health Service in England and Wales. First Class Delivery: Improving maternity services in England and Wales (National Report). Abingdon: Audit Commission Publications; 1997.
21 MacArthur C, Lewis M, Knox G. Health after childbirth: An investigation of long term health problems beginning after childbirth in 11,701 women. London: HMSO; 1991.
22 Glazener C, Abdalla M, Stroud P et al. Postnatal maternal morbidity: Extent, causes, prevention and treatment. British Journal of Obstetrics and Gynaecology 1995; 102(4):282–287.
23 Bick DE. Postnatal care cannot be ignored. British Journal of Midwifery 1995; 3(8):411–412.
24 Marchant S, Garcia J. What are we doing in the postnatal check? British Journal of Midwifery 1995; 3:34–38.
25 Cluett ER, Alexander J, Pickering RM. What is the normal pattern of uterine involution? An investigation of postpartum involution measured by the distance between the symphysis pubis and the uterine fundus using a tape measure. Midwifery 1997; 13:9–16.
26 Cluett ER, Alexander J, Pickering RM. Is measuring postnatal symphysis-fundal distance worthwhile? Midwifery 1995; 11(4):174–183.

How does it feel to you?

Uterine palpation and lochial loss as guides to postnatal 'recovery'

2 – THE BLiPP STUDY (BLOOD LOSS IN THE POSTNATAL PERIOD)

Sally Marchant   Jo Alexander   Jo Garcia

The lack of evidence of the value of routine fundal height measurement described in Part I, and the apparent wide range of 'normal' vaginal loss postpartum, led us to believe that this area merited further work. We therefore undertook a research study into the routine assessment by midwives of postpartum uterine involution and vaginal loss as recorded by the mothers. We identifed implications for clinical practice and resource management[1] but we also found that the records being kept by midwives were disturbingly inconsistent. Part III of this series will give the women's own descriptions of their postpartum uterus, and summarise the implications of the whole study for clinical practice.

Overview

The BLiPP study was a two-year project which took place in two districts in the South and West Region during 1995 and 1996. The study was funded by the South and West Research and Development committee.

The study had three parts:

- a case control study – the subject of this article
- a prospective survey of unselected new mothers (Part III of this series gives some of the results of this)
- a GP card notification study[2] (not covered here).

It included over 1000 women in two districts in southern England. Ethics committee permission was received for each element of the work. The study aimed to investigate:

- women's experiences of, and problems with, vaginal loss from 24 hours to three months after a birth
- risk factors for postnatal bleeding problems
- the value of routine midwifery observations in relation to predicting these problems
- treatment and referral patterns for women presenting with such problems in general practice.

The case control study

A case control study aims to compare one group of subjects who experienced a specific outcome with another group who did not. Comparison of characteristics of the two groups enables the identification of any which may have been associated with the outcome in question.[3]

The case control study reviewed medical and midwifery records over a two year period for women who were admitted to hospital for excessive or prolonged vaginal loss or uterine infection postpartum. Each case record was compared with two control records. Controls were identified from the delivery registers as those women whose deliveries occurred in the same place as, and next in time after, the case delivery. The research midwife (SM) conducted the majority of the data retrieval with the assistance of three other midwives. To explore any bias from the data retrieval, an inter- and intra-rater comparison for consistency over a series of key data items showed an acceptable agreement of not less than 97% with the majority of comparisons reaching 98% and 99%.

The hypothesis for the case control study was:

Routine assessment by midwives using abdominal palpation of uterine height and observations of vaginal loss in postnatal women, from 24 hours after delivery until the midwife discharges the mother from her care, fails to predict abnormal vaginal bleeding or uterine infection during the first three months postnatally.

The case control analysis examines the association between hospital admission for such problems and various antecedent factors, for example previous history of secondary postpartum haemorrhage. In addition, any association with the contemporaneous postnatal midwifery observations was explored. Full details of the methodology, sample size calculations and results have been given elsewhere.[4]

Table 6.5.1 Assessment of uterine involution by midwives on postnatal day 2

	District 1		District 2	
Assessment of involution	n = 439	%	n = 290	%
No visit that day	1	0.2	3	1
Of those visited	[438]	%	[287]	%
Uterus too tender	40	9	29	10
Measurement	67	15	208	73
Description	240	55	16	6
Other	83	19	32	11
Uterus just or no longer palpable	-	0	-	0
Visit made but no records	8	2	2	<1
Total	438	100	287	100

Table 6.5.2 Assessment of uterine involution by midwives on postnatal day 5

	District 1		District 2	
Assessment of involution	n = 439	%	n = 290	%
No visit that day	24	5	77	27
Of those visited	[415]	%	[213]	%
Uterus too tender	2	1	2	1
Measurement	52	12	157	74
Description	275	66	18	9
Other	71	17	20	9
Uterus just or no longer palpable	3	1	5	2
Visit made but no records	12	3	11	5
Total	415	100	213	100

Table 6.5.3 Assessment of uterine involution by midwives on postnatal day 10

	District 1		District 2	
Assessment of involution	n = 439	%	n = 290	%
No visit that day	119	27	133	46
Of those visited	[320]	%	[157]	%
Uterus too tender	0	0	1	1
Measurement	26	8	47	30
Description	144	45	10	6
Other	36	11	7	4
Uterus just or no longer palpable	87	27	72	46
Visit made but no records	27	9	20	13
Total	320	100	157	100

Descriptions from the midwives' records

Appropriate record keeping has always been an important aspect of midwifery practice,[5] but this may have been seen as having greatest priority for the events surrounding the labour and birth. The UKCC identifies the principles underpinning record keeping and its expectation of a standard which can 'demonstrate the chronology of events and all significant consultations, assessments, observations, decisions, interventions and outcomes'.[6]

The UKCC also maintains that inadequate and inappropriate record keeping negatively affects the overall wellbeing of the person being cared for. Examples quoted of this are disruption to effective communication between staff, creating the risk of medication or other treatment being duplicated or omitted and failure to focus attention on the early signs of deviation from the normal condition by the omission of recording significant observations and conclusions.[6]

The findings below relate to the routine assessment of postnatal fundal height recorded by midwives in the midwifery records of the 729 women in the case control study, who received their postnatal care between October 1993 and December 1995.

The position of the uterine fundus

The midwifery observations of fundal height were recorded on a data collection sheet and then coded according to pre-set criteria based on descriptions for assessment of uterine involution in current midwifery textbooks. This converted each clinical observation into a code that was entered onto the data sheet. Variables for the colour, odour and amount of vaginal loss, including a description of clots passed, were coded as described above but these data will not be discussed here.

The midwifery record of the state of the uterus was categorised according to whether it was:

- a measurement (with or without a description)
- a description without a measurement, or
- recorded in the form of abbreviations or symbols only (there being neither measurement nor description).

Also recorded was whether the uterus was too tender to palpate, no longer palpable or where although a visit had been made, there was no record of the state of the uterus. The categories which describe the midwifery records for the state of the uterus on postnatal days two, five and ten are given in Tables 6.5.1, 6.5.2 and 6.5.3. The findings are set out according to district in order to display the differences for discussion. All the women in these tables in whom the uterus had been recorded as being too tender to palpate had been delivered by Caesarean section. The relationship of such an observation to the development of pathology has been discussed elsewhere.[1]

The recording of uterine involution

These 'snapshots' of how involution was assessed by the midwives show some quite marked differences between the districts. In District 1, it was more common for midwives to record only a description of the involuting uterus rather than to assess it using some form of measurement. In District 2 the reverse was true. In District 1, more use was also made of symbols and abbreviations. This may suggest that different 'traditions' for recording have developed in the two districts, which are some distance apart. In a small proportion of women on each of the three days, a visit was made but no record of the state of the uterus. This may suggest that a more relaxed approach was being taken to what was formerly considered an essential part of every postnatal visit or perhaps the observation was made but not recorded.

Conclusions on midwives' record keeping

The pattern of normal involution has been demonstrated as varying widely amongst individuals[7] and to be assessed more accurately if there is continuity of observer.[8] However the majority of women in this study (83%) received home visits from more than one midwife. If there is benefit in assessing the uterine fundal height for postnatal women, and the case control study suggests that there is,[2] better quality record keeping is important to enable assessments by different midwives providing care to the same woman to be compared. It is suggested that the identification of potential morbidity requires consistency in both the method of assessment and the

Examples of the symbols and abbreviations used

Arrows alone:

Arrows and text:

↑umb or s p

↓ umb or s p

Arrows and circle with a dot
(this may represent the umbilicus?)

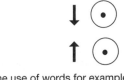

The use of words for example:

Going down

1f ↑umb

normal

n/p; p/p; j/p

↓ grapefruit (or orange, kiwi or plum)

12, 14, 15, 17 weeks size

The use of n/p was particularly difficult to interpret as this could mean not palpated or not palpable. There was also the dash, those that were not interpretable to the data collectors (even though they were themselves midwives) and the illegible.

subsequent recording of the observation made. Which method of assessment is best remains to be established.

Note: Some of the material included in this paper was first presented at the 1997 Research and the Midwife conference.

REFERENCES

1 Marchant S, Alexander J, Garcia J, et al. A survey of women's experiences of vaginal loss from 24 hours to three months after childbirth (the BLiPP study). Midwifery 1999; 15:72–81.
2 Alexander J, Marchant S, Garcia J. The BLiPP Study. Final report to the South and West Research and Development Committee, 1997. ISBN 1-85899-095-5.
3 Schlesselman J. Case control studies: Design, conduct, analysis. New York: Oxford University Press; 1982.
4 Marchant S. Routine midwifery assessment of postpartum uterine involution and vaginal loss and the relationship of these observations to morbidity. Unpublished PhD thesis. Portsmouth: University of Portsmouth; 1999.
5 UK Central Council for Nursing, Midwifery and Health Visiting. Midwives' Rules. London: UKCC; 1994.
6 UK Central Council for Nursing, Midwifery and Health Visiting. Standards for Record Keeping. London: UKCC; 1993.
7 Cluett ER, Alexander J, Pickering RM. What is the normal pattern of uterine involution? An investigation of postpartum involution measured by the distance between the symphysis pubis and the uterine fundus using a tape measure. Midwifery 1997; 13:9–16.
8 Cluett ER, Alexander J, Pickering RM. Is measuring postnatal symphysis-fundal distance worthwhile? Midwifery 1995; 11(4):174–183.

How does it feel to you?

Uterine palpation and lochial loss as guides to postnatal 'recovery'

3 – WOMEN'S ASSESSMENT OF THEIR OWN UTERUS

Sally Marchant   Jo Alexander   Jo Garcia

As part of our study into the routine assessment by midwives of postpartum uterine involution and blood loss as recorded by the mothers, postnatal women completed questionnaires and kept diaries of their experiences. This final article describes the survey, gives the results relating to the women's assessment of their own uterus and summarises the three articles.

The survey

The women were asked to complete a First Questionnaire during the first few days after the birth and then to keep a diary, daily from the second to tenth postnatal day, and then once a week for the next three weeks on postnatal days 14, 21 and 28. A Final Questionnaire was sent to the women three months after the birth. All data was anonymised: full details of the organisation of the survey have been described previously.[1] From a total of 660 women eligible for recruitment to the survey, 524 (79%) agreed to take part (263/354 (74%) from District 1, 261/306 (86%) from District 2). Of these, 67% returned their First Questionnaire, 162 women (62%) from District 1 and 188 (72%) from District 2.

The focus of the First Questionnaire was to gain insight into women's expectations about events associated with postpartum recovery, for example the duration of vaginal loss or occurrence of vaginal loss problems, as well as to record their experiences of actual events. Overall, findings from the study suggest that women's postnatal vaginal loss is considerably more varied in type, quantity and duration than suggested by textbooks. For example, for the duration of vaginal loss, the median number of days reported was 21 with an interdecile range (10th to 90th percentile) of 10 to 42 days. These results are fully reported elsewhere.[1] This article reports on two of the questions posed concerning the women's expectations about normal postpartum uterine involution, and their experiences of palpating their own uterus.

One question concerned the time it took for the uterus to return to approximately the same size as it had been before pregnancy. A range of categories was offered and these ranged from 10 days to six weeks; a 'don't know' option was also included. Forty-five percent (78/175) of primiparous women and 43% (75/175) of multiparous women thought it took six weeks for the uterus to 'return to normal' and 14% (25/175) and 19% (34/175) respectively said this took between two and four weeks. More multiparous (19%, 33/175) than primiparous women (10%, 17/175) said this occurred within 10 days. Primiparous women (55/175, 31%) were significantly more likely to report that they did not know how long it would take for their uterus to return to 'normal' (31/175, 18%, Odds Ratio 2.07 [95% CI 1.2-3.5]). Two multiparous women did not complete this question.

The second question asked whether the woman had felt for her uterus since the birth of her baby. The majority of women (234, 67%) said that they had not done this (see Table 6.6.1). Of those who had tried to do so, 36% (39/109) could describe how it felt. The descriptions of how this felt are given in Table 6.6.2. Some of their descriptions identified the position of the uterus in the abdomen, and some described its texture and size. It is of interest that the women's descriptions quite clearly identify key characteristics associated with the postpartum uterus. For example the descriptions suggest the uterus has intermittent contractions, resulting in a texture which is at times very firm and at others less so, and that the shape is generally oval or rounded in some way. These observations are strikingly like those in textbooks.

Postpartum uterus: women's perspective

During pregnancy, women appear be 'in touch' with and to touch their enlarging abdomen and there have been seductive images of pregnant film stars in magazines doing so. However, once the baby is born, the authors' general perception is that the mother shows little further interest in her uterus per se, although the desire to get 'back into shape' is common.[2] In some areas of Germany, midwives suggest women palpate their uterus after childbirth, in the same way that UK midwives undertake the postnatal uterine assessment (Reitz E, German midwife, personal communication). This appeared to the authors to be an area not often discussed with women in the UK. 36% of those who had tried to palpate their uterus could describe what they felt, even though it is not routine to explain to women what they might expect to find.

Summary of findings

The organisation and content of midwifery care in the postnatal period have recently received attention from policy makers and researchers. Women appear to be dissatisfied with this aspect of maternity care and midwives are questioning the role of assessments or observations which are performed on a routine basis for all women regardless of whether the women may need or benefit from them. There have been very few studies evaluating these routine aspects of care. Findings from the BLiPP study[1] have given a much clearer picture of the ranges for colour, amount and duration of postpartum vaginal loss. In addition the research demonstrated that women would like more information about this aspect of postpartum health. Perhaps we should also consider involving women in the assessment of their own uterine involution.

Data from the case control study[3] suggest that the assessment of uterine fundal height for postnatal women has value with regard to predicting subsequent readmission with secondary intrapartum haemorrhage and should not therefore be abandoned in the pursuit of reducing costs or saving time. It is arguable, however, whether there is any point in undertaking and recording an observation if the record cannot be unambiguously understood by others and used to construct an accurate chronological picture of events. Cluett and colleagues[4] clearly demonstrate the need to be sensitive to women's individual patterns of involution. This considerable

Table 6.6.1 Have you felt your tummy to feel the size of your womb since your baby was born?

		%
Total number of women who returned first questionnaire	350	
Had not felt for their uterus	234	67
Had felt for their uterus	109	31
Didn't answer the question	7	2

Of those who had felt for their uterus:

Tried but couldn't find uterus	17	15
Tried but unsure about what they felt	53	49
Could describe how it felt	39	36
	109	100

Table 6.6.2

Three women described where the uterus was in the abdomen:
- just below the umbilicus
- halfway between the umbilicus and pelvis
- a lot lower down

Other descriptions were of the shape:
- a pear
- melon
- tennis ball
- a fist

and of how it felt in texture:
- hard muscle
- hardening from time to time
- like jelly and floppy
- an empty balloon
- a tummy inside a tummy
- a soft lump

variability, alongside the likelihood that postnatal care is provided by a number of midwives, highlights the primary importance of accurate record keeping, both to improve outcomes for postnatal women and for the maintenance of professional standards in midwifery. It is interesting to reflect that the descriptions used by some women perhaps appeared to be more readily informative than the records of some of the midwives.

Note: Some of the material included in this paper was first presented at the 1997 Research and the Midwife conference.

REFERENCES

1 Marchant S, Alexander J, Garcia J, et al. A survey of women's experiences of vaginal loss from 24 hours to three months after childbirth (the BLiPP study). Midwifery 1999; 15:72–81.
2 Marchant S, Garcia J. What are we doing in the postnatal check? British Journal of Midwifery 1995; 3:34–38.
3 Alexander J, Marchant S, Garcia J. The BLiPP Study: Final report to the South and West Research and Development Committee, 1997. ISBN 1-85899-094-7.

4 Cluett ER, Alexander J, Pickering RM. What is the normal pattern of uterine involution? An investigation of postpartum involution measured by the distance between the symphysis pubis and the uterine fundus using a tape measure. Midwifery 1997; 13:9–16.

Reflecting on the postnatal experience

- What do you feel are the aims of postnatal care? Are these aims reflected in your practice? If they are not (e.g. because of time restraints) is there anything you can do to change this, or maximise your efforts?

- How have women you have worked with celebrated their postnatal period, or created individual rites of passage for their new baby and family? Do you feel this is helpful for families? If so, how could you gather and give information on this to the women you work with?

- Do you use the postnatal 'discharge' check (whether in hospital or home) to find out about women's perceptions of their experiences? Is this something you could use to evaluate your own practice? If you feel that verbal discussion with women might not result in accurate information being given, consider whether it would be worth asking a few women to fill out a short form about this anonymously.

- How can we frame the questions we ask women postnatally, to ensure that these are open enough to enable women to feel they can say what they need to, maximise their understanding and knowledge and ensure that we get enough information to be able to meet their needs?

- Do you encourage women to write their birth stories? If you have pregnancy and/or birth experiences of your own, have you written yours? How do women's stories compare with the birth story of the attending midwife, or the woman's partner?

Group exercise

Women and midwives can learn much from sharing their own and other people's birth stories, not only in the immediate postnatal period, but long after the event. Traditional midwives tend to tell birth stories to each other in circles, often in the evening, sometimes around a kitchen table or even a fire, while also sharing food and drink. Find a small group of midwives (between four and eight is probably optimal) who would like to share stories of their own births, and/or the births you have attended. If you need to find a way to get people talking, initially, you might ask for the funniest birth story, or the longest or shortest birth story, or the first or last birth each midwife attended.

Once you have experienced this kind of ritual story sharing, you might consider whether this is something that might be useful for women who you have attended, either at the end of their postnatal period, or even during pregnancy. You may want to have one or two midwives to facilitate the discussion, or invite women to organise this themselves. You might want to consider asking each woman if they would like to bring an older friend, mother or sister to share their stories of birth and mothering also. If you do this for pregnant women, you may want to ask the group to agree not to tell 'horror stories', as this will be uncomfortable and frightening for some women.

Focus on:
Abuse

SECTION CONTENTS

Child sexual abuse and pregnancy

A personal account

Khadj Rouf

I am a survivor of child sexual abuse. When raised as a topic, child sexual abuse gives rise to a range of reactions, including disbelief, anger and fear. It is a topic that is guaranteed to silence a room full of people, leaving many squirming with discomfort. Despite recent media coverage, there is still much ignorance and stigma about abuse. I was reminded of this when I became pregnant. I was shocked to find that there is very little material available to read, and some health professionals were not aware of the challenges that I was facing.

Abused by father

I was abused throughout most of my childhood by my father. He used a variety of tactics to ensure my compliance, ranging from terrorising me to affection and bribery. I was made to feel that I was a consenting party to the abuse and that it was all my fault. I tried to tell my mother about the abuse when I was seven years old, but I was not heard. It took me another eight years to pluck up the courage to tell her again. Thankfully, I was heard and believed. My mother divorced my father, and he was later prosecuted for what he had done.

It would be safer to think that stories like mine are rare. Sadly, child sexual abuse is all too common. Surveys reveal that at least 8% of girls are abused[1] and some estimate that it is as high as 38%.[2] It is also estimated that between 3 and 11% of boys are sexually abused.[3,4] Consequences of being sexually abused can include anxiety, depression, hostility, poor self-esteem and self-destructive behaviour.[5] Other research indicates that there is a link with psychiatric illnesses resulting in in-patient treatment[6] and with post-traumatic stress disorder.[7] For something that is so common and which can be so damaging, it is shocking that there is not more reference to it in pregnancy books and magazines. Its absence is a measure of the social pressure to keep silent about this hidden problem.

You may be thinking 'What has this got to do with pregnancy?' The answer is that pregnancy is a time of huge physical and emotional change, and one which brings women into contact with many people who are involved in giving intimate care. I was relatively lucky to have been believed as a child, and I was able to get excellent psychological support to help me recover from the trauma. I am now a qualified psychologist. Yet despite this, I found my pregnancy a time when many memories of abuse resurfaced and old fears returned. I felt vulnerable, emotionally raw. I felt scared by the medical interventions that I faced. I scoured books and magazines for help through this time but could come up with very little. I talked to my midwife and my active birth teacher who were wonderfully supportive. They agreed that there was a huge gap when it came to the information I was searching for. There were three areas in which I particularly needed support.

Coping with physical change

I, like many people who have been abused, have had a difficult relationship with my body. It took time to learn to like my body and staying in control of it became really important. During pregnancy, I found that I was changing each day and these changes were in the public arena. People who were passing acquaintances would pat my belly and comment on my size. This was very disconcerting, particularly as I had experienced so much uninvited attention earlier in my life.

Care during pregnancy also involved scrutinising my physical changes. My bump was regularly touched and measured. I was regularly asked to produce urine samples. Notes were written in jargon that I often did not understand. It was helpful to have a midwife who explained what the procedures were for, and what the jargon meant. She also recognised that I still owned my body, even though I often felt that I did not!

Choices during pregnancy and birth

I have always viewed pregnancy as a natural life event, not a medical condition. However, I found myself confronted by a world of technology and physical examinations. I found these procedures difficult and sometimes frightening. Some procedures reminded me of the abuse. There were professionals who did not seem to recognise how stressed I was, and assumed that I would be happy to have, for example, multiple vaginal examinations. The record was to have three vaginal examinations given by two different professionals in one morning, following a scare early in my pregnancy. I was made to feel that these examinations were all necessary for the good of my baby. I left the hospital drained and in tears because I felt, once again, that I had lost ownership of my body. I am sure some professionals perceived me as over-anxious or stroppy. From my point of view, I was trying to keep myself and my baby safe from invasive procedures.

I decided to take more control over my pregnancy by planning a home birth. I made a positive choice to labour where I was most comfortable, relaxed and in control. I was dismayed to find that some professionals very obviously disapproved of my choice and treated me as though I was being irresponsible. They did not understand how my history governed what I wanted during pregnancy and birth – that I needed to feel that I still owned my body, that I wanted real choices about my care, that what were routine medical procedures for them, were strange, frightening intrusions for me. There were some professionals who were excellent and I cannot fault their care. However, it seemed to be hit and miss whom I got caring for me. I do not think that this level of variability is acceptable.

It would have been helpful if medical procedures had been carefully explained, with the pros and cons discussed so as to allow me an informed choice. All procedures should be carried out in a sensitive manner, and only when necessary.

It was helpful to have a supportive, sensitive midwife whose consistent care during pregnancy and postnatally allowed me to build a strong relationship with her. I was able to discuss my history with her. She facilitated discussion about my concerns, rather than being too afraid to talk about them. She regularly asked me for feedback on her care. She believed that I had been abused. She was supportive, and had helpful attitudes towards the abuse, e.g. that victims are not to blame. She did not disappear quickly after my baby was born, but recognised that I needed extra support, rather than rapid transfer to a health visitor who barely knew me.

This strong, consistent relationship with my midwife meant that I could discuss fears openly, e.g. being touched by medical staff I did not know, having to undergo invasive procedures. I could also give her honest feedback, without fear that it would impact badly on my care, or my baby's care. She also encouraged me to write a birth plan and explored this in detail with me. She helped me to see where I needed to be flexible. This was important in helping me to feel in control.

By the time I went into labour I felt as positive and prepared for the birth as I could be. I felt that I had been listened to, and felt that my midwife was an ally who cared about what happened to me as well as my baby. At times, other professionals (unfortunately, some midwives included) had made me feel like I was nothing more than a rather second rate means of carriage for the precious being within me. They did not seem to recognise that I had my baby's best interests at heart too. However, that did not mean that I had automatically ceased to have my own needs. My welfare and my baby's welfare were inextricably linked.

Memories and fears

The medical interventions triggered memories of abuse, but memories were also triggered by the prospect of becoming a parent. I found myself remembering my own childhood and worrying about how I could protect my child from what I had suffered. My partner was very supportive and we talked through many issues. However, at times, I think he found it difficult to help me and I felt very alone with my worries, particularly as the birth approached.

I, like many women, had fears about the birth. These included coping with pain, losing control, becoming a mum… There is some evidence that such fears can block progress during labour. Sheila Kitzinger once said to me '…birth is not only a matter of physiology, but of what is going on in our minds. Anxiety and fear, feeling trapped in a hospital environment, or being rushed to perform, prevent spontaneity and interfere with smooth muscle function… Any woman who has been sexually abused is likely to distrust her body and want to guard and protect it – keep it safe from intrusion. When she is in the second stage of labour… the sensations she experiences may be specially threatening. It is vitally important for a midwife to understand this…' This highlights the importance of every pregnant woman having supportive, consistent care, with easy access to counselling services if needed. It is particularly important if the woman does not have a supportive partner, friends or family around.

Creating a positive experience

My daughter was born at home, with my partner and sister-in-law present. I had not previously met the midwife who came, but she read my birth plan and was sensitive and respectful. The fact that she read my birth plan was really helpful. It immediately established a rapport between us. She explained procedures during the labour. She was encouraging and reassuring at times when I was in a great deal of pain and when I was frightened. She helped with massage as a form of pain relief. She also stayed beyond her shift, when it was clear that my baby was well on the way, which spared me the disruption of working with another midwife for the last stage of labour. She did not even bat an eyelid when my language became a tad colourful during transition! Above all, she treated me with humanity and respect, never questioning my wishes, but obviously working within the bounds of her professional framework.

Despite the negative experiences I had during pregnancy, I can say that I am happy with how it went, and I might even contemplate it again one day!

I decided to write this article because more attention needs to be paid to how child abuse impacts on pregnancy. I think that there should be more material available to women about child sexual abuse, ranging from pregnancy and birth to thinking about childcare.

Sessions about child abuse in antenatal classes could be helpful. This could raise painful issues, especially if the woman has not disclosed abuse before. However, parents-to-be may already be struggling alone with these problems. There may also be current risks to the woman or child if the abuser is still in contact. To raise problems early might prevent difficulties later on, such as postnatal depression or the abuse of other children.

Sessions that involved discussion of child abuse could also benefit other parents, by educating them about danger signs that their child might be being abused, and teaching them how to handle any suspicion of abuse.[8]

Health professionals need to ensure that they are educated about abuse themselves. This raises issues about training and supervision. Good training and supervision networks could help women to disclose abuse, improve their satisfaction with, services and prevent possible problems in the parent-child relationship later on.

It may be difficult to think about further training in the current climate of diminishing resources. However, midwives have a key role to play in working with pregnant survivors of abuse, because they have most contact with women throughout the birth process.

All women should be able to enjoy pregnancy. Sadly, previous experiences that harm a woman's sense of self can interfere with this. Child sexual abuse is one such experience. Despite abuse being so common, its impact on pregnancy is neglected. Women may struggle with the trauma alone, and professionals may compound the problem through a lack of awareness. There is an urgent need for change here. Sensitive, informed care can help make pregnancy a positive experience, and may prevent problems between the parents and child later on.

Welcoming new life into the world is a privilege. Professionals could do more to acknowledge and support the integrity of the woman who is giving birth, and be aware that any one of the women whom they seek to serve may have suffered sexual abuse.

Acknowledgements
Many thanks to Sheila Kitzinger and Anne Peake for helpful comments. Thanks also to Ian, Ro, Beth Galloway, Marion Woodward, Anne Haynes and Kay Millar for support during pregnancy and birth. This paper is dedicated to my daughter, Yasmin.

REFERENCES

1 Fritz G, Stoll K, Wagner NA. A comparison of males and females who were sexually molested as children. Journal of Sex and Marital Therapy 1981; 7:54–59.
2 Russell D. The secret trauma: Incest in the lives of girls and women. New York: Basic Books; 1984.
3 Kercher G. Responding to child sexual abuse. Huntsville, TX: Criminal Justice Center, Sam Houston State University; 1980.
4 Bagley C. Child sexual abuse: A child welfare perspective. In: Levitt K, Wharf B (eds). The challenge of child welfare. Vancouver: University of British Columbia Press; 1985.
5 Browne A, Finkelhor D. Impact of child sexual abuse: A review of the research. Psychological Bulletin 1986; 99:66–77.
6 Craine LS, Henson CE, Colliver JA, et al. Prevalence of a history of sexual abuse among female psychiatric patients in a state hospital system. Hospital and Community Psychiatry 1988; 39:300–304.
7 Rowan AB, Foy DW, Rodriguez N, et al. Post traumatic stress disorder in a clinical sample of adults sexually abused as children. Child Abuse and Neglect 1994; 18:51–61.
8 Peake A, Fletcher M. Strong mothers. Russell House Publishing: 1998.

Domestic violence
A midwife's personal account

The recent report Confidential Enquiries into Maternal Deaths in the United Kingdom[1] describes domestic violence as 'a serious and very important, but often overlooked cause of maternal and infant morbidity and mortality.' It is said to affect one in ten women at any one time, and is associated with morbidity, fetal death, miscarriage, depression, suicide, alcoholism and drug abuse. The report states it not only affects the woman, but can also have profound and lasting effects on all members of the family. In the report six cases of maternal death caused by domestic violence were cited.

In a similar vein, another influential Government report[2] says that 'all healthcare and social service staff have a vital role to play, identifying and helping such women to disclose domestic violence, and to provide adequate support, practical advice and an awareness of the services and options available to the victims of abuse.' It is this author's experience that such help is not readily available.

Health care workers are not trained in, and do not want to face the issue of, domestic violence and so remain unaware of their clients' needs. According to one author: 'Midwives have an inclination to block out difficult situations, because we are ill prepared to deal with the realities of women's lives.'[3] It is the resulting failure in care that has prompted me to share my own very personal and distressing experience of domestic violence, and to describe how it affected me personally and professionally. My hope is that by bringing such issues into the open, midwives will be able to feel a deeper empathy with women in their care.

The incident

When I was physically abused by my husband, the incident was completely unexpected and severe in nature. It came as a total shock to me.

I had been in a stable and happy marriage for nearly 18 years, although I now recognise that a degree of emotional abuse had been occurring over the previous two years.

I find recalling the details of the incident difficult. I have buried the event deep within my subconscious, to enable me to rebuild my relationship with my husband. However, if I am to share this experience, then I should briefly describe what happened.

We had been to a family social event, a happy occasion, during which time we had all had a social drink. Looking back, it is true that my husband had appeared quiet and insular throughout the evening. A group of us went home in a minibus.

On arrival home, some family members remained in the minibus, while I left to go into the house. My husband followed, then he suddenly became angry, hurling abuse at me for no apparent reason. He began to shove and push me up the street and into the house. As his anger increased he became more violent. I remember thinking, 'Don't antagonise him. Just keep quiet and shield yourself, and his anger will subside'.

I remember the children screaming and crying 'Let her go'. This only seemed to fuel his anger. I recall him gripping me by the face and throat and pushing me into the wall. I was afraid that I would not survive. The rest of this trauma must remain private – I feel unable to delve any deeper.

I recall several police officers battling to restrain my husband. It all seemed so unreal, like a terrible nightmare. The children were taken to a place of safety by a family member.

I felt totally humiliated as I was transported by ambulance to hospital. My physical injuries included severe bruising to the majority of my body and a large haematoma to the back of my head. I could not make eye contact with any of the staff – the feeling of humiliation was harder to bear than the physical injuries. I did not really feel any pain until the following day, when the total shock I experienced began to subside. Although physical injuries heal, the emotional and psychological scars remain, for the whole family.

The initial trauma of such abuse was worsened by having to stay in a place of safety, away from the familiarity of my home and friends. I found this compounded my feelings of low self-esteem, and heightened the feelings of being degraded and unworthy. What had I done to cause such an attack?

I now know I had done nothing. As Horley observes in her book *Love and Pain*, women almost always look to themselves for the cause of the abuse, rarely do women accept that it is they who are the victims.[4]

The aftermath

Women are often discouraged from reporting crimes of domestic violence to the police, because the police view them with suspicion and contempt.[5] In direct contrast to this, I was received with sympathy by the local police force, perhaps because my partner was also violent towards several police officers as they came to my assistance.

However, mistakes were made; statements were not taken from me until after my husband had been released from court the following day. Delays like this can lead to the woman not obtaining an emergency injunction order, which would allow her and her children to remain safely in their own home until a court hearing is convened.

Also, it seems that the police overlooked my statement in their attempt to charge my husband with police assault. Mistakes like this fuel the stress of the whole situation, and do lead to women not pressing charges.

In fact I decided not to press charges, as I thought it would only serve to prolong the trauma for all the family. What also dissuaded me from pressing charges was that five weeks after the incident I was still waiting to hear whether the Crown Prosecution Service would support me.

I was also overlooked with regard to the support and counselling available from the police domestic violence team, as both the police and the accident and emergency department failed in their responsibility to inform them. As a midwife, I was aware that some support was available – consequently I referred myself to Relate and Victim Support. Through their counselling, and with further help from the police domestic violence team, I have started to come to terms with the incident.

I have also been fortunate to receive support for my children from friends and family. It is these people, and some of my work colleagues, who deserve my gratitude. They helped me through this experience, being there to listen when I needed to talk – but also sitting quietly while I cried and suffered feelings of humiliation. I felt isolated and alone; there are always some areas of abuse that cannot be shared. I would like to express my total gratitude to a close relative, whose support and advice helped me retain my sanity, and to my colleagues who accepted my mood swings throughout my recovery period.

Many of the emotions I have experienced during this personal crisis cannot be put into words. As the physical wounds heal, the psychological wounds continue to gape and I remain emotionally vulnerable. I feel that I now fully understand the reactions and feelings of an abused woman – having lived the experience of an abused person I can truly empathise with those who have suffered a similar fate.

From my husband's perspective the main factor which led to his violent outburst was undoubtedly stress. I now recognise that I had allowed my partner to gradually erode my self-esteem. I had fallen into the trap of giving him my total attention, selflessly putting him first, even before the children or myself. I had accepted the gradual onset of emotional abuse, although I cannot say when in our marriage this had began to occur.

Reflection

Reflection is an important human activity, one in which people recapture their experience, think about it, mull it over and evaluate it.[6] One concise definition states that: 'Reflective learning is the process of internally examining an issue of concern, triggered by an experience, which creates and clarifies meaning in terms of self, and which results in a changed conceptual perspective.'[7] Reflection has become part of my life, both in my working and in my personal life. To ensure a logical progression through my reflection on being the victim of domestic violence, I chose to use Johns's model[8] as a structural framework.

The primary reason for reflecting on this event is selfish; I needed to write it as a therapeutic measure. I have written several letters expressing my feelings of humiliation, worthlessness, anger at myself, my partner, the system. All have served a purpose, but then been posted to the bin, unread by anyone else. I find it difficult to accept, or describe, how I feel. Utter confusion best describes my inner turmoil. I feel changed by the experience – it is like pregnancy in that every cell in your body is affected. I feel as if everyone knows I have been abused, ostracised from the 'normal', almost as if I wear a collar which announces my abuse.

My second reason for reflecting on domestic violence is that it brought home to me my own snobbery, lack of knowledge and the shortcomings in the care I have given. I always assumed that domestic violence occurred in the lower social classes. Reading in-depth studies of all kinds of abuse, emotional, psychological and physical, has dispelled my ignorance. Domestic violence is not class related; wife abuse occurs in all walks of life and in all ethnic and religious groups. Professionals, tradesmen and all educational levels are represented, from the bin man to the consultant doctor.[4,9]

Women who are abused often deny to friends, relatives and professionals that it has occurred. I denied my abuse to myself. I could not come to terms with the fact that my partner could inflict such injuries on me. I found myself looking into the mirror several times a day to make sure it was not just a bad dream. I still cannot fully accept what has happened – perhaps it is nature's way of protecting me, a defence until I can face it. One researcher states that 'Victims may feel isolated, trapped, worthless, ashamed, have low self-esteem, and a profound loss of self-respect.'[4] I support her findings; my self-respect has plummeted to an all-time low, and I often wonder how I allowed this to happen.

Five months later, with the help of counselling, I have accepted my partner back and I am trying to rebuild my marriage. Marriage is based on trust, and the success of trying to rebuild a marriage following a violent episode depends on whether the trust and love factors can be rebuilt.

What midwives can do

As a positive outcome of my experience, I decided to become informed about abuse, so that I can improve the care I provide to women. A staggering one in three women, and one in five marriage partners, suffer physical violence at some stage in their life.[10] As midwives we owe it to these women firstly to help to identify abuse, then to offer skilled counselling, opening opportunities for women to talk through their experiences. We should then be able to offer support and up-to-date information, to allow them to choose their own way forward.

In our role of midwife, we must be sensitive to the signs of abuse and open conversations which allow women to feel safe and confident. We can make sure the woman knows the midwife will respect her confidentiality, so that she feels able to divulge personal information. The midwife's job is to support her and her family, inform her of the services available and what her rights are, valuing and respecting her as an individual at all costs. The midwife should never judge and never make decisions for her. Real midwifery requires intimacy and emotional commitment, but midwives will often take the easy road, and keep to a superficial interaction, to resist involvement.

It is important that as midwives we are aware of support groups and the correct procedure following a violent attack on a woman. Accurate advice is also

> ### Remember
>
> - Domestic violence is a serious crime.
> - Everyone has the right to live their life free of fear, threats and abuse.
> - If you are a victim you are not alone, there are people who can help you.
> - Your partner's violence is not your fault.
> - Contact Women's Aid, and/or the police for further help and advice.

important; for example, I was told three weeks after the attack that I needed photographs of my injuries for an appearance in court. By this time most of my bruising had faded. Groups such as Men of Violent Emotions can support both partners if they choose to get back together. Midwives must be aware that such a decision is the woman's own choice, and ensure that she feels supported in whatever decision is made.

Women should be helped to recognise that all violence is against the law; it is a criminal offence. Women need to know that they can take refuge, what procedures will be instigated, what they are entitled to by law. Help can be sought from the local police domestic violence unit – a plain clothes, female officer is available, and will arrange to visit at home, or a pre-arranged place. She is a source of help and guidance. It is important to inform the woman that such a visit does not have to lead to police charges, or direct police involvement.

Women need professional help from counsellors, such as the Victim Support Agency, Relate, the Samaritans. Victim Support can provide guidance, financial direction, and free counselling – they also have a wealth of information regarding housing and benefits. The Samaritans can provide a friendly ear. Women's Refuge Centres and social workers can provide help and support. Relate can offer guidance if the woman chooses to return to her marriage and they offer a place of neutrality which allows the couple involved to vent their feelings without fear of further attack. The telephone number for all local groups can be found in Yellow Pages.

There is legislation providing women with protection against molestation, and an injunction can be used to prevent her partner from entering the marital home, or contacting her. It is important that women of low income are informed of Legal Aid, as often they fear the cost of taking their case to court.

Personal change

I have learnt a great deal about the effects of violence on a woman and her family. The incident has made me a stronger person in some areas, and more vulnerable in others.

With regards to my role as a midwife, I have gained insight into the traumas some women suffer, and a fuller understanding of the subsequent feelings. I have more empathy with women and I am no longer afraid to become involved, to question women about their injuries, or delve into conversations which may be the woman's way of communicating her distress.

My care is no longer superficial. I am proud be an advocate for women and hold my head high as a midwife who is truly 'with woman'.

The author, who wishes to remain anonymous, is a midwife in the Manchester area.

REFERENCES

1 Department of Health. Why mothers die: Report on confidential enquiries into maternal deaths in the United Kingdom 1994–6. London: The Stationery Office; 1998.
2 Department of Health. On the state of the public health. Annual Report of the Chief Medical Officer of the Department of Health 1996. London: DoH; 1996.
3 Clarke R. Through a glass darkly. Nursing Times 1994; 90(48):58–59.
4 Horley S. Love and pain: A survival handbook for women. London: Bedford Square Press; 1988.
5 Gelles RJ. Family violence, 2nd edn. Newbury Park, CA: Sage Publications; 1987.
6 Boud D, Keogh R, Walker D. Reflection: Turning experience into learning. New York: Kogan Page; 1985.
7 Boyd EM, Fales AW. Reflective learning: key to learning from experience. Journal of Humanistic Psychology 1983; 23(2): 99–117.
8 Johns C. Professional supervision. Journal of Nursing Management 1993; 1:9–18.
9 Walker L. The battered woman. New York: Harper Row; 1979.
10 Borkowski M, Murch M, Walker V. Marital violence: The community response. London: Tavistock Publications; 1983.

Childbirth in women with a history of sexual abuse

Part 1: A case history approach

Maggie Smith

While working on the delivery suite of a large maternity unit in 1995, a situation occurred that made me realise that women with a history of sexual abuse may be especially vulnerable during pregnancy and childbirth.

A woman was being admitted to the labour ward and, although she consented to a vaginal examination as part of the routine admission procedure, every time I attempted to examine her, she closed her legs tightly, wriggled up the bed and repeated 'You'll go through me... you'll go through me' in a distressed and agitated manner.

As I was a student midwife at that time, my mentor took over, but the woman would not permit my mentor to examine her either. Various other members of staff became involved and tried to persuade the woman to be examined. Their approaches ranged from kindly reassurance and cajoling to reproaching her with comments like 'How are we supposed to know what's going on if we can't examine you?' Despite agreeing to let several other staff members try again, just as the examination was beginning, the woman lost control and her behaviour followed the earlier pattern. After a time the midwife who was in charge of the labour ward became impatient and told the woman that she would have to notify the medical staff. A male doctor made a further unsuccessful attempt but by this time the woman was so distressed that further attempts were abandoned.

Later that morning the woman's behaviour, which was perceived by some as non-compliance, was being discussed by a group of midwives in the staff coffee room. I had read a report relating to the sequelae of sexual abuse[1] and suggested to my colleagues that the woman's response to the attempted vaginal examinations may have indicated such a history. My suggestion was met with a variety of responses, and while some midwives gave accounts of women they had cared for where they suspected a history of sexual abuse, others seemed unaware of the links which the literature suggests exist between certain behaviour patterns and a history of sexual abuse.

One member of staff appeared to find the whole subject quite distasteful and dismissed it as being 'totally ridiculous' saying:

'... she's just being awkward and anyway, it's only the NCT types who won't let you examine them.'

At that time, I was studying for a BSc degree in Midwifery and decided that it would be worthwhile studying the subject in greater depth. My aim was to try to discover how childbirth affects women with a history of sexual abuse and in which ways midwifery practices might be improved to take into account the experiences of such women.

A review of the literature

A search of the midwifery literature identified very few references which related specifically to this subject. Insofar as midwifery textbooks are concerned, women with a history of sexual abuse are almost invisible, as very little has been written about the potential implications that such experiences might have on labour and childbirth. Other literature reviewed included material examining the nature of sexual abuse and the effects it can have upon women in general terms.

There have been very few studies examining the impact which a history of sexual abuse may have on pregnancy and childbirth, but those which are available suggest that abused women experience particular difficulties during labour and childbirth.[2-8]

A number of personal accounts written by 'survivors' of abuse describe their pregnancy and childbirth experiences.[9-13] One survivor described sexual abuse as 'a staggering problem' which is 'shrouded in silence'.[10] Another survivor recalls the trauma of being so brutally raped as a young child that she bears a scar from her clitoris to urethra.[9] Two women[9,13] had 'forgotten' their childhood trauma until their pregnancy; childbirth is believed to trigger the reawakening of memories of childhood abuse.[13] Describing the birth of her baby, one woman said '...I was screaming that it felt like the abuser's penis in me'.[9]

In telling their stories of childbirth, one survivor describes 'birth rape' and another speaks of being 'invaded from without by the obstetric procedures, and from within by devastating memories of the incest experience'.[10,12]

Following the birth of her baby, one survivor was moved to write about aspects of maternity care which she found particularly empowering, and her article appeared in the National Childbirth Trust publication *New Generation*.[11] She wrote:

'I saw the same midwife all the time... I was not asked to undress at all... It was understood that no-one else was to enter the room unless absolutely necessary... Throughout the whole of my labour, I had no internal examinations at all. The midwife said she could tell by the length and type of contractions I was having when I entered second stage'.[12]

All of these women reported connections between the pain and fear they had experienced while being sexually abused and the pain and fear of childbirth.

Jenny Kitzinger, one of the early researchers in the field, interviewed 39 women aged between 16 and 59, who were survivors of childhood sexual abuse. She concluded that obstetric/gynaecological encounters in which women are unable to control what happens to their body can reproduce the dynamics of sexual violence, bringing back 'overwhelming memories'. Obstetric procedures which combine 'nakedness, touching, intrusion, pain or discomfort and powerlessness' leave women with a history of sexual abuse feeling 'dirty and violated.'[2] Some women in Kitzinger's study explained that the 'rituals' used to desensitise the vaginal examination, such as lack of eye contact and isolated focus on the genitals, actually served to reinforce links with previous experiences. For many women, having to lie in a lateral position was particularly difficult, because it was in this position that they were abused 'while they lay facing the wall, pretending to be asleep'. The voyeuristic nature of the women's experiences of abuse were recaptured when medical or other students were present in an observational capacity during labour and childbirth.[3]

A large study on a self-selected sample of 500 women investigated the occurrence of post-traumatic stress disorder (PTSD) in women who had undergone obstetric/gynaecological procedures.[4] In common with Kitzinger's study, the author found that the women in her sample described the obstetric procedures and experiences in the same language as they used to describe sexual abuse. They included the following:

'degrading and distressing'; 'I came away hurting and feeling violated'; 'It felt undeniably like rape'; 'dehumanising and painful'; 'I cried and shouted but was held down and told to stop making a noise'; 'humiliation... as if it happened yesterday'; 'I felt abused... like a piece of meat on a slab'. The author concluded that a connection exists between obstetric and gynaecological procedures and the subsequent development of PTSD. However, she acknowledged that PTSD may already have been present in women who had been sexually abused and she made the point that 'this group of women may be particularly susceptible to obstetric/gynaecological trauma because of their past experiences, either because the vaginal examinations re-awaken repressed memories, or because the procedure in some way repeats, or is felt to repeat, the past trauma.'

Although it was not clear from Menage's study which women had undergone obstetric as opposed to gynaecological procedures, the themes relating to fear, pain, feelings of humiliation, powerlessness and perceived lack of sympathy are apparent throughout, and correlate with women's own anecdotal accounts.

The women in the limited number of studies which have been carried out connected being sexually abused with giving birth, as both experiences involved painful genital sensations and an invasion of body boundaries which caused them to feel objectified and depersonalised.

The participants in the studies reviewed here were self-selected and the retrospective data are naturally dependent upon their subjective recall ability. Nevertheless, this should not detract from what can be learned from them as it is a woman's own perception of events surrounding labour and delivery which will influence her long-term psychological well-being. These perceptions may not be congruent with that of the professional who cared for the woman.

Adult sequelae of child sexual abuse and rates of prevalence

It is important that those caring for childbearing women have an understanding of the effects of sexual abuse in order to be able to recognise indicators which may be suggestive of such a history.

Research generally supports the view that childhood sexual abuse is a significant trauma which is an important predictor of long-term mental health impairment.[14-18] Depression is the symptom most commonly reported, and a high incidence of suicide attempts among victims of child sexual abuse has been found.[14,19] A panoply of other mental health problems commonly includes: anxiety and low self-esteem, difficulties with interpersonal relationships, sexual dysfunction, eating disorders, needle phobias, substance abuse, self-destructive behaviours and symptoms of post-traumatic stress disorder.[20] These vary in prevalence and severity. Chronic pelvic pain, dyspareunia, vaginismus and urogenital or gastrointestinal complaints have also been reported.[21] Whilst all of these symptoms may be found in the non-abused women, the patterns are more severe in sexually abused women and particularly severe in survivors of incest.[22]

It is estimated that post-traumatic stress disorder develops in one in five incest survivors. It is characterised by intrusive re-experiencing of the traumatic event which can manifest itself as avoidance of stimuli associated with the event, dissociation and/or numbing of general responsiveness.[1] Situations which resemble or symbolise the sexual abuse, such as a vaginal examination, may provoke flashbacks to the original trauma and intensify the woman's psychological symptoms.[4] The effects of sexual abuse are significantly more traumatic when it involved the father, or a father figure, than when it was perpetrated by any other person.[14] Women with a history of childhood sexual abuse have a propensity towards revictimisation in later life, and studies indicate that they are at greater risk of rape and physical violence from their partners.[14]

There is immense variation in prevalence rates quoted within the literature, partly because of differing data collection methods, but also because there is no uniform definition of child sexual abuse. As one would expect, studies that have used a broad definition have found considerably higher prevalence rates than those using a restricted or narrow definition. Kelly quotes prevalence rates varying between 16% and 54% in the UK.[23] Sheldrick concludes that at least one third of adult women have had sexual contact with an older person as a child.[18] In a more recent review of the epidemiological research on child sexual abuse, Pilkington and Kremer report rates which range from 3% to 90%![20]

The reported cases may represent only the tip of the iceberg with up to 98% of incest cases going unreported.[14,24] The reasons for non-reporting of sexual abuse are complex. In order to survive psychologically, many victims successfully repress the memory of their abuse for many years.[25] Marked memory deficits typically occur in survivors whose abuse was characterised by early onset and violent or sadistic episodes.[26] Trigger factors in later life can provoke the return of the memories.[27] The abuser may use various strategies to coerce the victim to keep the 'secret'; shame and stigmatisation may prevent victims from speaking out.[22] Finally, even if the abuse is revealed, the revelation may be met with disbelief, so that no further action is taken against the perpetrator.[14,15]

Sexual abuse of children occurs within all socioeconomic and ethnic groups.[15] Whilst it is true that most abusers are males, Wilkins,[28] writing in the *British Medical Journal*, warns that sexual abuse should no longer be considered the exclusive domain of men, and states:

'the medical profession is slowly and reluctantly having to acknowledge that the prevalence of women who sexually abuse children is greater than previously thought, and that doctors need to become sensitised to the possibility.'

It is not only boys who suffer at the hands of female abusers. A therapist for survivors of sexual abuse refers to many women she has counselled who have been sexually abused by females in a brutal manner.[29] This is contrary to the popularly held belief that if women do abuse, it is gentle, unaggressive cuddling, fondling or kissing.

Summary of the literature review

The literature reviewed indicates that childhood sexual abuse is a common occurrence and is a subject which, in the words of one victim, is 'shrouded in secrecy' because of associated feelings of fear, guilt, shame and confusion. Severe psychological trauma frequently occurs at the time of the abuse. Victims may have no conscious memory of the sexual abuse but there are thought to be certain trigger factors which stimulate memory recall. Of particular significance for the midwife is that childbirth appears to be one such factor. Women who have a history of being sexually abused may experience particular difficulties during childbirth that are directly related to their abusive experiences and this may result in further psychological trauma.

The available data makes it clear that sexual abuse is so common that midwives are at some time bound to care for women who have been sexually abused.

The next article in the series tells the life story of a woman who was sexually abused by her father over a ten year period, beginning when she was three years of age. It is this woman's belief that her experience of being sexually abused had a profound effect upon her childbirth experiences.

REFERENCES

1 Mayer L. The severely abused woman in obstetric and gynaecologic care: Guidelines for recognition and management. The Journal of Reproductive Medicine 1995; 13–18.

2 Kitzinger J. Recalling the pain. Nursing Times 1990; 86(3):38–40.

3 Kitzinger J. The internal examination. The Practitioner 1990; 234:698–700.

4 Menage J. Post-traumatic stress disorder in women who have undergone obstetric and/or gynaecological procedures: A consecutive series of 30 cases of PTSD. The Journal of Reproductive & Infant Psychology 1993; 11:221–228.

5 Rhodes N, Hutchinson S. Labor experiences of childhood sexual abuse survivors. Birth 1992; December.

6 Parratt J. The experience of childbirth for survivors of incest. Midwifery 1994; 10:26–39.

7 Burian J. Helping survivors of sexual abuse through labor. MIDIRS Midwifery Digest 1996; 6(3).

8 Smith R. Childhood sexual abuse: Sexuality, pregnancy and birthing. New Zealand: Inside-Out Books; 1996.

9 Rose A. Effects of childhood sexual abuse on childbirth: one woman's story. Birth 1992.

10 Lipp D. Mothering after incest. Mothering 1992; Spring:115–120.

11 Anonymous. Abuse. New Generation 1993; June:48.

12 Christensen M. Birth rape. MIDIRS Midwifery Digest 1993; 3(3):304–305

13 Heritage C. A burden to share. MIDIRS Midwifery Digest 1995; 5(4):431–432.

14 Browne A, Finklehor D. Impact of child sexual abuse: A review of the research. Psychological Bulletin 1986; 99(1):66–77.

15 Bachmann G, Moeller T, Nenett J. Childhood sexual abuse and the consequences in adult women: A review. Obstetrics and Gynaecology 1988; 71(4):631–642.

16 Hooper P. Psychological sequelae of sexual abuse in childhood. British Journal of General Practice 1990; 40: 29–31.

17 McClelland L, Mynors-Wallis L, Fahy T, et al. Sexual abuse, disordered personality and eating disorders. British Journal of Psychiatry 1991; 158(10): 63–68.

18 Sheldrick C. Adult sequelae of child sexual abuse. British Journal of Psychiatry 1991; 158(10):55–62.

19 Herman J, Hirschman L. Families at risk for father-daughter incest. American Journal of Psychiatry 1981; 138:967–70.

20 Pilkington B, Kremer J. A review of the epidemiological research on child sexual abuse: Clinical samples. Child Abuse Review; 4:191–205.

21 Rapkin A, Kanes L, Darke L. History of physical and sexual abuse in women with chronic pelvic pain. Obstetrics & Gynaecology 1990; 76(1):92–96.

22 Doob D. Female sexual abuse survivors as patients: avoiding retraumatization. Archives of Psychiatric Nursing 1992; VI(4):245–251.

23 Kelly L. Surviving sexual violence. Cambridge: Polity Press; 1988.

24 Russell D. The secret trauma: Incest in the lives of girls and women. New York: Basic Books; 1986.

25 Couirtois C, Riley C. Pregnancy and childbirth as triggers for abuse memories: Implications for care. Birth 1992; December:222–223.

26 Draucker CB. Counselling survivors of childhood sexual abuse: Counselling in practice. London: Sage Publications; 1992.

27 Burgess A. Biology of memory and childhood trauma. Journal of Psychosocial Nursing 1995; 33(3):16–26.

28 Wilkins R. Women who sexually abuse children: Doctors need to become sensitised to the possibility. British Medical Journal 1990; 300:1153–1154.

29 Longdon C. A survivor's and therapist's viewpoint. In: Elliott M (ed). Female sexual abuse of children. Essex: Longman Group; 1993.

Childbirth in women with a history of sexual abuse

Part 2: A case history approach

Maggie Smith

The first article in this series discussed the mental health problems which women with a history of sexual abuse encounter in adult life. These include anxiety, depression, difficulties with interpersonal relationships, sexual dysfunction, eating disorders, needle phobias, substance and alcohol abuse as well as self-destructive behaviours. The fear and pain experienced during childbirth has been described by some women as reminiscent of sexual abuse. Many women are unable to articulate these feelings, as feelings of guilt, shame and stigmatisation are universal.[1,2]

Mary

In 1996, I began to study the experience of childbirth for women with a history of sexual abuse. A friend who was aware of the subject I was studying introduced me to 'Mary', who had been sexually abused by her father over a ten-year period. Mary's motivation for volunteering to take part in this study was the hope that disclosure of her experiences might help to heighten awareness and enhance understanding among health professionals as to the nature of this 'invisible' problem and how it can affect pregnancy and childbirth experiences.

Before contacting Mary, I sought advice from a psychologist as to whether such a meeting might have a detrimental effect on Mary's psychological well-being.[3] I was concerned that talking to me about her past experiences might stir up feelings of anxiety which I was not qualified to deal with. The view of the psychologist, which was subsequently borne out by the available literature, was that generally women welcome being provided with an opportunity to speak freely about sexual abuse, as simply telling their story provides some sense of cathartic release.[4,5,6] Furthermore, the fact that Mary volunteered to speak with me rendered her less vulnerable than had the approach been the other way around.

Giving voice to those who have been abused by 'allowing' them to speak out is believed to contribute to the process of empowerment, especially for those women who may never have been heard. Jill Astbury, a feminist psychologist, believes that research into childhood sexual abuse has beneficial effects for the women studied because it indicates that the subject is being taken seriously by medical and social scientists. Astbury further points out that asking women relevant questions assures them that it is safe to disclose, and that their accounts will be accepted as true and meaningful.[2]

This view is shared by Dijkstra[6] who suggests that speaking out can be seen as a validation, or a way to seek support which can contribute to the process of recovery.

Mary agreed that our conversations could be tape recorded and that her life history could be used in my dissertation. In recognition of the fact that telling one's story can be a painful process[7] I told Mary that she need not discuss anything she was not comfortable with, that she could withdraw from the study at any time, and that a psychologist would be available for consultation following the interviews should Mary feel the need for this.

The confidential nature of the interview process was stressed to Mary, who was assured that any identifying details would be changed and that she would have the opportunity to peruse and amend the transcripts of tape recordings before they were incorporated into the dissertation. I interviewed Mary at her home for approximately five-and-a-half hours in total over a six-week period during January and February, 1997. We had barely exchanged names when Mary began pouring out her life story. She subsequently explained that her urgency to begin her story arose from a sense of 'getting it over with – just like the abuse'.

The interviews yielded a substantial quantity of data, and the midwifery, medical and psychosocial literature was used as the conceptual framework for analysis of the transcribed data. A transcript of the first tape recorded interview was prepared and shown to Mary who made a number of amendments before validating the contents. Following analysis of the data, I met for a third time with Mary to ensure that she was happy with what had been written about her, before the work was submitted to the academic staff at the University.

The life history study

Mary is an articulate 36-year-old professional woman, married with two children. She has one brother and they were brought up in a fairly affluent household by professional parents who are both alive and live nearby.

Mary was sexually abused by her father for a period of about ten years, and it is her belief that her mother was aware of the abuse. She thinks it began when she was very young, probably around three years of age. Fear was a key aspect of Mary's relationship with her father whom she described as: 'very, very domineering and quite, quite frightening'. To Mary's knowledge, her brother was not abused.

Mary's childhood was fraught with problems of one sort or another. An example of this was the difficulties she encountered with schoolwork, particularly learning to read and write. It was suggested by an educationalist that Mary should go to a special school, but her mother would not allow this. Mary hopes this decision reflected her mother's feelings for her, but she also believes that she was used to satisfy the sexual needs of her father as she explains:

'I think she was put on, you know, sexually, and that I was some kind of trade off.'

Reflecting on how this has affected her feelings towards her mother she says:

'...I've struggled a lot with my mother. I suppose it would have been very difficult for her in the 1960s if she had confronted the abuse. She might have faced destitution and I might have ended up in a children's home and not had the opportunities I have had.'

Mary spoke of various psychological ploys which were used to ensure that she kept the 'secret', and explains:

'The mechanisms that were used against me were that I was accused of being a liar, and also, that I was ever so slightly mad. Though it seems a funny thing to say, I grew up thinking that I was actually mad.'

By the time she was ten, Mary was exhibiting very disturbed behavioural symptoms and remembers being taken to the family general practitioner. She expressed surprise that the GP did not pick up clues relating to her disturbed behaviour patterns as she recalls:

'The doctor asked me how my nerves were at ten! [years of age] Didn't he think that meant anything? Then it was back and forth [to the doctor's]. My Mum took me – I was very stressed having total panic attacks spilling over everywhere. Finally at 15 [years old], the doctor gave me Valium. I flushed them down the loo, and staggered along.'

Mary describes entering her teenage years in a 'fog' explaining that she had no conscious memory of the abuse at that time. She began having intercourse with boys of her own age when she was about twelve years old, and had a number of sexual partners by the time she was 15 years old. She felt as though she had some control over the relationship if she had sex with a boy:

'... I could give him the sex and that ensured that he would probably still go out with me, but it [intercourse] was just something that was done to me.'

Mary remembers feeling bewildered that her teenage friends 'made such a fuss about boys and intercourse' as she thought 'What's the matter with them, after all, it's only sex?'

Eating became a problem for Mary, who developed anorexia when she was about 16 years old. She can pinpoint the very day her eating disorder began:

'I remember there was a girl in our sixth form, and she once said to me, 'oh, you look nice today, you look slimmer' and that was it. Just that, and I just lost and lost weight. I didn't really have to be that secretive because my parents didn't seem all that bothered really.'

Mary also abused diuretics. She said:

'What I would do was have a meal, then use the pills to get water out so I would be immediately thinner. Then I would starve myself again until I really was that thin.'

She remembers that she loathed menstruating and thinks this was possibly to do with the realisation that the woman in her was beginning to emerge. During her teens, the relationship between father and daughter was 'appalling'. Mary began shouting a lot, and in this way, found she had some control and could stop her father from coming into her bedroom.

At 16 years of age, Mary left home to live with a friend but she 'couldn't manage' and was effectively forced to return home. However, she did not live with her parents for very long because as soon as she had taken her 'A' levels, she left home again and found work. After working for one year, she returned to study as a self-supporting student and graduated at degree level with honours. She married her first husband when she was 20 years old, a marriage which was to last only one year before ending in divorce. Following this, Mary had a nervous breakdown.

Throughout her life, Mary has suffered continuously with depression and anxiety and has had various periods of counselling with a clinical psychologist. Referring to her state of mind at various times, she explains:

'I've never had ordinary, uncluttered feelings about anything... I grew up being told that firstly, I was a liar, and secondly that I was mad, and through a vast amount of my counselling, I believed "you lied, you were that vile child" because it was easier to believe that I was lying than to face the truth, and then I could cope with it again ... I've felt totally different to others and my ambition for the last ten years has been to be like other people.'

Mary is now married to Adrian, and in describing their relationship, Mary says:

'I suppose I survive in my relationship with Adrian because in a nice way, I'm the one in control because he almost always says to me "What do _you_ want to do?"'

Although they have a good relationship in general terms, they have had considerable difficulties with the sexual side of their relationship. Following the birth of their first child, Adrian and Mary consulted a sex therapist. Mary explains:

'...It was when I had Andrew [her first child], something happened to me and although I didn't understand why, I just knew I couldn't have another [baby]. I just could not deal with it. This caused problems with our sex life so we went to a therapist. The therapist said "I want you to go home and lie on the bed together and practise stroking each other" and I couldn't do it, I just could not do it. She [the therapist] was so angry with me for not even trying and so was my husband. She [therapist] said to me "Well, what can you do Mary?" and I said "I can hold his hand" and that was about as far as I could go.'

Despite all the problems, Mary did become pregnant again a further three times. Sadly, she miscarried twice, once at 12 weeks and the second time at 20 weeks' gestation before giving birth to their second child, Steven. After Steven's birth, Adrian decided to have a vasectomy in the belief that it was Mary's fear of another pregnancy which was preventing them from having a 'good sex life'. By this time, Mary was aware that there was more to her sexual dysfunction than just the fear of a pregnancy and was beginning to realise something else was preventing her from being what she describes as 'a proper woman'. She said:

'I went to see my GP and said "Look, I'm really worried that in the end he'll leave me because he's going to find out that it isn't anything to do with worrying about getting pregnant" and I just said to her "I can't let anybody touch me" I said "I don't even mean... [pause in conversation] I just mean I can't let people touch me. I can let women touch me, but I can't let men".'

She was referred to a clinical psychologist with whom she had counselling for approximately two years. During this period, Mary faced up to the memories of her sexual abuse. She explained 'It all came out, bit by bit and it was like reliving it.'

Counselling helped Mary to understand that there were elements of re-living the abuse during her childbirth experiences. Here Mary poignantly describes the similarities:

'...The feeling of powerlessness was there because in labour, you can't get out of bed in the same way as I could never escape as a child. It was the feeling that this was being done to you and you would get through it by adopting the same strategies, it was only the passage of time. Also, during my labours, I had to have a catheter and that was very much the feeling of just being messed about with down there. So like with all my other experiences during the abuse, I mean, I remember vividly as a child there was one particular piece of wallpaper and I knew it so well, and like that, I was in control during labour and I remember focusing on the clock and it was the same feeling by taking your mind out of your body. Although I did get through it, I was unprepared for it, it was so shocking.'

Mary believes her choice of pain relief was most definitely influenced by her experience of sexual abuse. Although she feels she has a high pain threshold and ideally would have opted for a more 'natural birth', she chose instead to have epidural anaesthesia. Her reason for this decision was that she was 'absolutely terrified' of an instrumental delivery and believed that without an epidural, she would be worn out by the pain of the first stage of labour and therefore unable to push the baby out herself. Based on this conviction, she made the decision to conserve her energy for what she regarded as the most important part, the pushing, and thus prevent her 'worst nightmare – forceps delivery' from being realised.

Reflecting further on her feelings about the birth, Mary said:

'... I didn't understand it at the time, but you know, I didn't have any stitches or a cut and when I came away from it, [the birth] I just felt this by anybody's standards was an easy birth. So why did I feel that I was being raped? Why did I feel that? You know, because that was what I re-lived, that feeling of penetration.'

Referring to her carers in labour, Mary recalls her feelings of concern about what they would think of her:

'I was worried that the midwives might not like me or that they might think I was mad. I didn't think it mattered so much what happened to me, but what mattered to me very much, was that the midwives should find me acceptable.'

After the birth of her first baby, Mary suffered badly with depression. She recollects:

'... After Andrew was born, I didn't really cope very well at all. I remember I used to push him out in his pram and will him to go to sleep, and my mother-in-law started to look after him for a couple of hours a day because she realised I was so depressed.'

The sex of her children was extremely important to Mary, who was concerned that the birth of a daughter would remind her of herself as a vulnerable child. She said:

'...I've been lucky that I've had two boys because I think seriously that I would not have coped with a girl. It would have just been too much to watch myself grow up again.'

At the present time, Mary is employed full-time in a professional capacity and has recently completed a Master's Degree in Education, and she feels she has begun the process of recovery. Her self-determination combined with counselling has helped her to feel that she has resolved much of the grief and anger surrounding her experiences of abuse. Commenting upon the situation, she says 'One thing my counsellor made me understand, is that it is only my strength of character that has got me through and kept me looking for help, some women don't. Although I'm free in many respects, I'm not totally free but at least I've finally come to like myself.'

Discussion

Mary's life-story may be viewed as a classic portrayal of a woman with a history of sexual abuse. Clearly, her history of sexual abuse had a profound effect upon her during her childbirth experiences.

Children who are sexually abused frequently experience impaired learning[8] and Mary was no exception. As a teenager, she developed anorexia nervosa. A number of studies have found evidence of childhood sexual abuse in women with an eating disorder.[5] The fact that she abused diuretics is not surprising, given that self-destructive behaviour is frequently reported in the literature.[9]

It is noteworthy that Mary began to have sexual intercourse in her early teens with a number of partners. Ainscough and Toon report that survivors of sexual abuse frequently follow this pattern.[10] Many lack self-worth and become 'promiscuous' believing that it no longer matters what happens to their body.

In adulthood, Mary experienced sexual dysfunction, which is extremely common among survivors of sexual abuse.[8] Depression, the symptom most commonly reported by survivors of childhood sexual abuse,[8,11] has plagued Mary over the years, especially following childbirth. There are two possible explanations which link her history to the episodes of postnatal depression. The first is that sexual abuse in itself has been highlighted as a risk factor which significantly increases the chances of developing postnatal depression.[12] The second is that her birth experiences, which were shaped by her history of sexual abuse, were not perceived as 'good' or 'positive' and this in turn can affect long-term psychological well-being and satisfaction with motherhood.[13,14]

In common with other survivors of sexual abuse[15,16] Mary used denial, repression, rationalisation, minimisation and dissociation, which are psychological defence mechanisms to cope with sexual abuse at the time it occurred, and at other times throughout her life when psychologically vulnerable.

It can be seen that the process that helped Mary to cope whilst she was being sexually abused – dissociation – was evident again during her childbirth experiences. Mary was unable to get out of bed during labour in the same way, she tells us, that she could never escape as a child during the abuse. She uses the metaphor of taking her mind out of her body and describes how she focused on the clock, in much the same way as she fixed her gaze on a piece of wallpaper as a child.

Dissociation, which is also referred to as psychological escape, is a reaction to trauma and is said to be a primary psychological process in response to overwhelming experiences.[17] Victims abused before the age of 13 years, as Mary was, demonstrate a markedly higher level of dissociative symptoms.[17]

The literature reviewed in the first article in this series, confirms that other survivors employ techniques acquired whilst being sexually abused to help them to 'get through' labour and delivery.[16-21] The strategies which protect victims from emotional distress at the time of the sexual abuse can become habitual coping mechanisms throughout life.[22]

A trigger factor for memory recall

A number of authors have expressed the view that childbirth has the capacity to stimulate memory recall of childhood abuse.[23-26] This view is supported by Mary's comments 'I just felt this, by anybody's standards, was an easy birth. So why did I feel that I was being raped? Why did I feel that? You know, because that was what I re-lived, that feeling of penetration.'

During her labour, Mary was particularly concerned that the midwives should have a good opinion of her and was concerned in case they thought she was 'mad'. It is not uncommon for labouring women to be anxious to please their caregivers,[27,28] but in this instance, it is likely that Mary's concern stemmed from an internalised belief that she was stigmatised. Stigmatisation is indicated by her comment that her ambition for many years had been to be like other people as she had a sense of being 'totally different'. Herman[29] reported that all of the women in her study who experienced father-daughter incest had a sense of being branded, marked or stigmatised.

There are definite psychological connections between having been sexually abused and labour and childbirth, which is why survivors link the two experiences. One example of this referred to by Mary was the *powerlessness* which she experienced during sexual abuse, that was recreated during childbirth. '...The feeling of powerlessness was there because in labour, you can't get out of bed in the same way as I could never escape as a child. It was the feeling that this was being done to you and you would get through it by adopting the same strategies, it was only the passage of time.'

The influence of sexual abuse on the choice of pain relief

The idea of a forceps delivery was totally abhorrent to Mary who feels her choice of pain relief was directly related to her experience of being sexually abused. She chose to have an epidural in the belief that it would reduce her risk of an instrumental delivery. Studies show that epidural block is actually associated with an increased risk of instrumental deliveries;[30] therefore, she could have unwittingly caused the very thing she most feared; being penetrated by forcep blades.

REFERENCES

1 Doob D. Female sexual abuse survivors as patients: Avoiding retraumatisation. Archives of Psychiatric Nursing 1992; VI(4):245–251.
2 Astbury J. Crazy for you: The making of women's madness. Australia: Oxford University Press; 1996.
3 Jowitt M. Personal communication. 1997.
4 Meiselman K. Incest: A psychological study of causes and effects with treatment recommendations. San Francisco, CA: Jossey-Bass.
5 McClelland L, Mynors-Wallis L, Fahy T, et al. Sexual abuse, disordered personality and eating disorders. British Journal of Psychiatry 1991; 158(Supp. 10):63–68.
6 Dijkstra S. Two mothers abused as children on raising their children: Making a plea for a differentiated approach. Child Abuse Review 1995; 4:291–297.
7 Streubert H, Carpenter D. Qualitative research in nursing. Philadelphia, PA: Uppencott & Co; 1995.
8 Browne A, Finklehor D. Impact of child sexual abuse: A review of the research. Psychological Bulletin 1986; 99(1):66–77.
9 Bachmann G, Moeller T, Nenett J. Childhood sexual abuse and the consequences in adult women: A review. Obstetrics & Gynaecology 1988; 71(4):631–642.
10 Ainscough C, Toon K. Breaking free: Help for survivors of child sexual abuse. London: Sheldon Press; 1993.
11 Sheldrick C. Adult sequelae of child sexual abuse. British Journal of Psychiatry 1991; 158(Supp. 10):55–62.
12 Buist A, Barnett B. Childhood sexual abuse: A risk factor for postpartum depression? Australian & New Zealand Journal of Psychiatry 1995; 29:604–608.
13 Oakley A. Women confined: Towards a sociology of childbirth. Oxford: Martin Robertson; 1980.
14 Ball J. Postnatal care and adjustment to motherhood. In: Robinson S, Thomson A (eds). Midwives, research and childbirth, vol. 1. London: Chapman and Hall; 1989.
15 Bass E, Davis L. The courage to heal: A guide for women survivors of child sexual abuse. London: Cedar Press; 1988.
16 Smith P. Childhood sexual abuse. Sexuality, pregnancy and birthing. New Zealand: Inside-Out Books; 1996.
17 Zlotnick C, Shea M, Peadstein T, et al. Differences in dissociative experiences between survivors of childhood incest and survivors of assault in adulthood. Journal of Nervous & Mental Disease 1996; 184(1):52–54.
18 Rose A. Effects of childhood sexual abuse on childbirth: One woman's story. Birth 1992; 19:4.
19 Lipp D. Mothering after incest. Mothering 1992; Spring: 115–120.
20 Christensen M. Birth rape. MIDIRS Midwifery Digest 1993; 3(3):304–305.
21 Heritage C. A burden to share. MIDIRS Midwifery Digest 1995; 5(4):431–432.
22 Drefucker CB. Counselling survivors of childhood sexual abuse: Counselling in practice. London: Sage Publications; 1992.
23 Menage J. Post-traumatic stress disorder in women who have undergone obstetric and/or gynaecological procedures: A consecutive series of 30 cases of PTSD. The Journal of Reproductive & Infant Psychology 1993; 11:221–228.
24 Rhodes N, Hutchinson S. Labor experiences of childhood sexual abuse survivors. Birth 1992; 19:4.
25 Parratt J. The experience of childbirth for survivors of incest. Midwifery 1994; 10:26–39.
26 Abrahams C. Hearing the truth: The importance of listening to children who disclose sexual abuse. Rochester: Chapel Press/NCH Action for Children Publication Unit; 1996.
27 Kirkham M. Labouring in the dark: Limitations on the giving of information to enable patients to orientate themselves to the likely events and timescale of labour. In: Wilson-Barnett J (ed). Nursing research: Ten studies in patient care. Chichester: John Wiley & Co; 1983.
28 Kirkham M. Midwives and information-giving during labour. In: Robinson A, Thomson A (eds). Midwives, research & childbirth 1. London: Chapman Hall; 1989:117–138.
29 Herman J, Hirschman L. Families at risk for father-daughter incest. American Journal of Psychiatry 1981; 138:967–970.
30 Dickersin K. Pharmacological control of pain during labour. In: Chalmers I, Enkin M, Kierse M (eds). Effective care in pregnancy and childbirth. Oxford: Oxford University Press.

Childbirth in women with a history of sexual abuse

Part 3: A case history approach

Maggie Smith

The previous articles in this series provided a summary of a literature review on the subject of childbirth for women with a history of sexual abuse. Possible indicators of sexual abuse were highlighted and the life history of a woman who had been seriously abused over a ten-year period by her father was described.

The life history study correlates well with other qualitative research which has looked at sexual abuse and subsequent childbirth experiences. It is acknowledged that the findings are limited by reason of it being a retrospective life history study which relies totally on the participant's subjective recall. Nevertheless, it highlights a number of important issues which are relevant to those providing care to childbearing women.

The trauma of childbirth for women with a history of sexual abuse

There is substantial evidence to suggest that for many women, childbirth can be a traumatic experience which can have long-term implications not only for the woman herself, but for her whole family.[1-6] The literature reviewed, together with the findings of this study, indicate that women with a history of sexual abuse may be particularly traumatised by childbirth as a direct consequence of the abuse. This is especially so during procedures which expose the genitalia, and include penetration of the vagina by hand, speculum, suction cap or forcep blades. These examinations may be reminiscent of the abuse and evoke feelings of powerlessness and vulnerability. Furthermore, the procedures may be undertaken by caregivers who are, unfortunately, unaware of the psychological effects of their actions.

Research indicates that when stress and anxiety occur during the active first stage of labour, the response of the body is the production of higher plasma cortisol and adrenaline levels which lower uterine contractile activity and may result in a prolonged first stage.[3] On this basis, it may be possible to reduce complications and medical interventions and prevent further trauma, by the provision of sensitive psychological care.

How should the needs of survivors of sexual abuse be met?

In order to tailor care which is appropriate to the specific needs of survivors of sexual abuse, some authors have suggested that attempts should be made to identify survivors in the antenatal period by taking a history which includes questions about past sexual experiences.[7,8,9]

Those who advocate incorporating questions about sexual experiences into a medical/obstetric history warn that professional failure to initiate discussion of the subject conveys a message to women either that such abuse does not occur or that it does not matter.[8] This is thought to confirm the woman's belief in the need to deny the reality of the experience, or its importance in her life. Not asking these questions contributes to society's long-standing practice of minimising the enormous emotional, financial and physical toll taken by childhood sexual abuse.[8]

During the early months of pregnancy, women are questioned about many aspects of their medical and social life. These enquiries touch on sensitive and personal areas, for example, maternal smoking and alcohol consumption. Enquiries are made about obstetric history, including questions relating to whether there have been any previous pregnancies which ended in therapeutic abortion. Given such scrutiny, one can understand the logic of the assertions made by those in favour of routine questioning; that psychological damage may occur if a woman is not asked about past sexual experiences. If it is accepted that women would benefit from enquiries which provide an opportunity to discuss their history, one must then consider who should make these enquiries, at what time, and in what manner?

The 'booking' interview is the time when a detailed medical and social history is taken. However, Rosemary Methven's research indicated that it is often no more than an impersonal, ritualised, 'form filling exercise', which is not conducive to the all-important task of establishing a relationship.[10] It is acknowledged that, since the time of Methven's study, there have been moves to improve the context of the booking interview, for example, by seeing women in their own homes. However, the recent clinical experience of the author confirms that many midwives suffer from time constraints which prevent them being able to devote as much time as they would like to taking a history. The very worst scenario would be for the subject of sexual abuse to be included as part of a booking interview and relegated to a tick box on a 'booking' form.

Given the profoundly sensitive nature of the topic, and the problems which have been identified following disclosure which has been inappropriately handled,[11,12,13] it could be argued that questions about sexual abuse metaphorically represent a can of worms which most midwives are probably not qualified to open. Furthermore, in view of the rates of prevalence, it should be borne in mind that some midwives may find it very painful to speak about sexual abuse as they too will have a personal history.

Specialist midwife counsellors

Rather than directly inviting disclosure, an alternative approach might be to inform women that a specialist midwife counsellor was available to whom they could self-refer. This information could be given out routinely, perhaps in the form of a booklet issued at the same time as other health promotional literature at the start of pregnancy. The benefits of this would be two-fold. Firstly, it would help to break the secrecy which surrounds sexual abuse and may help reduce feelings of stigmatisation which are known to occur, and secondly, it would provide a resource for the woman if and when she felt ready to access it.

The role of the specialist midwife could include the provision of social support during pregnancy, which may help to foster a relationship of trust. The midwife could be on call to provide intrapartum care, in the same was as caseload carrying midwives. This would provide for continuity of carer, the benefits of which are well documented throughout the midwifery literature. The initial investment of resources required to provide these specialist midwives could result in more favourable outcomes for women with a history of sexual abuse both in terms of physical and mental health. This could be extremely cost effective.

The recommendation is made taking into account the work of Ann Oakley, who demonstrated the importance of the social support component of midwifery care in terms of improved outcomes.[14] The research midwives in her study became trusted by the women and were not regarded with suspicion – unlike social workers or health visitors, who were seen as agents for surveillance and monitoring. It is of particular significance that the midwives were trusted with information that was not made available to those involved in the woman's routine antenatal care. A similar finding was made in another study which evaluated the effect of midwifery support for socially disadvantaged women.[15]

From this current study the importance of providing sensitive psychological care for the distinct needs of women who have been sexually abused has emerged. As we have seen, it is likely that these women will not have disclosed their experiences to their caregivers. Therefore, one of the main aims of care should be to help all women retain a sense of dignity and control throughout pregnancy, labour and childbirth. To this end, caregivers should strive to ensure that women are fully involved in decision making by adopting a 'partnership in care' philosophy. By altering the balance of power dynamic, women may be assisted to overcome the destructive feelings of helplessness which may have been established many years before. The intrapartum experiences described by the anonymous author in *New Generation*,[16] referred to in the first article in this series, provide an excellent illustration of this and suggest some fairly simple measures which may help women to feel that they remain in control.

It has been noted that vaginal examinations, which are disliked by most women,[17] are particularly anxiety-provoking for women with a history of sexual abuse. Many would argue that routines surrounding birth are often carried out with no clear rationale, and the frequency with which they are performed is determined by ritualistic and routine protocols, which are not necessarily in the best interests of childbearing women and their babies.[18,19] A move towards a less medicalised, more woman-centred model of care which reduces the number of vaginal examinations, and indeed any other interventions, to the absolute minimum, is required for all women. If, however, an examination cannot be avoided, caregivers can do a great deal to help empower individual women by adopting strategies which promote a feeling of control.[20]

Midwives are in a unique position to influence not only the experience, but also the outcomes of childbirth for women. If midwives are to take advantage of this and assist women to optimise childbirth experiences, a shift in emphasis with regard to caregiving is required. Although caring for the physical needs of childbearing women is of paramount importance, of equal importance is the need to treat women with sensitivity and respect in order to enhance their psychological wellbeing. The essence of midwifery practice is those skills which ensure the woman feels safe and strong.[21]

In order to nurture, protect and strengthen women, the subject of sexual abuse needs be included on all midwifery education programmes so that practitioners are equipped to recognise and meet the distinct psychological needs of survivors. Care given during pregnancy and childbirth cannot be effective unless those providing it are sufficiently aware of the particular problems experienced by individual women, and informed about the wider social circumstances in which these are occurring.[22] In addition, there is a great need for continuing professional development courses to heighten awareness and understanding among qualified practitioners.

I conclude this article by referring to the work of Jean Ball. Following her research into the effects which midwifery care may have upon the emotional needs of women, she wrote:

'Midwives, doctors and all other staff who are privileged to share in the care and experiences of parents at the birth of children have a great responsibility to enhance and enrich the experience, and this is particularly important when the mother is vulnerable to distress because of predisposing factors and events over which she has little or no control.' [23]

Based on the findings of my study, there would appear to be little doubt that a history of sexual abuse renders women extremely vulnerable, especially during childbirth. It is therefore hoped that those who provide care to childbearing women will recognise this, and will develop strategies for providing sensitive, holistic care in order to meet their needs.

REFERENCES

1 Raphael-Leff J. Psychological processes of childbearing. London: Chapman & Hall, 1991.
2 Kitzinger S. Childbirth and society. In: Chalmers I, Enkin M, Keirse M (eds). Effective care in pregnancy and childbirth, vol. 2. Oxford: Oxford University Press; 1989: 827–832.
3 Niven C. Psychological care for families before, during and after birth. Oxford: Butterworth-Heinemann; 1992.
4 Ralph K, Alexander J. Borne under stress. Nursing Times 1994; 90(12):28–30.
5 Sherr L. The psychology of pregnancy and childbirth. Oxford: Blackwell Science; 1995.
6 Hoiden J, Sagovsky R, Cox L. Counselling in a general practice setting: A controlled study of health visitor intervention in the treatment of postnatal depression. British Medical Journal 1989; 298:223–236.
7 Courtois C, Riley C. Pregnancy and childbirth as triggers for abuse memories: Implications for care. Birth 1992; 19(4):222–223.
8 Hoiz K. A practical approach to clients who are survivors of childhood sexual abuse. Journal of Nurse-Midwifery 1994; 39:13–18.
9 Sang J, Petersen B. Incorporating routine screening for history of childhood sexual abuse into well-woman and maternity care. Journal of Nurse-Midwifery 1995; 40(1):26–30.
10 Methven R. Recording an obstetric history or relating to a pregnant woman? A study of the antenatal booking interview. In: Robinson S, Thomson A (eds). Midwives, research & childbirth. Oxford: Oxford University Press; 1991.
11 Longdon C. A survivor's and therapist's viewpoint. In: Elliott M (ed). Female sexual abuse of children. Essex: Longman; 1993.
12 Elliott M (ed). Female sexual abuse of children. Essex: Longman; 1993.

13 Weaver P, Varvara F, Connors R, et al. Adult survivors of childhood sexual abuse: Survivors' disclosure and nurse-therapist's response. Journal of Psychosocial Nursing & Mental Health Services 1994; 32(12):19–25.
14 Oakley A. Social support and pregnancy outcome: A report of a randomised trial. British Journal of Obstetrics and Gynaecology 1990; 97:155–162.
15 Davies J, Evans F. The Newcastle community midwifery care project. In: Robinson S, Thomson M (eds). Midwives, Research & Childbirth. Oxford: Oxford University Press; 1991.
16 Anonymous. Abuse. New Generation 1993; June: 48.
17 Raid M, Garcia J. Women's views of care during pregnancy and childbirth. In: Chalmers I, Enkin M, Kierse M (eds). Effective care in pregnancy and childbirth. Oxford: Oxford University Press; 1989.
18 Chalmers I, Enkin M, Kierse M (eds). Effective care in pregnancy and childbirth. Oxford: Oxford University Press; 1989.
19 Walton I. Sexuality and motherhood. Hale: Books for Midwives Press; 1994.
20 Kitzinger J. The internal examination. The Practitioner 1990; 234:698–700.
21 Kirkham M. A feminist perspective in midwifery. In: Webb C (ed). Feminist practice in women's health care. London: John Wiley & Co; 1986.
22 Elbourne D, Oakley A, Chalmers I. Social and psychological support during pregnancy. In: Chalmers I, Enkin M, Kierse M (eds). Effective care in pregnancy and childbirth. Oxford: Oxford University Press; 1989.
23 Ball J. Reactions to motherhood: The role of postnatal care, 2nd edn. Hale: Books for Midwives Press; 1994.

Sexual assault and flashbacks on the labour ward

Jo Desborough

I have been sexually assaulted. There. I've said it. For so long that was the difficult bit, but now I realise that it is the coming to terms with what happened, learning to live with myself, my grief, my fears and my emotions, and desperately trying to meet people's expectations and find the coping mechanism that people tell me I must in order for my life to move on, that is difficult.

From the time the assault took place, people, including my assailant, have told me what is best for me – whom I should tell, what I should do. Others have simply shut off, not knowing how to deal with it. An amazing few support me, and one person in particular has given me great courage and strength – how can somebody really appreciate what it means to have just one person there for you at a time when you feel so alone?

I am writing this now because it feels right. People advise me whom I should tell to get the support I need, but far more important is the sudden realisation that I must tell everybody, so that the women in our care get the support they need.

My story

I am not a naive person; I know of events that happen in 'the real world'. I have had boyfriends but had chosen to remain a virgin until last summer at the age of 24. It was good, it felt safe, it was my choice. Then one night in October I met a guy. We talked as though we had been friends for years. You talk to some guys and you know the score – thanks, I'm flattered but I'm not interested in 'one-night stands'. But this was different. He spoke of his fiancée, the conversation naturally flowed, we were relaxed. I was not drunk nor did he appear to be. There were no signs for me to suspect his intentions. We went for a walk to his house nearby for a drink. The atmosphere was light and easy – until he turned.

His hands went round my neck and he pushed me down. He changed his grip so that he had one arm round my neck with his hand applying heavy pressure to my throat. He lay on top of my right side. He was strong. I could barely breathe, I was trapped – but he had a free hand.

My mind went into overdrive. The pain was excruciating. I thought I was going to die. In response to my gasps for air and pathetic pleas for him to stop came his reassurance that it was okay, he knew what he was doing. He seemed convinced for his own reassurance that I was enjoying it.

As quickly as he became violent, he relaxed again and acted as if nothing had happened. I was able to pick myself up, dress and leave. I made my way back to the club to find my friends. I was hysterical, they were supportive, we went home. One friend tried to convince me to go to the police but I couldn't do that. At 3.30 in the morning I showered until after the hot water ran out but I still felt so dirty. I was sore internally for a good week after and prayed for my cycle to return so that I might feel clean and somehow normal again. It did, two weeks late.

Picking up the pieces

I am lucky. I am alive, I am not pregnant, I was not raped – well, not with his penis, anyway. The only physical scar that remains is inside my mouth where my tooth went into my lip in the initial struggle. I am left with enormous shame, feeling that I am to blame for what happened, although people tell me I shouldn't.

I normally have the strength to be an advocate for women and for my peers, yet I had complied with his demands. He is only a human being, certainly no better that me or anyone else – yet I complied. I thought I knew myself, but I am now having to undergo a huge process of self-discovery as I desperately try to regain some self-respect.

Moving on

My heart pounds as I write this, but I am determined to learn whatever I can from this experience and share it with other midwives. What makes me so troubled is the connection that I now see so clearly between what happened to me and what so often happens to the vulnerable and trusting pregnant women in our care. Many of the midwives I work with have extraordinary strengths in communication, clinical skills and compassion, and yet my experience has made me question the necessity and appropriateness of many of the activities they undertake in their role as midwives. The events I see on the labour ward on a daily basis in the name of midwifery care can often trigger flashbacks for me to that October night, which tells me that this correlation is true.

The most obvious issue is that of vaginal examinations. As a midwifery student, I understand the indications for occasional VEs, but I seriously challenge their frequency and the way in which they are undertaken. Just as I felt no reason not to trust my attacker, midwives quickly gain the trust of women in their care. Our identification badges, our uniforms, our titles and the labour ward routine and environment, so alien to women, all imply our power, which we use to gain compliance with the many procedures which we instigate. Modern childbirth includes some very invasive techniques, and yet women are never informed that they are entitled to refuse these procedures. In this we abuse our power and their trust in us.

Many VEs are performed simply to comply with hospital policy; why is the concept of informed choice not appropriate here? We use hollow phrases to try and reassure women that the VE is in their interests, that it will not hurt, that they are safe and that they must trust us. It is the language of abusers. I personally have been present during VEs where senior midwives have used these words, seemingly oblivious to the woman's pleas to stop. Just as my attacker was relaxed about his actions as if they were routine, midwives so often fall into the same dangerous trap of thinking that vaginal examinations are routine. They are certainly never routine for women. After my experience, should I ever become pregnant, I cannot imagine complying with a VE.

Breastfeeding support is another area where something that is routine for midwives can seem like an assault to women. I have seen many a breast grappled with in the name of what is natural and best.

A large percentage of women we care for during childbirth will have suffered abuse, as will a large number of midwives. But disturbingly many women relate stories of how they felt abused by midwives and doctors during childbirth itself. Surely the last thing we want is for women who do not have a history of abuse leaving our labour wards feeling victims of assault – feeling as I felt after my attack. The vitally important message is not just to improve care for those women who have been abused, but to prevent others from feeling or being abused by us.

Who's in control?

Control in giving birth needs to be returned to the women themselves. Vaginal examinations and breastfeeding may seem the most obviously intimate areas of midwifery care but underlying everything is the fundamental issue of control. Even the best midwives I see still control and manipulate women. Following my assault, so many times people have tried to take over and tell me what I must be feeling, rather than simply asking me how I feel and giving me enough respect to wait and then listen to my answer. Midwives need to stop telling women what to do and take the time instead to listen carefully to each individual's story and respect her as a fellow human being. We must take time to ask women how they are feeling, listen, and then formulate our response carefully and individually.

Too often on our labour wards the impersonal 'care' we give seems more to protect us (think of regimented four-hourly VEs, monitors, enforced pushing, drips) than to benefit the women. It is no excuse to say that childbirth, like sexual assault, is one of life's experiences, and therefore whatever happens between the first contraction and the final push is somehow acceptable. 'Put it down to experience' is what many well-meaning people have said to try to reassure me. That is not good enough.

Conclusion

My experience is mine; I am sure that many others have experienced worse. How we as individuals deal with our experiences, our emotions and the lessons they teach us is unique to each one of us. Even with the best of intentions, others should not attempt to control them. I ask for patience and understanding as I put myself back together and learn to feel safe again.

What is midwifery about if it is not about trust? Women need to feel safe in order to let go of conscious control to give birth. They must trust their midwives – with their naked bodies, their sexuality, the lives of their babies. They trust us with their fear of failure, their fear of humiliation, their vulnerability. They must trust us to protect them while they abandon themselves to the experience of giving birth, and they trust us to help and care for them while they slowly and gently put themselves back together, as whole bodies, as whole women and as new mothers ready to go back into the world.

That precious gift of trust is what a good midwife can give to a woman, who will perhaps experience it for the first time in her life. And so what immeasurable and profound harm we do to that vulnerable new mother if we abuse her trust and her body, take control, ignore her cries and leave her humanity and self-respect in tatters. She learns very quickly, as I did, that she is not good enough, that it was her fault or deficiency in some way, and loses all sense of self-worth. She begins her life as a mother, not at the height of her creative power but full of inadequacy, perplexing grief and confused emotions. All this is in the hands of the midwife.

It took the experience of sexual assault for me to start to understand this. I share it in the hope that we can all begin to think about what being a midwife really means.

Practice check

- Question the need for every VE – your overall aim should be to do as few as possible. Is the VE absolutely essential, or is it just labour ward routine? Is there any other method of gaining the information you need, such as general observation or abdominal palpation? Do you have confidence in your diagnostic ability in these less invasive midwifery skills?
- In your own practice, do you offer women a genuinely informed choice about whether to have a VE? How might you change your practice to do this?
- Review the language that you personally use around VEs. Does it embody genuine respect for your clients' autonomy or is it full of empty, shallow phrases?
- Could you do VEs with the woman in positions other than passively lying down? Have you ever considered doing them while she is standing up – a more assertive position in which she is more in control of what is happening?
- Although they have no physical sensation, remember that women with epidurals can still feel 'invaded', penetrated and abused. They may even feel more violated as they are powerless and paralysed. Stop the practice of using them as 'learning opportunities' for students, without gaining their genuine, informed consent.
- Have you developed the skill of 'hands off' breastfeeding support? Handling and manipulating a woman's breasts should always be your last resort, and must always take place with a woman's complete, genuine, informed consent.
- Think back honestly over your practice through the years. Have you ever done anything that a woman might have considered abusive? Are you sure? How would you know?

Breastfeeding

In spite of ever increasing evidence to support the benefits of breastfeeding for baby, mother and society, the matter of providing nutrition for our young would appear to be more complex and contentious than ever. Without a doubt, the profile of breastfeeding in the UK has increased somewhat in the past decade. Much of this heightened awareness may be attributed to UNICEF and the success of the Baby Friendly Initiative (BFI). The practice of promoting early mother/baby contact highlighted in Kate Olsen's article is no longer an espoused theory, having generally become accepted as good practice. Yet five years ago who, except perhaps those within the neonatal unit, had heard of skin-to-skin contact?

No one can deny the impressive gains in those units seeking to achieve BFI accreditation or the philosophical intention to normalise breastfeeding in favour of artificial feeding. However, I have a concern that the BFI may be in danger of losing momentum by adopting an unyielding approach. Whilst attending a BFI training course last year, I challenged the requirement of a breastfeeding policy as one of the Ten Steps. I explained that I felt that we had battled to replace the authoritative stance of policies with guidelines in maternity services, and felt that this insistence was a volte-face, utilising authoritarian tactics in order to gain compliance. I was informed that introducing a breastfeeding policy within trusts was the only way in which the Baby Friendly Initiative was going to make a major difference, and a breastfeeding policy was therefore mandatory. I fear that this somewhat dictatorial approach of UNICEF may actually prove to be counterproductive, and this may be what Sue Battersby reflects in her piece.

Perhaps we need to consider winning over mothers as well as offering kudos to those units achieving BFI status. It is conceivable that we have been sitting on the fence for too long and that this has rendered us incapable of supplying women with the information that they require in order to make informed decisions about feeding their babies. Perhaps, as Maureen Minchin states so eloquently, we need to address the risks of artificial feeding openly. And, as Jeremy Dearling suggests, we may need to consider our marketing skills. It is known that the infant formula industry spends millions of pounds per annum on advertising in the UK alone. If midwives are to attempt to counterbalance this onslaught from the industry, then perhaps we need to consider offering a marketing component within our education programmes to provide midwives with such skills.

The matter of what our breast milk contains is one of escalating concern, and the article by Michel Odent clearly outlines the problems and discusses actions to ameliorate if not eliminate the threats that PCBs, dioxins and other environmental toxins represent to the health of our children. These problems need to be addressed and debated; if we ignore the issues then the only access that mothers may have to information is found within the popular press who publish stories of mothers poisoning their babies with their breastmilk.

Breastmilk represents a mother's diet on a microcosmic scale, which in turn reflects the content of our local and global environment. Midwives and mothers need information about how they can best afford to minimise any risks and to place the risk in context.

The increased chances of survival of very pre-term and low birth weight babies has introduced a whole new episode into the breastfeeding debate. We have many gaps in our knowledge about the nutritional needs of these babies and need far greater understanding about how their needs are catered for in the composition of breastmilk. Elizabeth Jones has worked tremendously hard at North Staffs Hospital to ensure that babies with special needs are receiving the optimal nutrition available, and increasingly her work suggests that breastmilk provides everything that a very gestationally immature baby requires. Every neonatologist and neonatal nurse should heed her pioneering work on the value of hind milk before reaching for the fortifier as a prescribed requirement for every baby within the neonatal unit.

Finally, what goes around comes around, and in the light of ever-changing evidence, we should be aware of trends and fashions in breastfeeding, and how these influence our practice. Sally Inch and Chloe Fisher's article on dealing with nipple damage brought this home to me. After a decade or so of advocating dry healing methods we are now being advised to use white paraffin products to encourage healing. This example serves as a salutory message for me of recognising that research evidence should guide our practice but not dictate it. There are very few absolutes in midwifery and that applies equally within the practice of breastfeeding. We should be reminding ourselves as much as the women that we serve to 'never say never; and never say always'.

Lorna Davies

The carrot and its role in the promotion of breastfeeding

Jeremy Dearling

Prostitution is popularly believed to be the oldest profession in the world. This is a fallacy. The oldest profession in the world is selling.

The first chapter of Genesis clearly demonstrates that salesmen have the edge over prostitutes when it comes to longevity. The Genesis account describes how Eve was engaged in conversation with a salesman (the snake) in the full knowledge that she could do whatever she wanted except eat the apple. The snake persuaded her of the benefits of eating the apple. It is generally understood she found this not to be one of her better decisions.

The snake convinced Eve that eating the apple would enhance her quality of life, and that is basically what a salesmen does. A salesman sells by finding out what motivates his customers and tailors his pitch to show them how his product will enhance their quality of life.

As an ex-salesman I am often amazed by the frequent use by health professionals of the stick when the carrot would do a far more effective job. Patients' decisions are often influenced by penal arguments rather than by rational ones. Take breastfeeding for example. Those midwives who are interested enough and committed enough both to promote the practice and to give support to those who elect to breastfeed often use the stick to influence mothers' decisions rather than the carrot. And the stick used is guilt. I've spoken to many mothers about what motivated them to choose their method of feeding their infant, and I found it disturbing that so many of them were motivated to breastfeed by guilt. Their guilt was generated not solely by health professionals, but also by their family, culture, and society. Influencing behaviour by creating a climate of guilt is not only poor practice, but it is arguably unethical, and certainly ineffective.

There is an alternative method of promoting breastfeeding but it is not a method that midwives, or for that matter any health professional, are currently taught. It is a big secret, known only to the formula milk companies and every industry and business in the world who employ salesmen. Salesmen have locked into this secret for years but midwives are oblivious to it. Salesmen know how to motivate people by making them feel good about using their products.

For years breastfeeding has been promoted with the stick method; it is 'natural', it is best for the baby, QED give baby the breast. The subtext to all this has been: you are unnatural if you don't breastfeed, if you really want to be a good mother then you will breastfeed your baby, and any other decision makes you a pariah. The success of this method can be seen in the annual report and accounts of companies such as Cow & Gate, Nestlé etc.

The point I want to get across here is that, despite the reality that there are many who will always breastfeed and don't need persuasion, there are also many who will never breastfeed no matter what. The undecided thousands are targeted by formula milk companies successfully. Infant formula companies market their product. Midwives don't market theirs. Midwives know about a superior product but don't sell it. Why? Because they do not know how to. Communication may well play a part in modern midwifery training but selling skills don't. But if you want to change any behaviour of your client group, the lessons are there to be learned from salesmen, who have been changing the behaviours of their client group from time immemorial.

Lesson one

So! Here is lesson one from the Carrot School of Health Promotion. When you first meet a salesman, what happens is so subtle you probably don't realise what is going on. Salesmen start by talking and listening; they gather information from the moment you meet them. What they are looking for are clues as to what will motivate you to buy from them. No conversation with any salesman is ever idle. In the trade this is described as seeking your 'Hot Button'.

Take double glazing for example. People will buy double glazing for a variety of reasons: security, soundproofing, old windows are falling out, low maintainance, appearance, product design, ventilation benefits, and so on. You may go to a company wanting to choose a product that will save you having to paint, because you hate decorating, but unless a salesman asks why you want to change your windows he will never know. Almost certainly he will never make a sale if, instead of telling you about the maintainance-free benefits of the product, he rambles endlessly about the security aspect of the design.

What has this got to do with breastfeeding? Women make their breast/bottlefeeding decisions for a variety of reasons as well. Factors involved include: partner involvement, time, cost, preparation, self-image, peer pressure, family expectations, perceived role in society, and many more. Why then is it so suprising that the message fails when it has been so consistently put forward without tailoring it to the woman's concerns?

The critical thing to bear in mind, whether in selling or health promotion, is that we are all selfish beings. Salesmen home in on what the client will see as a benefit to themselves, known in the trade as WIIFM. What's In It For Me? is the clue to changing behaviour. Midwives often promote breastfeeding by getting the mother to focus on the benefits to the baby. Formula milk companies sell bottlefeeding by focusing mothers' attention on the benefits to them. If midwives want to change behaviour they would do well to drop the promotion in favour of the sell, and focus more on the needs of the mother than the needs of the baby. It's simple.

Up and down the country I can hear the worried mutters: 'I can't do it. If I wanted to be in sales I wouldn't have become a midwife'. It's a fair point but frankly, I don't believe those who say they can't do it. Look at any selling textbook and you will read the same message. Anyone can sell.

Use your time with mothers to establish what is important to them in whatever role they see themselves; mother, wife, lover, woman or employee. It won't be hard. You are powerful people and they will tell you one way or another. Look at how they present themselves: professional, earth mother, down-trodden, happy, frightened, supported, 'mumsy', enthusiastic – the list is endless. Learn how to use this information to make them feel good about themselves in deciding to breastfeed. Are they worried about their shape or figures? Then discuss how breastfeeding will shrink their uterus and use up fat deposits. Is money a worry? Discuss the economic benefits of breastfeeding. Use whatever argument you wish to motivate the mother to breastfeed *provided you*

and your colleagues are going to be there to support her in that decision. If you cannot be there when she needs you, don't bother to persuade her in the first place.

Need to listen

The critical thing is listening. Too many sales are lost by salesmen trying to make the sale because they believe that the customer will buy from them because of what they say, and that if the customer doesn't buy it was because the customer wasn't listening in the first place. In fact the reverse is true. Sales are lost because the salesmen were not listening.

The same goes in health promotion. Too many health promotion messages are lost because the health promoter believes that the patient wasn't listening to them, when in fact it was because the health promoter wasn't listening to the patient. This happens either because we haven't time to do so with the pressures of the job, or because we haven't the skills to spot what the patient is really saying, and what is motivating the patient.

The last part of a sale is called 'closing the deal'. It comes in the form of asking for a commitment. For example: 'So Mrs Smith, you have expressed an interest in our product. Now, if I tell you that this gadget comes in leopard skin bakelite with mains adaptor and removable handles, do we have an agreement to buy?' How does this translate into promotion of breastfeeding? Once you have found what will motivate a woman to decide to breastfeed and demonstrated that deciding to breastfeed is going to be the best decision for her quality of life, you then need to ask her if she will agree to give breastfeeding a try. When you have asked this question there next comes the most difficult bit of this whole easy business. Be silent until she answers. It is important not to fill this space with your need to revisit what has gone before in your discussion, and let the silence speak. You may then get another 'objection' in the form of another question. In which case deal with that objection as you have done all the others. When you have done this, close again. Ask for a commitment. If she says, 'Let me think about it', ask her what is it she wants to think about and then close again. When you have got a commitment congratulate her, even ask her to sign her calendar to mark the occasion, and then remind her from time to time of her decision in subsequent visits.

Different approach

This has been a whirlwind tour round the carrot patch. Some may not feel comfortable with this approach. Some may not feel it is ethical. But if you believe that breastfeeding is the best option for mother and child and agree that traditional methods of changing behaviour have had only limited impact up to now, perhaps it is time for a different approach, by motivating women through helping them see that it has a benefit to them in real terms. If you always do what you have always done, you will always get what you always had.

If the goal is to increase the number of women who decide to breastfeed, it is time to look at what works as a means of changing health behaviours. We should not be so isolated and superior as to believe that the world of commerce has nothing to teach us. There is scope for health professionals to improve their listening and communication skills. The critical thing however, is that if you succeed in increasing the number of women who breastfeed who are under your care, you have a duty to support them. Fail them in this support and you do a generation and your profession a disservice.

Breastfeeding and bullying
Who's putting the pressure on?

Sue Battersby

The increasing use of the terms 'pressure', 'guilt', 'bullied' and 'coercion' used in association with breastfeeding is a phenomenon that should raise concern amongst those involved in the promotion and support of breastfeeding. As a researcher involved in four independent breastfeeding research projects, I have noted something unexpected in my research findings: the ever increasing frequency of the use of these terms, not only by childbearing women but also by midwives. A growing portfolio of incidents and quotes has been compiled during the research process which bears witness to the problem. Midwives openly discuss the dilemmas they have encountered, both within their own personal experiences and also as part of their professional practice.

Mothers express that they feel pressurised and coerced into breastfeeding. More recently, the media has presented articles about breastfeeding in which again mothers are using the term 'pressure'.[2]

The term 'pressure' is defined as a 'moral force that compels' whereas to coerce means 'to compel... by force or authority without regard to individual wishes or desires'.[3] Midwives have a tendency to use the terms 'pressure', 'bullied' and 'guilt' whilst mothers talk of 'pressure' and 'coercion'.

Midwives' personal experiences

The majority of midwives choose to breastfeed their infants but there are a few that feel pressured to do so against their wishes. Comments like 'I initially wanted to bottle feed my first baby but because I was a midwife I felt I should breastfeed' and 'With my first child I had just qualified and felt pressured', are examples of how some midwives feel they must comply with the demands of their peers and their profession.

These midwives are fully informed of the benefits of breastfeeding and their wish to bottle feed is rooted in something far deeper, their cultural upbringing. It must be acknowledged that midwives belong to the same cultural identity as that of other breastfeeding women, and that societal and professional demands may make them feel pressurised to conform against their wishes.

Midwives' professional experiences

The fear of conformity can also be identified within midwives' professional practice. They are aware that they should be promoting and supporting breastfeeding but do not always feel they are supporting the mother by discussing breastfeeding, especially when mothers have expressed their desire to formula feed. The support they wish to provide for bottle feeders is hindered by hospital policies that are too entrenched in breastfeeding and are too 'narrow'. Some midwives express how 'We don't give enough support to bottle feeders. I feel I should give demonstrations but feel under pressure not to do so!' They also feel that their professional judgement is in jeopardy because they are unable to 'use their own initiative' when caring for women.

When talking about professional practice, some midwives express how they are even reluctant to discuss the benefits of breastfeeding. As one midwife explained: 'Midwives are reluctant to explain clearly the health benefits of breastfeeding and the potential health problems associated with bottle feeding for fear of offending women or appearing to be forcing breastfeeding. This would not be the case with other health choices, for example vaccinations.'

This was not an isolated comment. Within other maternity units midwives have expressed similar feelings. Another midwife explained: 'I feel that many midwives (myself included) are hesitant in fully informing women of physiological benefits to the baby – for fear of putting increased pressure on them.' This hesitancy had been fuelled by comments the midwife had overheard from women who were attending the maternity unit in which she worked.

Guilt was a word that was also linked with breastfeeding. Guilt is defined as the 'fact or state of having done wrong or committed a crime'.[3] Are mothers made to feel that they have committed a crime if they have made a conscious decision to formula feed their infant? Is this not contrary to Changing Childbirth[4] which advocates that women should be given control and choice within maternity services?

This view was expressed by a midwife who thought that women 'have too much pressure to breastfeed and may do so out of guilt and be unhappy – this is wrong.' Comments related to guilt were frequently made; there are many more examples. Another midwife expressed very similar feelings by saying 'the client has a right to choose the method by which to feed their baby without the need for guilt or recrimination'.

Why do midwives feel guilty for trying to persuade a mother to breastfeed, but do not hesitate to persuade her that that her baby should really have Vitamin K? Part of the reason for this is perhaps that breastfeeding is seen as an emotive and controversial subject, and also the benefits of breastfeeding are not so easily recognisable for many in a developed country; as one midwife did explain, 'bottle fed babies do thrive'. Another reason is that there is a strong emphasis within midwifery care that there should be a partnership between the midwife and the woman and that by discussing breastfeeding, midwives feel that it could make women 'hostile towards us'.

Mothers' experiences of 'pressure'

At a recent two-day Surestart workshop where plans for the introduction of a 'peer support' programme were discussed, there were mothers who stood up on both days to describe how they had felt coerced and pressurised into breastfeeding. They asked us to consider our methods of breastfeeding promotion to make it more sensitive to mothers' needs. However, one mother who had chosen to breastfeed supported the midwives by saying that she too had been presented with a list of advantages of breastfeeding but in no way had she felt pressurised. Are mothers actually pressurised, or is it their sense of guilt that makes them feel pressurised? Many mothers know the benefits of breastfeeding but have external or psychological pressures that deter them from adopting it as their choice of infant feeding.

Mike Woolridge[5] proposed a further explanation during his presentation at the national conference 'Barriers to breastfeeding: Time for a new approach'. He discussed how some mothers who smoke may opt to bottle feed as they are aware that they will pass on harmful substances to their infant if they breastfeed. Can this really be true? Many mothers who smoke during pregnancy know the harmful effects smoking can have on an unborn child but take no positive steps to remedy this.

Recently The Daily Mail published an article on breastfeeding which examined 'both sides of this controversial subject'.[2] A mother was interviewed who explained that she 'was put under a lot of pressure from the midwives at the hospital to breastfeed her son'.

Are mothers being coerced into breastfeeding? When conducting interviews with new mothers the author asked one mother why she had decided to breastfeed.[1] She said she had not. She explained:

'I was going to bottle feed but while I was waiting for the epidural to wear off the midwife just put her on, just gave her to me and said 'put her on'. I think because I was so woozy and wasn't aware of what the hell was going on at the time I just fed her.'

For this mother the outcome was positive: she actually liked the feeling of breastfeeding and went on to successfully breastfeed her daughter. But what a different tale it could have been. It could be classed as assault and an official complaint could have resulted. That would have been a backward step for the promotion of breastfeeding.

Removing the pressure

How do we take the pressure out of breastfeeding, not only for women but also for midwives? It has been recognised that excessive zeal in the promotion of breastfeeding can be counterproductive[6] and therefore there needs to be a balance between informing women of the advantages of breastfeeding and not coming across as coercive. A midwife said that 'perhaps some training in how to encourage and promote breastfeeding without 'scaremongering' and pressuring women is what is required'.

When implementing the Baby Friendly Initiative the involvement of more midwives in the process may help to make them feel valued and feel that they are instrumental in their hospital achieving the Baby Friendly Award. This would give them ownership of the policies rather than a sense that the policies had been imposed from above.

Many midwives feel it is difficult to promote breastfeeding as by the time the midwife comes into contact with the woman the decision about infant feeding has already been taken. This has been identified as the case in the literature.[7,8,9] What many midwives have suggested is that breastfeeding should be more supportively promoted in the media. This unfortunately is not the case. When breastfeeding is presented, it is either as a controversial issue or in the case of famine where a starving mother is shown breastfeeding her infant. Neither of these help to positively promote breastfeeding. Should something that is normal and natural be presented as controversial? Even the health professional, Dr Rosemary Leonard who presented the 'ultimate breastfeeding guide' in *The Daily Mail* came across as very negative about breastfeeding. Reading her list of the negative aspects of breastfeeding was enough to put any prospective mother off.[10]

One midwife felt that asking midwives to promote breastfeeding was too much. She strongly believed that the only way to increase breastfeeding rates is to change the underlying culture. This requires an effort by society as a whole not just focusing on health professionals. This would surely be the best way of removing the pressure both from midwives and the women!

There is certainly evidence that both midwives and mothers perceive that undue pressure is exerted at times when attempts are made to promote breastfeeding. If the advantages of breastfeeding are to be recognised by society then this problem must become an urgent issue for future multidisciplinary debate.

REFERENCES

1 Battersby S. Midwives' experiences of breastfeeding: Can the attitudes developed affect how midwives support and promote breastfeeding? Proceedings of the International Confederation of Midwives 25th Triennial Congress, Manila, 1999: 52–56.
2 Hope J. To breastfeed or not? The Daily Mail 2000; Wednesday April 26:24–5.
3 McLeod WT, Hanks P (eds). The new Collins concise dictionary of the English language. London: Guild Publishing; 1987.
4 Department of Health. Changing Childbirth. London: HMSO; 1993.
5 Woolridge M. Infant feeding and inequalities. Presented at the National Conference 'Barriers to Breastfeeding: Time for a new approach'. Monday 15 May 2000.
6 Department of Health and Social Security. Report on Health and Social Subjects 32. Present day practice in infant feeding: Third report. London: HMSO; 1988.
7 Battersby S. Breastfeeding: A dying art. Unpublished thesis. Sheffield: Sheffield City Polytechnic; 1992.
8 Jones DA. The choice to breast or bottle feed and the influences upon that choice: A survey of 1525 mothers. Child care, health and development. London: Blackwell Publications; 1986.
9 Thomson A. Why don't women breastfeed? In: Robinson S, Thomson A (eds). Midwives, research and childbirth, vol.1. London: Chapman and Hall; 1989.
10 Leonard R. The facts and myths about breastfeeding your baby. The Daily Mail 2000; Wednesday April 26:25.

Artificial feeding and risk

The last taboo

Maureen Minchin

Artificial feeding of the young baby is a risk behaviour, like smoking or heavy drinking in pregnancy, shaking a baby, driving with a child unrestrained in a car, or many other things that humans sometimes do out of choice or necessity. Like all risk behaviours, it is not always or immediately and obviously harmful to everybody exposed to the risk. Some shaken babies have not been permanently brain damaged, many smoked-over children have grown up apparently normal, millions of children have been driven in cars at high speeds without the slightest damage occurring.

Reducing risk

Despite the statistics, we try to reduce or eliminate risk behaviours wherever possible when it comes to raising our children. Why? Because some children are seriously or permanently harmed, and we can never control or predict which children it will be. So Governments and community agencies tell parents that all children are at risk, by running (often fear-inducing) campaigns. These campaigns certainly create great guilt and hurt in those unfortunate enough to have damaged their children by taking the advertised risk. The campaign does not aim to do this, but accepts it as a by-product of trying to prevent other children being damaged in future. Public health messages are about prevention and the good of the whole community, not the feelings of the minority already affected by having taken risks.

Why is there such a taboo on talk of the risks of artificial feeding? Why do health campaigns talk of the benefits of breastfeeding, rather than telling parents plainly that there are risks to artificial feeding? Do we try to stop smoking by extolling the joys of clean air, or do we talk of the risks of smoking? Do we try to stop babies being shaken by talking about the benefits of a calm handling technique, or do we talk about the risks to the brain of being shaken? Western society does not want to face the fact that artificial feeding is risky, so babies must be sacrificed to current social convenience, the smallest victims of the marketplace.

Childhood diseases

Health authorities around the world, from the World Health Organisation to the American Academy of Pediatrics, are now well aware of the scientific evidence that children who are not breastfed for at least four to six months, or who are exposed to foreign proteins too early in life, have a much greater chance of developing disease in childhood and adulthood, and a lesser chance of realising their full cognitive and physical potential. Diseases that cost this society fortunes – ear infections, juvenile diabetes, asthma, allergic disease, orthodontic problems, speech and learning difficulties, adult gastrointestinal disorders, obesity – are all more common in those not solely breastfed from birth to at least four months. These outcomes remain constant regardless of socio-economic status. That some children are lucky, or have good genes, or are not exposed to trigger factors for disease, and/or aren't obviously affected, does not alter the fact of risk and cost to all. Informed choice becomes a joke when parents are never told the whole truth.

Let's be very clear about a few things. Where artificial feeding is concerned, no one knows what the best recipe for formula is. Much of the content of formula is based on studies in pigs and rats. Formulae are rarely tested comparatively to see which brand, or version of a brand, results in fewer health problems for babies. Companies add different ingredients based on what is affordable and available at the time. Peanut oil was used for decades; it is now banned because it has been shown to cause allergic reactions and even deaths. Marine algae (truly) are now being used as fat sources, along with fish heads and eggs, with no studies of allergy being done yet again. Genetically modified ingredients have been used already in some infant formulae. Even if we knew exactly

- What to put in (which we don't: breastmilk has thousands of components and is still being researched)
- how to put it in (which we can't: many of breastmilk's ingredients are unique bioactive factors that are destroyed by processing; cows' milk analogues are not equivalent in any case)
- How to avoid making processing mistakes (which we can't: there have been many accidents and mistakes in design, manufacture, transport, storage etc. in this industry as in any other)
- How to make sure it is all still there so that there is neither excess nor deficiency throughout the shelf-life of the product (which we can't: companies begin with 'overages' (excesses) in order to ensure that there is not a deficiency by the end of the period; rate of decline of nutrients varies with storage conditions)

…we still don't know exactly how the baby's body uses what we put in, in any but the crudest measures: external size. Yet two babies can be identical weights and heights, but the breastfed baby boy will have on average more lean muscle mass and less fat than the artificially-fed boy, and the fat in his body will be of a different composition. Fats are critical not only to brains (IQ, learning ability) but to central nervous system development and myelination. Demyelinating disease, like so much else, is more common in adults not breastfed as children.

Production problems

Are parents comfortable in the knowledge that an Australian infant formula company apparently considers it excessive to spend Aus$1,300 on assays of aluminium levels in its infant formula?

Are parents happy that the proposed new standard for infant formula will now prescribe maximal levels only for ingredients already shown to be toxic in excess, after industry objected to the setting of maximal levels for all ingredients?

Do parents know whether the litre of water their bottle-fed child will drink each day comes from house or community pipes contributing lead, asbestos, nitrates or dioxins? The breastfeeding mother's body substantially shields her young baby from such risks.

It is literally true that artificial feeding is an avoidable health risk, and many babies are harmed by it. The later in the first six months that babies are exposed to infant formula, or any other food, the better they will cope. What is tolerable or even useful as part of a weaning diet is very different from what is tolerable as the sole food of the newborn.

Enabling breastfeeding

If we take this avoidable risk to our children seriously, what this means, of course, is that we must provide the quality care and support for women that enables them to breastfeed. (Physiologically almost all can, and we could provide the rest with breastmilk if we understood its value.)

It is not enough, as some Governments do, to exhort women to breastfeed in a society where most of the important supports for women have been eroded or destroyed, and in which the pressures on young families have never been greater. We need to address problems which arise from the current timing of hospital discharge, cuts to maternal and child health services, and modern workplace conditions, all of which conspire to make it unlikely that all women can carry through their informed choice to breastfeed.

Knowing that it is better, but not being able to breastfeed, will add extra layers of anxiety or guilt or pain for many women, unless and until women are helped to understand why they did not succeed at breastfeeding.

Giving up does cause enormous grief for many, and for some that pain is healed only when they have successfully breastfed a subsequent child. We who work with women know all those feelings, and do our best to help women deal with them honestly. We know that while they feel guilt at not having achieved the best for their child, rage would be more appropriate. They have been betrayed.

Denial of dangers

Alas, some people live in a state of denial of such truths, because they are painful. Older mothers, some dealing with children's health, behaviour or learning problems, angrily reject all information that suggests that these problems might be related to premature weaning. Some even consider that society must not publish any such facts if they make parents feel anxious or guilty, and until recently that was the understood self-censoring role of the media.

But science is finally catching up with commerce, and asking the questions about infant feeding that should have been asked before formula use was ever widespread.

The powerful emotions generated by breastfeeding failure can be transmuted into anger at society's role in undermining breastfeeding, and a commitment to work so that other women and children do not have to suffer, because they are helped to succeed. Let's not patronise parents and deny truth by attempting to conceal three inescapable facts:

- Artificial feeding is risky, probably the largest uncontrolled in vivo experiment in human history, and the costs to society and the planet beggar belief. A Jewish rabbi called it a Holocaust every year: 1.5 million child deaths annually for want of breastfeeding. Infant formula is a fallible, second-rate, industrially-manufactured substitute that can never hope to match breastmilk, even if it could be safely produced, afforded, stored, prepared and used.

- Lactation is powerful and almost all women can breastfeed. Women fail to breastfeed for avoidable and manageable social reasons which are beyond their control and overdue for change.

- Children, families and society pay the price of artificial feeding, while multinational companies – and the rich who own them – profit from their misery.

Successful preterm breastfeeding

Elizabeth Jones   Andy Spencer

There have been enormous advances in both technology and neonatal expertise in the last decade. It is no longer unusual for infants born as early as 24 weeks' gestation to survive, leaving both neonatologists and parents with innumerable problems.

The birth of a premature infant is a frightening crisis for parents. The decision to breastfeed may be directly influenced by the birth of a sick neonate, since the provision of breast milk is often the only tangible contribution to infant care a mother can make, when all other care is performed by nurses and physicians.[1]

Success at North Staffs

Despite the enormous importance of lactation to this vulnerable population, many women fail to sustain lactation in the stressful environment of a neonatal unit. Lactation failure not only deprives infants of the benefits of their mother's milk, but also may reinforce negative maternal feelings of inadequacy and guilt.[2] Breastfeeding failure is not inevitable following preterm birth; it is perfectly feasible to sustain lactation for many weeks using manual milk expression. The establishment of successful preterm breastfeeding is also achievable, if mothers are supported by expert guidance and support.

In 1995, an internal audit on the North Staffs Neonatal Unit revealed that 65% of babies were discharged breastfeeding. The aim of this paper is to outline the specific lactation management guidelines and breastfeeding interventions which we have found to be helpful in supporting a positive feeding outcome[3] and which we consider led to this high success rate.

The special qualities of preterm milk

Preterm mothers' own milk differs in composition from that of a mother who has delivered at term. Specifically, preterm milk has significantly higher concentrations of lipids, protein, sodium, calcium and selected immunoglobulins.[4] The low osmolarity of human milk and the presence of immunoglobulins are thought to help an immature gastro-intestinal tract to adapt to enteral nutrition.[5]

Human milk also contains growth factors, hormones and lipases which all contribute to both the tolerance and utilisation of nutrients. The type of fat that is fed to the preterm infant is thought to be important in terms of growth and development.[6] Human milk contains long chain polyunsaturated omega-3 fatty acids, which are suggested to be essential for the myelination of neural membranes, retinal function, and brain development.[7] Although preterm formulas now contain a supply of long chain polyunsaturated fatty acids, their absorption is less than that for infants fed human milk.[8]

Preterm infants have a reduced ability to utilise dietary lipids, due to a reduction in pancreatic lipases. The enzymes in human milk help to improve the efficiency of fat breakdown, leading to better absorption.

Meeting energy requirements

When enteral feeds are commenced, tiny babies are often fed by feeding tubes, which are passed from the mouth or nose to the stomach. Fat globules often adhere to the sides of feeding tubes, which reduces significantly the quality of the milk received.[9] Furthermore, if milk ejection is not sustained, an infant may be fed primarily on fore-milk, which can lead to sub-optimal nutrition. Preterm babies require a good energy source both for growth and development, and to maintain an adequate body temperature.

If an infant's energy requirements are not met by expressed breast milk there is often a practical solution. It is important to observe a mother while she is expressing. Her technique may be poor, or she may have unrealistic expectations about the time required. If her technique is good, and the volume of milk is adequate, the baby can be fed on 'hind milk'. In samples of expressed milk obtained from mothers on the neonatal unit, the fat content increased by two-thirds from the start to the end of the feed.[10]

Sometimes, to achieve adequate growth, it is necessary to supplement human milk with a nutritional fortifier. The use of human milk fortifiers should not be used routinely, but can be useful when other measures fail. Human milk is low in protein and a low urea and albumin level in the baby indicates the need for supplementation.

Many women feel disappointed by the suggestion of milk fortification, but should be reassured that additives are usually only needed as a short-term measure. The nutritional and immunological advantages of expressed milk are important, and supplementation is only needed temporarily, to help an infant become strong enough to successfully breastfeed. All low birth weight infants need supplementation with vitamins, iron, and minerals.[10]

Starting lactation

The most appropriate time to initiate lactation is in the immediate postpartum period. It is thought that early milk removal creates the optimum impetus for the development and sensitivity of prolactin receptors, which ensure early milk production.[11] In reality, early preterm milk expression can be very hard to achieve, particularly if infant survival is in doubt. It is almost as if making a feeding choice forces a strong commitment to the future – a commitment which is impossible to make. Also, many of the women who deliver preterm infants are forced to do so due to obstetric complications, and are often unwell in the immediate postpartum period. On our unit there is often a time lag from delivery to the first milk expression, and the expression schedule may be erratic during the early days.

The earlier a mother delivers the more difficult it appears to be to sustain lactation. Mammary development may be poor,[12] and fatigue, stress and anxiety are all powerful inhibitors of lactation.[1] The performance of oxytocin in promoting milk ejection is easily inhibited, and without a strong trigger, its pulsatile action is difficult to sustain. Locally active suppressor peptides are also thought to reduce the volume of milk produced if they are allowed to concentrate through infrequent or inadequate breast emptying.[13] Sadly, a poor milk volume followed by declining production is often associated with preterm delivery.[14]

We discussed earlier the importance of prolactin in the establishment of a milk supply. However, the role of prolactin is thought to be crucial not only as an impetus to milk production, but in all areas of mammary development. Both oestrogen and progesterone in pregnancy have long been recognised as important hormones in the preparation of mammary tissue for lactation. However prolactin also appears to aid antenatal mammary development by ensuring ductal growth.[13] During the early postnatal period it then provides the trigger for milk production. Thus prolactin appears to be active throughout the course of lactation;[15] efficient prolactin cycling may well prove to be the key to sustaining lactation following maternal/infant separation.

Techniques to increase supply

A study to compare the effect of different methods of manual expression on prolactin levels suggests that double pumping produces significantly higher prolactin levels than other methods of milk removal.[16] A recent randomised controlled trial at the North Staffs in which single (sequential) pumping and double (simultaneous) pumping were compared on a population dependent on manual expression to sustain lactation, showed very significantly that women allocated to use a double pump produced both higher volumes of milk and fat concentration than those using a single pump.[17] Women using a double pumping system often produced milk in excess of infant requirement, which avoided the sequelae of anxiety and frustration that a poor milk supply often causes.

Erratic or delayed oxytocin response is a common problem associated with long-term pumping.[18] Many studies from the dairy industry support the importance of eliciting milk ejection prior to milk removal.[19] Although animal studies can only provide a frame of reference, lactation experts in the United States suggest that if milk ejection is not triggered prior to pumping, both nipples and breast tissue may be exposed to high levels of vacuum, resulting in mammary tissue trauma.[20] In our recent trial in which women acted as their own control for breast massage, paired data suggested that massage was highly effective in promoting milk ejection, especially when single (sequential) pumping was utilised. Milk removal time and milk yield were also improved.[17]

The technique of milk expression is also very important. Women should be advised to sit comfortably with a straight back. Before positioning the milk collection set it may help to support the breast from underneath, with fingers flat on the ribs, and the index finger at the junction of the breast and ribs. This will support the breast tissue forward into the funnel, which should be placed with the nipple central. The funnel should be held close enough to mammary tissue to obtain a patent seal, but not so firmly to the breast that milk flow is inhibited. Women must be advised to use only as much suction as is needed to obtain milk flow, since unnecessary pressure may cause mammary trauma. Frequent expression is essential, and we advise at least six to eight sessions in 24 hours, including at least one night expression.

Preterm breastfeeding

Mothers of preterm infants should be encouraged to touch and caress their tiny babies. As soon as an infant is stable, skin-to-skin contact between mother and baby should be started, since it encourages a mother to gain confidence in handling her tiny infant, and allows the baby access to the breast. Tiny babies respond favourably to tactile and olfactory stimuli, and often surprise both parents and neonatal staff by their innate ability to feed. Preterm infants are only able to tolerate limited sensory stimulation, and the desire to sleep may override the ability to feed. Mothers have to be very patient during this transitional period.

It is often very helpful for a mother to stimulate milk flow by expression prior to a breastfeed so that energy can be conserved by the provision of post-ejection milk. An underarm breastfeeding position works very well, since the baby's body is in a position of flexion, which promotes a coordinated oral response. His head can also be easily controlled by his mother's hand, and an underarm position provides eye contact between mother and infant.

By using hand expression, a stream of milk can be expressed to provide olfactory and sensory stimuli. Preterm babies often exhibit extreme excitement by nuzzling closer and licking the milk with their tongues. Sometimes they simply open their mouths and swallow the milk, which is expressed directly into their mouth. When the stimulation becomes overwhelming, they abruptly go to sleep.[10]

The disparity between breast and mouth size does not seem to be a significant problem. Nipple tissue is very elastic, and even when very tiny, the infant appears to be able to draw the nipple deep into the mouth so that it is wedged between the tongue and the palate. The photograph at the beginning of this article shows an infant born at 27 weeks' gestation enjoying a breastfeed when only 31 weeks old. What can take some time to develop is a rhythmic suckling pattern. Initially, due to poor suck/swallow/breathe coordination, the sucks may appear in isolation. Later, there may be long pauses between bursts of sucks. Positive steps should be taken at this stage to ensure an early transition from non-nutritive to functional suckling.

Cup feeding

Cup feeding can be a very useful tool to promote the early acquisition of oral skills. Cup feeding accelerates the transition from naso-gastric to established functional breastfeeding by providing a positive way to learn suck/swallow/breathe co-ordination.

Cup feeding also provides a way to supplement poor breastfeeds, without the introduction of feeding bottles and teats. It is important to remember the pulsatile nature of oxytocin. Unless an infant has the ability to accomplish nutritive suckling, the flow of milk will be inhibited, compromising both the quality and volume of a feed.

The transition to home

The period immediately following discharge from the neonatal unit is a time of extreme vulnerability for mothers, and may precipitate a breastfeeding crisis. A major problem for the mother of a premature baby is that breastfeeding advice given in hospital and at home by community midwives and health visitors may be in conflict. A discharge plan involving breastfeeding should be made in conjunction with parents to provide continuity of care and anticipatory advice.

Giving a mother telephone support numbers and open access to hospital breastfeeding coordinators can also make an enormous difference to parents by providing a help line for emergency situations such as refusal to feed or significant weight loss.

Planning well in advance, often in conjunction with voluntary help organisations, will help to alleviate parental anxiety by providing a raft of practical breastfeeding support.

REFERENCES

1   Meier P, Brown L. State of the Science: Breastfeeding for mothers and low birth weight infants. Nurs Clin North Am 1996; 31(2):351–365.
2   Jones E. Strategies to promote preterm breastfeeding. MIDIRS 1995; 5(2):8–11.
3   Spencer SA, Jones E, Woods A. Breastfeeding: A multimedia resource for healthcare professionals. Matrix Multimedia; 1998.
4   Gross SJ, Slagle TA. Feeding the low birth weight infant. Clin Perinatol 1993; 20:193.
5   Lucas A, Cole TJ. Breast milk and necrotising enterocolitis. Lancet 1990; 336:1519–1523.
6   Lucas A, Morley R, Cole T, et al. Breast milk and subsequent intelligence quotient in children born preterm. Lancet 1992; 339:261–264.
7   Uauy R, Birch D, Birch E, et al. Effect of dietary omega-3 fatty acids on retinal function of very-low-birth-weight neonates. Pediatr Res 1990; 28:485–492.

8   Morgan C, Stammers J, Colley J, et al. Long chain polyunsaturated acids (LCP) absorption in preterm infants. Early Hum Dev 1994; 39:153–156.

9   Spencer SA, Hull D. Fat content of expressed breast milk: A case for quality control. BMJ 1981; 282:99–100.

10 Jones E, Spencer SA. Promoting preterm breastfeeding. New Generation Digest 1998; June: 4–6.

11 Neifert M, Seacat J, Gobe W. Lactation failure due to insufficient glandular development of the breast. Pediatr 1985; 76(5):823–828.

12 Ellis L, Picciano MF. Prolactin variants in term and preterm milk: Altered structural characteristic, biological activity and immunoreactivity. Endocrine Regulation 1993; 27:193–200

13 Prentice A, Addey C, Wilde C. Evidence for local feedback control of human milk. Biochem Soc Trans 1989; 17:489–492.

14 Hopkinson J, Schauler C, Garza C. Milk production by mothers of preterm infants. Pediatr 1974; 18:815–820.

15 Yuen BH. Prolactin in human milk. The influence of nursing and duration of postpartum lactation. Am J Obstet Gynecol 1988; 158:583–586.

16 Zinnamen M. Acute prolactin, oxytocin response and milk yield to infant suckling: Artificial methods of expression in lactating women. Pediatr 1992; 89:437–440.

17 Jones E, Spencer SA [unpublished data]

18 Walker M, Driscoll M. Breastfeeding your premature or special care baby. Weston MA: Lactation Associates; 1989.

19 Gorevit R. Current concepts on the role of oxytocin in milk ejection. J Dairy Sci 1983; 66:2236–2250.

20 Walker M, Auerbach K. Breast pumps and other technologies. In: Riordan R, Auerbach K (eds). Breastfeeding and human lactation. Jones and Bartlett; 279–332.

Intrauterine pollution and human milk pollution

Michel Odent

The effects of pollution during the 'primal period' represent one of the most serious threats to health that humanity has to face at the turn of the century. The primal period includes fetal life and the year following birth. Any event during these critical phases of development can have irreversible effects.[1]

Midwives, and all those interested in the health of the unborn generations, need to be aware of a few facts:

- We all have in our bodies between 300 and 500 synthetic industrial chemicals that would not have been there 50 years ago, because at that time they did not exist.[2]
- Most of these synthetic chemicals collect and accumulate over the years in the fatty tissues (they are fat soluble). They are passed on to the next generation across the placenta and via breast milk.
- These chemicals interfere with fetal growth and development through a multitude of mechanisms.

Although the same fat-soluble chemicals are present at different phases of the primal period, the issues of intrauterine pollution and of human milk pollution are somewhat different. Intrauterine pollution occurs at an earlier stage of human development and is therefore potentially more serious. Also, the transfer of pollutants through the placenta is unavoidable, whereas, after birth, there is a choice between human milk and formula. In formulae milk lipids are replaced by lipids of vegetable origin with a negligible content of fat-soluble chemicals.

Midwives would benefit from an increased understanding of the main families of pollutants that can interfere with the development of human beings:

- The term 'dioxin' encompasses a family of 219 different, toxic, chlorinated chemicals. They are by-products of the manufacture of organochlorine chemicals and may be emitted by garbage incinerators.
- PCBs (polychlorinated biphenyls) are a group of more

than 200 related compounds which have been used in the manufacture of electronic equipment. In spite of strict regulations in the 1970s, they are still present in human adipose tissues.
- The APEs (alkylphenol polyethoxylates) are the second biggest group of non-ionic detergents in commercial production.
- The chemical biphenol-A forms part of the epoxyresins group, which are used to coat tins.
- The phtalates (pronouced 'thalates') are added to polyvinyl chlorine plastics (PVC) to make them soft (many medical plastics are made from phtalates containing PVC).
- Trans fatty acids represent another group of fat-soluble pollutants. These artificial molecules (almost unknown in nature) were introduced into the human diet during the 20th century with the processing of oils; today they are abundant in such food as cakes, biscuits, French fries, fast foods etc.
- Heavy metals, in particular mercury.

Some new aspects of ill health in the population born after 1950 seem to be specifically related to intrauterine pollution. The best known example is the spectacular fall of the average sperm count since the middle of this century.[3,4] During the same period the number of abnormalities of the penis (in particular hypospadias) has increased,[5] and also the number of undescended testicles.[6] Another concomitant phenomenon is the increased incidence of testicular cancer. The current interpretation for the greater frequency of such ill-health problems is that many artificial chemicals disrupt the endocrine system during important phases of fetal development. More precisely many of them are deemed 'oestrogen mimics'.

Certain questions are specifically related to infant feeding. The main one is undoubtedly: Do the well-known benefits of breastfeeding outweigh the theoretical risks associated with human milk pollution? Such an unpalatable question has to be asked at a time when the high degree of milk pollution is well established.[7] For example, according to a WHO survey, the daily estimated dietary intake of dioxins and PCBs by breastfed infants in 1993-94 was 170pg per kg body weight at two months, and 39pg at ten months.[8] The tolerable daily intake according to the WHO is 10pg (the tolerable levels are based on lifetime exposure). The most authoritative answers to such questions are provided by two Dutch studies.[9,10] According to these 18-month follow-up studies, for the time being the conclusion is that the advantages of breastfeeding outweigh the risks. In the near future the results of follow-up studies among school age children will be published.

There is no advantage in reducing the duration of breastfeeding since the milk becomes less polluted as lactation progresses.

It would be more logical to try to renew the adipose tissues in which fat-soluble chemicals accumulate over the years before conceiving a baby. This is the objective of our newly-established 'preconceptional fat renewal' sessions. The programme includes a series of short, semi-fasting sessions, so that each fast weight loss is immediately followed by a fast weight recovery ('the accordion method').

Recommendations

If pregnant and lactating women follow these recommendations they will minimise the effects of intrauterine pollution and milk pollution:

- Wash fruit and vegetables. Peeling may be safer.
- Eat organic food whenever possible.
- Limit the consumption of fatty dairy products.
- Prefer lean meat to fat meat.
- When eating poultry, avoid the skin.
- Avoid freshwater fish. Prefer fish from the sea. If you take supplements, avoid fish liver oils. Prefer fish oils (made from the flesh of the fish).
- Go for products from the beginning of the food chain rather than those at the end; taking the example of seafood, sardines are not polluted whereas sharks are highly polluted and tuna fish are moderately polluted.
- Avoid losing weight too fast when breastfeeding. In 1990 I described the 'slimming nursing mother syndrome'[11] after hearing breastfeeding mothers report that their babies became unwell whenever they lost weight.

These recommendations can only have limited effects if they are followed after conception.

REFERENCES

1 Odent M. Primal health. London: Century-Hutchinson; 1986.
2 Howard V. Synergistic effects of chemical mixtures – can we rely on traditional toxicity? The Ecologist 1997; 27(5):192–195.
3 Carlsen E, Giwercman A, Keiding N, et al. Evidence for decreasing quality of semen during the past 50 years. BMJ 1992; 305:609–613.
4 Auger J, Kunstmann JM, Czyglik F, et al. Decline in semen quality among fertile men in Paris during the past 20 years. N Engl J Med 1995; 332:281–285.
5 Giwercman A, Skakkeback NE. The human testis – an organ at risk? Int J Androl 1992; 15:373–375.
6 Jackson MB. John Radcliffe Hospital cryptorchidism research group. The epidemiology of cryptorchidism. Horm Res 1988; 30:153–156.

7 Lyons G. Chemical trespass: a toxic legacy. World Wildlife Fund – UK Toxic Programme Report. Godalming: WWF; 1999.
8 Wise J. High amounts of chemicals found in breast milk. BMJ 1997; 314:1505.
9 Huisman M, Koopman-Esseboom C, et al. Neurological condition in 18-month-old children perinatally exposed to polychlorinated biphenyls and dioxins. Early Hum Dev 1995; 43:165–76.
10 Koopman-Esseboom C, Weisglas-Kuperus N, et al. Effects of polychlorinated biphenyl/dioxin exposure and feeding type on infants' mental and psychomotor development. Pediatrics 1996; 97:700–706.
11 Odent M. The unknown human infant. J Human Lact 1990; 6(1):6–8.

Breastfeeding: early problems

Sally Inch   Chloe Fisher

Among the most common problems for new mothers are engorgement, sore nipples, difficult attachment, babies that are difficult to settle – and babies who do not want to feed at all!

Sore, damaged and blanching nipples

These are almost always the result of incorrect attachment. If the baby has not been enabled to take a good mouthful of breast so that the nipple reaches the junction of his hard and soft palate, his tongue will compress the nipple against his hard palate as he feeds. Repeated compression of the nipple will usually result in damage. Depending on the design of the breast, the damage may be at the tip or the base. Some women experience intense nipple pain after a feed, accompanied by an obvious change in the nipple from its normal pink to a pinched, white colour. This occurs more often in women who have a history of Raynaud's phenomenon (fingertips going 'dead' in cold weather) but is usually a sign that the nipple is being traumatised during the feed as a result of incorrect attachment.

What works

- Exactly which aspect of the process of attachment needs attention is most easily determined by watching the mother put the baby to the breast. The clinic's 16-point checklist, reproduced here, encapsulates the positive aspects of the process, and the mother will have her attention drawn to the particular point to which she needs to pay attention. However, on the opposite side, the checklist records what we are actually seeing (see Table 8.6.1). Some mothers find it useful to know what specifically they were doing wrong, as well as what they need to do to put it right. The information on the checklist can also be shared with her midwife or health visitor.

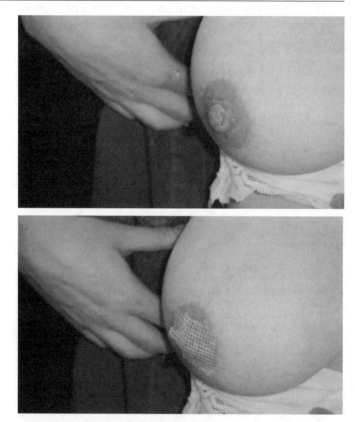

Figure 8.6.1 Cracked nipple, and dressing

- If the mother cannot tolerate the idea of feeding, we would suggest that she express her colostrum/milk for a day or two until her nipples have healed and then help her to improve the attachment when she is ready. Breast pumps, if not used judiciously, may make the damage worse, in which case hand expressing is preferable.
- If the nipple is so damaged that it has formed a scab which will crack and bleed when the nipple is stretched, small squares of sterilised gauze

The clinic checklist

Information for the health professional caring for:

Name:...

This mother and baby were seen in the Breastfeeding Clinic today:

Date:...

The presenting problems were:

....

The following recommendations were made (tick as appropriate):

☐ to find somewhere to sit at home that will reproduce the posture adopted in the clinic, i.e. straight back and almost flat lap

☐ to use a pillow to take the baby's weight while learning

☐ to sit with her back well supported and straight, and her trunk facing forward

☐ to support the baby or place him on a pillow in such a way that his nose (not mouth) is in line with the nipple before the feed begins

☐ to lay the baby's body in such a way that the baby comes up to the breast from below, so that the baby's upper eye could make contact with the mother's

☐ to support the breast by placing the fingers flat on the ribcage at the junction of the breast and ribs, with the thumb uppermost, thus firming the inner tissue

☐ to support the breast with a tubigrip 'sling' as well as the fingers before feeding

☐ to move the baby against the breast so that his mouth touches the nipple in order to elicit the gape

☐ having elicited the gape, to move the baby quickly to the breast so that his mouth makes contact with the breast at the height of the gape

☐ to support the baby's head and shoulders in such a way that the head is free to extend slightly as the baby is brought to the breast, so that the chin and lower jaw reach the breast first

☐ to bring the baby towards the breast, with slight pressure behind his shoulders, so that he is 'uncurled'. This will have the effect of bringing his tongue closer to the breast

☐ to aim the baby's bottom lip and jaw as far away as possible from the base of the nipple when he gapes, so that he scoops in as much breast as possible with his tongue

☐ to wrap the baby so that his arms are lying parallel with his body before he is brought to the breast, so that he can be closer to the breast

☐ to change hands, and hold the baby with the hand opposite the breast being fed from, while learning

☐ to hold the baby under her arm on the less easy side, so as to do the same job with the same hands for both breasts

☐ to use a small piece of paraffin gauze to prevent the damaged area of the nipple from forming a hard scab which sticks to the pad or clothing.

impregnated with yellow paraffin over the nipple (and under a breast pad) will prevent the damaged area from drying out. This is available, over the counter or on prescription, as 'Jelonet', 'Unitulle' or 'Parartulle'. Alternatively, a tube of soft white paraffin, kept just for the nipple and applied with clean fingers, will do just as well and is much cheaper. There is evidence that a superficial, clean wound will heal more rapidly if it is kept moist, and this is now the basis of modern superficial wound healing.[1]

What may work

Nipple shields are sometimes helpful and may reduce nipple pain for some women. Others find that shields make the pain worse. Their use does nothing to improve attachment.

They should never be used before the milk is in, as in this situation it is unlikely that the baby will be able to draw enough colostrum through the shield to satisfy his requirements.

(Before the milk is in, the mother would do better to express colostrum and give that to her baby.)

Nipple shields are essentially a way of marking time until the mother can get the help she needs to resolve the underlying problem. Their main disadvantage is that they often interfere with the transfer of milk and this may affect the baby's weight gain. If nipple shields are used for any length of time the mother's milk supply may start to diminish. Alternatively inefficient milk removal may result in engorgement and sometimes even mastitis.

(Although we do occasionally use nipple shields in the clinic, we never recommend them for sore/damaged nipples.)

What doesn't work

- Proprietory creams, lotions, sprays and so on do not, on their own, heal damaged nipples, regardless of the claims of the manufacturers. Greasy creams may help in the same way that paraffin gauze does, but only in conjunction with improving attachment.
- The frequently-repeated advice to expose damaged nipples to the air in a bid to aid healing, or to apply breastmilk to the nipples after the feed. Both of these measures will almost certainly result in the formation of scabs.[1]

Engorgement

Engorgement usually affects both breasts and is generally the result of inefficient milk removal, secondary to poor attachment (or infrequent expression, if the baby is not

Figure 8.6.2 Mother's eye view of breastfeeding

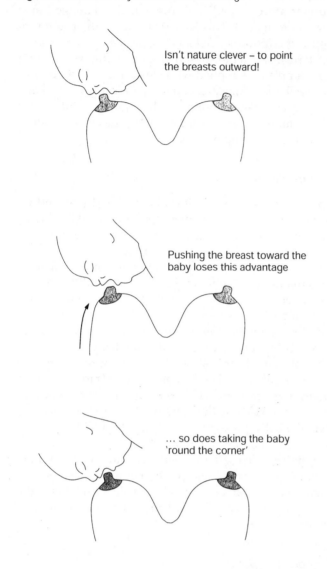

Isn't nature clever – to point the breasts outward!

Pushing the breast toward the baby loses this advantage

… so does taking the baby 'round the corner'

Table 8.6.1 The clinic checklist – observations

The mother's feeding technique was studied. She was:

☐ not placing the baby in front of the breast

☐ placing the baby square to her body instead of her breast

☐ trying to aim the nipple to the 'centre' of the baby's mouth

☐ putting the breast into the baby's mouth instead of bringing the baby to the breast

☐ flexing the baby's head as he comes to the breast (see diagram 'Isn't nature clever…')

☐ bringing the baby to the breast with the nose instead of the chin making the first contact (see diagram 'Isn't nature clever…')

☐ not eliciting a proper gape before moving the baby to the breast

☐ not bringing the baby to the breast quickly enough having elicited the gape

☐ twisting her body towards the baby instead of slightly away

☐ pushing her breast into the midline (see diagram 'Isn't nature clever…')

☐ 'chasing' the baby with her breast

☐ 'flapping' her breast up and down

☐ using a scissor grip to hold the breast

☐ providing no breast support

☐ holding the breast away from the baby's nose

☐ pushing the baby's chin down to open the mouth

☐ trying to attach the baby while he was crying.

What may work

• Cold compresses, cabbage leaves, cold flannels and anti-inflammatory drugs – to reduce swelling.
• Warm flannels, immersing the breasts in warm water (shower or bath) – to encourage milk flow.

There is no good evidence to guide practice, so the mother should do whatever she finds most helpful to relieve her discomfort.

What doesn't work

• Treating only the symptoms for fear of 'over-stimulating the supply'.

Untreated engorgement is a self-limiting condition – if the pressure in the breasts is raised and milk accumulates, milk production will be switched off and the swelling will subside. However the mother's milk supply may by that time be a long way behind her baby's needs, which will cause other problems.

Difficult attachment

If attachment is difficult for the mother it is most likely to be because she has not had sufficient practice. Talking

going to the breast). The areola is often oedematous, which makes attachment difficult. It is essential to encourage milk flow and milk removal, as prolonged engorgement will cause milk production to begin to be suppressed.

What works

• Attaching the baby well – if possible.
• Softening the breast by gently pushing away the oedema with the fingers may enable the baby to attach well and he will then relieve the breast.
• Gentle expressing, by hand or with a pump, may also soften the breast so that the baby can attach.

If it is not possible to attach the baby, attempt gentle expression every two to three hours until the milk begins to flow or the baby can be attached.

her through it may be all that she needs. If she needs to be helped, we would explain what we were doing and why. (An often-repeated complaint from women is that the helper 'just attached the baby and left'.)

If attachment is difficult for the mother because the breast tissue is inelastic but we are able to attach the baby well, we could reassure her that breast tissue changes quite dramatically during the first week and a few good feeds may be all that are necessary before she can attach her baby herself.

If we are not able to attach the baby either, we would show the mother how to hand express, how to give her colostrum to her baby and how to use the electric pump.

In the first 24-48 hours the value of the pump is mainly in its effect on the nipple and breast tissue – colostrum is usually best expressed by hand.

We would never use a nipple shield as part of the management unless the mother had an established milk supply. Nipple shields are not a substitute for good attachment and they are usually a poor substitute for a breast pump.

If the mother did not seem to be able to express enough to meet her baby's needs in the first 72 hours, her baby could be given banked EBM or 10% dextrose – with the mother's written consent. Women's Centre staff try to avoid giving a breastfed baby formula as they know that any formula at all is enough to sensitise susceptible infants. This is explained to the mother if she requests formula.

Great care should be taken when dealing with a baby who is difficult to attach. Repeated failed attempts may produce either frustration or lethargy in the baby. If the health professional applies pressure to the back of the baby's head as she tries to attach the baby, the baby may start to associate the breast with unpleasant experiences. Any other means of satisfying the baby's hunger may then be preferred by the baby who will 'refuse' subsequent attempts to attach him to the breast.

In these circumstances we have found it preferable to stop attempting to attach the baby and give expressed colostrum/milk before the baby manifests distress, and try again later.

We feel it is more important to enable the mother to feed the baby (with her expressed colostrum/milk) and to establish her lactation (by expressing) than to struggle to get the baby directly to the breast.

If attachment continues to be difficult but the mother wants to go home, she will need to borrow a pump (unless she can hand express adequate volumes). This is in order to maintain her lactation and feed her baby while she is learning. For some women, a hand pump may be adequate; we use the Avent Isis.

Electric pumps can be borrowed from the Breastfeeding Clinic, the mother's local health centre or hospital, or in

Table 8.6.2 Breastmilk production from birth

Age of the baby	Volume per day		Volume per feed	
	Range	Average	Average	Refs
Day 1 (0-24 hours)	7-123ml	37ml	7ml	1,3,5
Day 2 (24-48 hours)	44-335ml	84ml	14ml	3
Day 3 (48-72 hours)	98-775ml	408ml	38ml	1,2,3
Day 4 (72-96 hours)	375-876ml	625ml		1,3
Day 5 (96-120 hours)	452-876 ml	700ml	70ml	1,3
3 months	609-837ml	750ml		4
6 months		800ml		

References

1 Saint L, Smith M, Harmann P. The yield and nutrient content of colostrum and milk from giving birth to 1 month postpartum. British Journal of Nutrition 1984; 52:87–95.

2 Neville M, et al. Studies in human lactation: Milk volumes in lactating women during the onset of lactation and full lactation. American Society for Clinical Nutrition 1988; 48:1375–1386.

3 Houston MJ, Howie P, McNeilly AS. Factors affecting the duration of breastfeeding: 1. Measurement of breastmilk intake in the first week of life. Early Human Development 1983; 8:49–54.

4 Butte N, Garza C, O'Brien Smith E, et al. Human milk intake and growth in exclusively breastfed infants. Journal of Pediatrics 1984; 104:187–195.

5 Roderuck C, Williams HH, Macy IG. Journal of Nutrition 1946; 32:267–283.

some circumstances from SCBU. They can also be hired from the NCT/La Leche League at a daily rate, or from the manufacturers (Medela or Egnell-Ameda) at a monthly rate. (All clinical areas have these details.)

The mother will also need to know where she can obtain on-going help with attachment – in our area this is done by ensuring that before she goes home she is given a small white postcard on which are written all the details that she needs.

Unsettled baby

A baby that is crying again soon after he has been fed may not have been well attached. We would watch what the mother was doing and apply all the information in 'Breastfeeding... getting the basics right'.[2]

If the attachment is good, then the baby may be reacting to being removed from the closeness of his mother's body. If the mother needs to sleep, we would suggest that she feeds lying down and help her if necessary. (The short edge of a pillow placed under her ribcage at the junction of her breast and ribs may make attachment easier, as her breast is raised from the mattress.) The use of cot sides will ensure that the mother and baby can safely be left to sleep in a hospital bed.

Some babies will appear unsettled even if they have fed well at the breast. Their discomfort may not be caused by hunger and other means could be used to comfort them.

Wrapping the baby comfortably but securely and providing rhythmic motion, such as walking, may help to settle the baby.

The baby can be returned to the breast, with attention paid to the quality of attachment, if the baby remains unsettled.

The mother might try to express some colostrum/milk to give to the baby if she is concerned that the baby has not received all that he might from the breast.

Sleepy baby

The Women's Centre policy has recently been revised to bring it into line with *National Guidelines on Hypoglycaemia of the Newborn*. A copy of this document has been supplied to every clinical area and to each of the community hospitals.

It is acknowledged that these guidelines do not apply to the 10% of all babies who are at increased risk of developing hypoglycaemia.

Babies at increased risk include:

- preterm babies (< 37 weeks' gestation)
- small for dates babies
- babies weighing less than 2.5kg
- infants of diabetic mothers
- infants who are 'sick', e.g. birth asphyxia or infection.

However most of these babies will already be receiving special or intensive care, and all will be under paediatric surveillance.

The remaining 90% will be healthy term infants, many of whom will feed infrequently in the first 24 hours of their life. As few as three feeds in 24 hours is within the normal range and they may take, on average, as little as 7ml per feed (see Table 8.6.2). It has been shown to be unhelpful and unnecessary to measure the blood sugar levels of a healthy term infant, and this practice has now been abandoned in the Women's Centre.

The guidelines require that the feeding history of all babies is reviewed at eight hours of age, taking into consideration the notes made by the midwife caring for the mother and baby in the labour ward in relation to the baby's first feed, if one has taken place.

If there is concern about the infrequency of the feeds in the first 24 hours, attempts can be made to rouse the baby, perhaps by changing the nappy or by giving a gentle massage and then the baby can be offered the breast. If it is not possible to interest the baby in breastfeeding, hand expressed colostrum can be given to the baby by syringe or cup.

If at any time the condition of the baby causes concern, or if the baby had shown no interest in feeding for 16 hours, regardless of whether it has received colostrum, a paediatrician would be asked to see the baby to exclude any underlying pathology.

REFERENCES

1 Huml S. Sore nipples: A new look at an old problem through the eyes of a dermatologist. The Practising Midwife 1999; 2(2):28–31.

2 Inch S, Fisher C. Breastfeeding: getting the basics right. The Practising Midwife 1999; 2(5):35–8.

Stop taking the baby!

Kate Olsen

As a student midwife in my final year I remember being ushered into delivery rooms by scary labour ward sisters as they announced that it was high time I learned to 'take the baby'. And so I did. There was no policy or job description from which to learn, but from observing other, more senior, midwives I gathered that the role of the baby-taker went something like this:

- Come into the room without introducing yourself and enthusiastically join in the second stage exhortations to push, whilst peering at the CTG with a frown.
- Draw up the syntometrine, ready to inject into the woman's thigh at the appropriate point in the proceedings.
- As soon as the baby is born, the cord is clamped and the mother has glimpsed its genitalia, briskly and efficiently wrap it in several layers of tightly and cunningly folded hospital towels, as all newborn babies are at great risk of hypothermia. If he or she needs resuscitating, they will be at even greater risk of hypothermia, so do whatever resuscitation is necessary (on the resuscitaire, of course) and wrap the vulnerable baby in twice as many towelling layers as usual.
- The 'baby-taker' then has the great privilege of ceremonially presenting this precious parcel to its eagerly waiting mother. How I loved that part!

Ever keen to be a good student I watched and learnt. There was a great art to this towel folding and wrapping; my first few attempts had the towel flapping loosely around the baby as it wriggled both arms free and it ended up looking more like a roman toga around the baby's navel. This would never do. But I persisted and soon became very gratified by my neatly-swaddled babies, safely protected from the cold air and all its dangers.

I qualified at last, and over the next few years proudly passed on my technique to students following on behind me. I was a proper midwife. Now I look back, aghast, as I realise what damage I've (unwittingly) done.

Separating all those babies from their mothers over the years has put them at greater risk of the very things I was trying to protect them from. Babies who are taken away from their mothers at birth, to be wrapped up by a well-meaning midwife, are prevented from receiving skin-to-skin contact with their mothers in their first hour of life. Wrapping babies at birth, so much a part of everyday hospital routine, puts them at greater risk of hypothermia and hypoglycaemia, and significantly reduces their chances of breastfeeding successfully. The research findings in this area are clear:

- Newborns find their mother's breast partly by smell – clothing, wrapping in hospital towels and separation interferes with this instinctive natural process.[1,2]
- Newborns are much less likely to show the unique behaviour of gradually becoming more active, beginning to root and then successfully suckling within the first hour of life. They are at least three times less likely to suckle successfully.[3-7]
- Babies who are separated from their mothers and left in cots (e.g. during suturing) display distressed behaviour and cry more.[5,8,9]
- Mothers whose babies have touched their nipples and areolae within the first half-hour of birth show increased nurturing behaviour – they talk to their babies for longer and leave them alone less. So mothers who plan to bottlefeed could still enjoy and benefit from this instinctive interaction.[5,10,11]
- Babies who are wrapped are more likely to get cold; the best way to warm a baby is for it to have skin-to-skin contact with its mother. This is an effective measure against hypothermia and hypoglycaemia, and has been shown to be more effective than being wrapped and put in a heated cot.[8,12,13] Left alone in a crib, babies are more at risk of getting cold and having low blood sugar levels. Skin-to-skin contact is

particularly important for babies who have had a traumatic birth, required resuscitation and who need to get warm. It needs to be resumed as quickly as possible after any resuscitation is complete.

- The blood chemistry of babies who have been acidotic or had a period of 'fetal distress' rectifies itself more quickly if a baby has skin-to-skin contact. Any negative base excess returns more rapidly to zero, and their blood glucose will be higher one or two hours following birth.[8]
- Early contact and suckling stimulate the uterus to contract and thus reduce the likelihood of postpartum haemorrhage.[14]
- Babies who have uninterrupted skin-to-skin contact at birth are much more likely to be breastfed for longer (with all the health benefits for mother and baby that breastfeeding brings). This effect can still be seen three months after the birth.[15]
- Mothers who are able to enjoy this first hour of uninterrupted contact with their new babies feel higher levels of satisfaction with motherhood and have more positive feelings overall.[16]

It seems that the first hour or so following birth is a magical, never-to-be-repeated time in which the baby and mother are exquisitely attuned to each other through their mutually high levels of oxytocin and endorphins. The baby intuitively knows how to find the nipple and latch on; and the mother who has nipple stimulation instinctively knows how to respond to her baby. Odent has explained how this oxytocin exchange is a biochemical code that creates nurturing behaviour.[17]

Every midwife knows that a successful feed in that first hour is worth ten feeds later on. A separation of even 20 minutes – say while a woman is being sutured – can have a detrimental effect which then may take hours of midwives' time and mothers' angst to undo. Skillful management of this time – it has been called the fourth stage of labour – is part of our role. So what might the assisting midwife usefully do when asked to go and 'take the baby'?

- Perhaps she could quietly ensure that the room is warm for the baby and that the primary midwife has everything she needs within reach.
- She might check that a warmed blanket is ready to wrap around the mother and her new baby.
- She could gently support and encourage the mother as she scoops her new baby into her arms, help her to dry the baby and then wrap a blanket around them and let them get to know each other in peace.
- At a traumatic instrumental birth where resuscitation has been necessary, she could help the mother resume calming, skin-to-skin contact as soon as practical.

Suturing, cups of tea, bathing, baby weighing and telephone calls can all then take their rightful place as supporting cast to this main event.

We are all familiar with the idea that you never separate a cat from its newborn kittens or disturb a new litter of puppies with their mother. It is rather bizarre that we needed to spend so much research time and money to convince ourselves that it is also a bad thing to do to human beings! Some women seem to know already: in a large survey about women's experiences of waterbirth, women answered 'I liked it because no one took my baby away from me when it was born'.[18]

My own practice in this area is evolving, and now I talk about it in antenatal classes and at birth preparation discussions with prospective parents, so they too can understand how special and unique the first hour or so after birth is. Then at the birth itself, midwives and fathers can both simply sit back in awe as nature works her magic between a woman and her baby.

Acknowledgment
Much of the research to support this article has been taken from: World Health Organisation. Evidence for the ten steps to successful breastfeeding. Geneva: World Health Organisation, 1998.

REFERENCES

1 Porter RH, Makin JW, Davis LB, et al. Breastfed infants respond to olfactory clues from their own mother and unfamiliar lactating females. Infant Behavioural Development 1992; 15:85–93.

2 Varendi H, Porter RH, Winberg J. Does the newborn baby find the nipple by smell? Lancet 1994; 344:989–990.

3 Righard L, Alade MO. Effect of delivery room routines on success of first breastfeed. Lancet 1990; 336(8723):1105–1107.

4 Sosa R, et al. The effect of early mother-infant contact on breastfeeding, infection and growth. In: Ciba Foundation Symposium 45: Breastfeeding and the mother. Amsterdam: Elsevier; 1976: 179–93.

5 de Chateau P, Wiberg B. Long-term effect on mother-infant behaviour of extra contact during the first hour postpartum: A follow up at three months. Acta Paediatrica 1977; 66:145–151.

6 Thomson ME, Hartsock TG, Larson C. The importance of immediate postnatal contact: Its effect on breastfeeding. Can Fam Physician 1979; 25:1374–1378.

7 Ali Z, Lowry M. Early maternal-child contact: Effects on later behaviour. Dev Med and Child Neurol 1981; 23:337–345.

8 Christensson K, et al. Temperature, metabolic adaptation and crying in healthy fullterm newborns cared for skin-to-skin or in a cot. Acta Paediatr 1992; 81:488–493.

9 Christensson K, et al. Separation distress call in the human neonate in the absence of maternal body contact. Acta Paediatr 1995; 84:468–473.

10 Rosenblatt JS. Psychobiology of maternal behaviour: Contribution to clinical understanding of maternal behaviour among humans. Acta Paediatrica Suppl 1994; 397:3–8.

11 Widstrom A-M, et al. Short-term effects of early suckling and touch of the nipple on maternal behaviour. Early Hum Dev 1990; 21:153–163.

12 British Association of Perinatal Medicine, National Childbirth Trust, Neonatal Nurses' Association, et al. Hypoglycaemia of the newborn: Guidelines for appropriate glucose screening and treatment of breastfed and bottlefed babies in the UK. London: NCT; 1997.

13 Fardig JA. A comparison of skin-to-skin contact and radiant heaters in promoting neonatal thermoregulation. J Nurse Midwifery 1980; 25(1):19–28.

14 Chua S, et al. Influence of breastfeeding and nipple stimulation on postpartum uterine activity. Br Obstet Gynaecol 1994; 101:804–805.

15 Perez-Escamilla R, et al. Infant feeding policies in maternity wards and their effect on breastfeeding success: An analytical overview. Am J Public Health 1994; 84(1):89–97.

16 Ball J. Reactions to motherhood: The role of postnatal care, 2nd edn. Hale: Books for Midwives Press; 1994.

17 Odent M. The scientification of love. London: Free Association Press; 1999.

18 Harris H. Women's experiences of waterbirth. Unpublished masters' dissertation; 1994.

Reflecting on breastfeeding

- Think about your own philosophical stance in relation to breastfeeding. How do you honestly feel about breastfeeding? Have you ever breastfed or would you choose to breastfeed? How might your philosophy affect the guidance and support that you offer to women?
- How much do you know about the Baby Friendly Initiative? Is it something that has been introduced or is planned within your area of practice? What factors do you feel would facilitate the successful introduction of the initiative, and which might militate against it?
- How might you advise a mother who asks you about the wisdom of breastfeeding when she lives within the vicinity of an industrial waste incinerator?
- If you were asked to produce a marketing policy for breastfeeding within your area, how would you carry out your market research? What sort of questions would allow you to obtain the kind of information necessary to formulate a marketing strategy?
- Does your practice area have guidelines for hand expression and cup/alternative feeding methods? Imagine that as a practice development midwife you have been asked to produce evidence-informed guidelines to support the practice within your workplace, as part of an initiative to increase the breastfeeding rate. What would you include?

Group exercise

This exercise will not only provide food for reflection on attending breastfeeding mothers, but on communication skills in general. One midwife/student acts as the breastfeeding mother, with a suitable doll playing the part of her baby, while another plays the midwife. The 'midwife' needs to verbally interact with the 'mother', but with her back turned – so without looking at what the mother is doing. The 'midwife' should describe the process by which the baby can be put on the breast, while the 'mother' follows her instructions, asking any questions as she needs to.

This exercise not only leads to reflection on how to assist women verbally as well as through non-verbal, touch and other forms of communication, but enables reflection on any differences between 'what we say' and 'what we mean'. Other midwives in attendance can watch and reflect on the interaction. If each person takes a turn in each role, deeper reflection can be achieved, as lessons learned from the first interactions are put into practice and further issues are raised.

Lorna Davies

Alternative therapies

If a traveller from another galaxy looked at the range of healing modalities used on Earth, they might be surprised at the relative weight of trust being put in Western medicine in relation to other theories of healing. If this space traveller also had access to the history of healing modalities which had been used on Earth since time began, they might wonder why it was that Western medicine, a relative newcomer to the range of tools we have for health improvement, was not labelled as the 'alternative' system. It is sometimes easy to forget that modern medicine has reached the prominence it has in the Western world as much through political and historical chance as because it has systematically enjoyed greater success at healing than other modalities.

Yet within the current context, it is these mostly older modalities of healing which have come to be described as 'complementary' or 'alternative' to Western medicine. Having set itself up as the Gold Standard, this medical system then imposes upon other modalities the need to prove themselves through the tools and trials of the medical system rather than by whatever means are considered appropriate with the original philosophy of the modality itself. Jilly Rosser explores issues linking the historical introduction of medical interventions with the use of alternative therapies within a framework of evidence-based practice, and highlights some of the paradoxes which should cause all midwives to pause for thought.

Myra Parsons and colleagues have grasped the challenge to evaluate alternative therapies within a quantitative framework, by setting up a placebo-controlled, randomised trial to evaluate products containing red raspberry leaf. Their small-scale study has led to the initiation of a larger Australian trial and demonstrates one way in which such therapies can be researched. Linda Kimber carried out a survey of women who experienced massage in labour and found that this was positively evaluated not only by women, but also by their partners – some of whom felt it helped them become more involved during labour.

The past few years have seen both the development of specific guidelines for midwives in relation to the use of alternative therapies (UKCC, 1994) and a significant increase in the number of midwives who are undertaking additional training in the use of alternative therapies. These midwives are experiencing differing degrees of success in their efforts to introduce alternative therapies within the current system of maternity care. Mandy Curry describes the way in which Sonia Gent's ideas and determination, coupled with support from midwifery management, enabled the ideal of complementary therapies being offered to women to become a reality in Peterborough Maternity Unit. Joyce Reid discusses the baby massage classes offered by a health visitor in Forfar.

Midwives are also working to reflect upon different therapies and their possible uses for childbearing women. Jenny Green investigated the use of osteopathy with experts in this field, and presents their ideas as a trigger for midwives to find out more about this service. Jo Hartley asked a range of midwives and alternative therapists for their suggested treatment for women experiencing piles, and presents these results in her article. It is interesting to note the wide range of ideas raised, which suggests that there may not be one answer, but rather a number of solutions which work for different women. Is this true not only of specific treatments within healing systems, but also of the range of healing modalities themselves? As our knowledge of different types of therapy and healing philosophy continues to increase, so too will the possibilities for helping women.

Evidence-based practice – the new dogma?

Jilly Rosser

Imagine the following scenario. At Modern Times Maternity Unit it is part of labour ward policy to perform 20 minutes of reflexology on all primigravid women at 4cm dilatation. If a woman questions this intervention, pressure will be put on her to conform to the unit policy. If she insists on refusing this form of care, senior midwives and medical staff are brought into the room to issue dire warnings about the hazards to which she is exposing her baby. If she still refuses to comply she will be required to sign a disclaimer and the consultant will be informed. A record will be made in the woman's notes that she refused the treatment and that she is taking responsibility for this decision.

Ridiculous? Possibly, but this is a fairly accurate description of how interventions and forms of care have been introduced into practice in the past. Could it happen with complementary therapies?

The article by Mandy Curry (reprinted in this book as chapter 9.5) describes the setting up of a complementary therapies (CT) service within the maternity unit at Peterborough hospital. This is, to our knowledge, the most comprehensive and systematic introduction of CTs into midwifery practice that has occurred to date – a trail-blazing achievement of much interest to midwives throughout the UK.

Mandy Curry describes her intention, as manager, to take real steps towards providing a service which responds to women's expressed wishes. She has also been undertaking a thorough evaluation of the introduction of the CTs into practice and the results of that evaluation will be published later this year.

Caution

But there are some voices raised in protest at the introduction of this kind of service, sounding a note of caution. In a letter to *Changing Childbirth Update*[1] there is a warning against operating double-standards when introducing innovations in care. If midwives espouse the value of evidence-based practice (EBP), the writers argue, then they should look for the same level of evidence of efficacy for CTs as for other interventions in maternity care.

While this argument deserves to be taken seriously, there is something troubling about it. EBP is certainly an essential part of the approach to safe and effective care. It has been so enthusiastically received by midwives, because for so long we have watched (and participated in) practices being adopted into maternity care without any rational basis. Years later the practice is properly evaluated and found to be ineffective, or harmful, or with mixed benefits. The list of such practices is long and oft-rehearsed: pubic shaving, episiotomies, routine ultrasound scanning, electronic fetal monitoring (EFM) in labour and so on. What is so reprehensible about the use of these practices is that they were introduced into routine care with the implicit or explicit assurance to women that they would – in one way or another – make their births safer. More often than not, there was no choice offered to women; these interventions were policy, and the only way women could avoid them was by being well-informed, articulate, assertive and lucky.

This is the context into which the seed of EBP was sown; small wonder then it has flourished so – plenty of manure for it to feed on!

EBP is about identifying which aspects of care have been evaluated, determining whether they have been found to be effective, useless, or harmful, and using this information to enable professionals and service users to make better informed choices. But we must beware of making EBP the new orthodoxy and becoming inflexible in new and, perhaps, more subtle ways.

Choice

There are two fundamental differences between the way complementary therapies are being introduced into the maternity services in Peterborough and the way, say, EFM was introduced. The first is that complementary therapies are being introduced in response to women's expressed preferences. These preferences may be expressed by individual women or by one of the organisations which represent women's interests. Secondly, they are offered to women as a genuine choice and without ill-founded claims of their efficacy or benefit.

Let us look at these two points in a little more detail. Responding to the expressed preferences of consumers is an important element of women-centred care. If we were to decide that we would not respond to women's wishes about care unless there was substantial evidence to support that form of care, our hands would be tied. In a very helpful article on EBP which appeared recently in the *British Medical Journal*[2] this and other shortcomings of EBP as a new orthodoxy were explored:

'Evidence-based medicine may introduce a systematic bias, resulting in allocation of resources to those treatments for which there is rigorous evidence of effectiveness, or towards those for which there are funds available to show effectiveness (such as new pharmaceutical agents). This may be at the expense of other areas where rigorous evidence does not currently exist or is not attainable (such as palliative care services). Allocating resources on the basis of evidence may therefore involve implicit value judgements, and it may only be a short step from the notion that a therapy is "without substantial evidence" to it being thought to be "without substantial value."'

Women's requests

There is a genuine and important ethical difference between a practice being provided in response to women's requests, and a practice being adopted into unit policy and provided as a routine part of care, which women have to opt out of if they wish to avoid it.

Very similar arguments apply to the use of water in labour. The limited amount of evidence available to date shows no clear advantages or disadvantages to mother, baby or caregiver of immersion in water in labour. There are two possible responses to this evidence. Either one can say that, in the absence of evidence of its effectiveness, immersion in water should not be available as an option for women, or one can say that there is no

evidence on which to oppose a woman's request for immersion in water. It is difficult to see how we can move towards providing more flexible, women-centred care if we adopt the first position. There are so few aspects of care in normal labour which have been adequately evaluated that midwives would be hopelessly restrained if these were all we could offer. We would not be able to offer women choices or respond to their requests.

Which brings us back to the second difference mentioned earlier; that at Peterborough the complementary therapies are offered as an option to women without any promises of benefit, and as a genuine choice. No pressure is brought to bear on women to accept CTs and to decline them they do not have to opt out of unit policy or risk staff disapproval. This is an entirely different approach to that which has characterised the introduction of interventions into maternity care in the past. There are innumerable examples one could use to illustrate this. For example, the routine sucking out of the newborn. This has been done routinely, without informing – let alone inviting a choice from – the woman, without any evidence of benefit and seemingly with a total disregard of any possible harmful consequences.

Conclusion

Evidence-based practice is an important tool in the midwives' repertoire. It will enable us to base our care on a more rational footing and to avoid the appalling mistakes which have been made in the past (and continue to be made today). But EBP is a part of the philosophy of good care , it is not itself the definition of good care. Were we to allow it to become the new dogma, then even well-considered innovations which are welcomed by women, introduced after consultation and discussion, and evaluated thoroughly – such as complementary therapies in Peterborough – would be stifled.

As long as complementary therapies are introduced with this amount of caution, midwives cannot justifiably be accused of operating double standards. Instead we can be proud of moving towards an innovative, flexible and responsive approach to care.

REFERENCES

1   Smith I, Renfrew M. Correspondence. Changing Childbirth Update 1998; 11:18.

2   Kerridge I, Lowe M, Henry D. Ethics and evidence based practice. British Medical Journal 1998; 316:1151–1153.

Labour and the raspberry leaf herb

Myra Parsons   Michele Simpson   Kenneth Wade

The general belief in the community is that raspberry leaf, taken in tablet or herbal tea form during pregnancy, shortens labour and makes labour 'easier'. Many pregnant women take raspberry leaf in some form during pregnancy, following advice from family and friends, magazine advertisements, naturopaths, their midwife or their doctor. The effect of raspberry leaf, consumed during pregnancy, on the labour, birth and postpartum period has never been examined, except in laboratory studies, to the investigators' knowledge. All information has been anecdotal to date. The purpose of this study was to explore the safety and efficacy of raspberry leaf herb products, consumed by women during their pregnancy, prior to conducting a placebo-controlled, randomised trial.

Literature review

The raspberry leaf plant (Rubus idaeus Linn., Family: Rosacea) has been used medicinally for centuries – certainly as early as the sixth century.[1] It is said to be the best known and oldest of all the herb infusions and to be included as a proved aid in maternity in the most ancient of herbal books.[2] It is a common practice for women to use an infusion of dried raspberry leaves to allay the pains of labour.[3]

An experiment on cats by Burn and Withell found that an intravenous injection of raspberry leaf extract had a relaxant effect on the uterine muscle.[2] This 'relaxant effect' was later interpreted as 'producing more coordinated uterine contractions' in labour.[4] As Bamford et al explained, a major problem in obstetrics 'is incoordination of uterine action, and it may be that raspberry leaf extract is able to modify the course of labour favourably to produce more coordinated uterine contractions'.[4] Whitehouse noted that uterine contractions in postnatal women diminished in frequency and strength, and secondary contractions were eliminated, in women given 20-40 grams of raspberry leaf extract (fragarine) in the first few days after birth.[3]

The only side effect noted by Burn and Withell and Whitehouse was an accompanying change in blood pressure.[2,3] However, Burn and Withell found a 'slight' rise in blood pressure in some of the animals studied while Whitehouse noted a 'slight' decrease in systolic blood pressure in the postpartum women he studied.

In naturopathic literature, raspberry leaf is said to have many remedial effects. Castleman described its use for morning sickness, uterine irritability, and threatened miscarriages. According to Hoffman, if raspberry leaf is ingested regularly throughout pregnancy and also during labour it will 'strengthen and tone the tissue of the womb, assisting contractions and checking any haemorrhage during labour', a statement supported by Mills.[6,7]

Others take the view that raspberry leaf may cause or augment miscarriage, or premature labour. This opinion is based on a study conducted in 1970 and reported by the Pharmaceutical Society of Great Britain which found that raspberry leaf, when injected into strips of human uteri at 10-16 weeks of pregnancy, initiated contractions.

Although much is written of the benefits of raspberry leaf for pregnancy and childbirth, there is a paucity of research-based references and those found are dated and based on laboratory studies or postpartum women.[2,3,4]

Research questions

Compared with a control group, does the intake of raspberry leaf during pregnancy:

- have adverse effects on the mother or baby? Is it safe?
- demonstrate differences during the prebirth period, particularly gestation and during labour?
- reduce the likelihood of medical interventions during labour and birth?

This observational retrospective study compared a group of women who had used the raspberry leaf herb during

Table 9.2.1 Gestation period in days

	Raspberry leaf group	Control group	t	df	F	p
Mean (in days)	283.93	281.47	1.25	106	(50, 56)	.215
Standard Deviation	8.20	12.10			3.43	.067
Range (in days)	41 (260-301)	71 (230-301)				

Table 9.2.2 Length of labour in minutes

	Raspberry leaf group			Control group			t	df	p
	N	Mean	SD	N	Mean	SD			
First Stage	52	301.6	212.5	43	387.8	349.8	1.41*	93	0.17
Second Stage	44	49.2	47.9	34	40.4	32.2	0.92	76	0.36
Third Stage	52	12.1	26.3	43	10.6	18.1	0.33	93	0.74

*(Assuming unequal variances)

their pregnancy, with a group of women who had not. Variables were measured to assess safety:

- Blood loss <600 mls considered safe
- Apgar score at 5 minutes >6 considered safe
- Prelabour diastolic bp <90 considered safe.

The following variables were collected to examine the impact of raspberry leaf ingestion on gestation, labour and birth outcomes:

- Occurrence of known or suspected side effects of raspberry leaf (e.g. diarrhoea)
- Gestation at birth
- The occurrence of syntocinon intravenous infusion
- The occurrence of artificial rupture of membranes
- Length of first stage of labour measured from the onset of regular contractions in combination with dilatation of the cervix >2cm
- Epidural anaesthesia rate
- Length of second stage labour
- Forceps or ventouse extraction delivery
- Caesarean birth rate
- Length of third stage of labour
- The occurrence of meconium liquor
- Admission to Neonatal Intensive Care Unit or Special Care Nursery within the first 24 hours after birth.

Method

Participants in this research (n = 108) were a convenience sample. Women who had consumed raspberry leaf products during their pregnancy (n = 57) and who had given birth at Westmead Hospital between January and July 1998 were recruited to the study. The control group (n = 51) consisted of women who had given birth at Westmead Hospital during the same period but had not

taken raspberry leaf products during pregnancy or labour. Only data available in the medical records were collected on mothers and babies in the control group.

All women who gave birth during this period were approached regarding their consumption of raspberry leaf products in pregnancy. Those who responded in the affirmative (n = 57) were given a questionnaire which requested information regarding the type and amount of raspberry leaf consumed, the duration of consumption of the product during their pregnancy and labour, the person who recommended the herb, and any side effects noted. Approval from the participating Ethics Committee was obtained, along with written consent by all women in the study for access to their medical records. Data for the entire sample were obtained from the hospital obstetric database or the women's medical records and the information provided on the questionnaire.

The data in this paper were analysed using the PC version of the Statistical Package for the Social Sciences. Chi-square (X^2) tests were used to compare proportions and the F-test used to compare variances (Levene's Test for Equality of Variances). The level of satisfaction by the data of the assumption of homogeneity of variance was considered. If no significant difference was found between the variances of the measures from the two

Table 9.2.3 Delivery outcome

	Raspberry leaf group	Control group	Total
(n = 57)	(n = 51)	(n = 108)	
Normal Delivery	44	34	78
Forceps/Ventouse	8	9	17
Caesarean Section			
Elective	1	3	4
Emergency	4	5	9

(X^2 = 1.48, df = 1, p = .22)

groups using the F-test, the t-test of difference between means assuming equal population variance was used. If the F-test reported a significant difference between the variances of the two groups, the t-test of difference between means assuming unequal population variance was used. The paper explicitly reports application of the latter approach to the t-test.

Results

Data were analysed for the two groups, and findings are regarded as statistically significant if $p < 0.05$.

Equivalence of groups

The sample consisted of a majority of Caucasian women and was relatively equivalent for age, weight and parity. The average age was 28.72 years (sd = 4.46) for the raspberry leaf group and 30.35 years (sd = 5.347) for the control group. Statistically there is some difference between the groups on this variable (t (106) = 1.73, p = .086). This was a function of the sampling procedure. The average weight of the raspberry leaf group was 67.75 kg (sd = 12.43) and 67.25 kg (sd = 13.41) for the control group. There was no statistical difference between the groups on this variable (t (98) = .19, p = .85).

The raspberry leaf group (n = 57) consisted of 59.6% primiparous women and 40.3% multiparous women while the control group (n = 51) consisted of 51.0% primiparous women and 49.0% multiparous women. There was a slightly greater proportion of primiparous women and women birthing their second babies in the raspberry leaf group and a slightly greater proportion of women birthing their third and fourth babies in the control group than expected by chance ($X^2(2)$ = 3.49, p = .17). This result was not statistically significant.

Raspberry leaf consumption

In the raspberry leaf group the largest proportion of women drank raspberry leaf tea, 56.1% (1-6 cups of tea per day), while 40.4% ingested tablets (1-8 tablets of varying dosages per day) and 3.5% of women consumed a combination of raspberry leaf tablets, tea or tincture (4-6 tablets and 1 cup of tea or 1 dose of tincture per day). Women commenced raspberry leaf as early as 8 weeks gestation with 13% commencing at 8-28 weeks, 59% at 30-34 weeks and 28% at 35-39 weeks. The duration of consumption of the raspberry leaf products was over a 1-32 week continuous period. Six women chose to cease the consumption of raspberry leaf during their pregnancy for the following reasons:

- 2 women did not like the taste of the tea

- 1 woman stated she 'took castor oil instead' (this was in the week preceding labour)
- 1 woman stated she had 'early labour pains' (this was the onset of full term labour)
- 1 woman experienced an 'increased frequency of Braxton-Hicks contractions'
- 1 woman experienced an episode of diarrhoea after consuming raspberry leaf tablets for one week at 32 weeks gestation.

The women in the raspberry leaf group identified midwives (31.6%, n = 18) and their doctor (29.8%, n = 17) as most responsible for recommending raspberry leaf products during their pregnancy. Only one woman was advised by her naturopath. 29.8% (n = 17) of women were influenced by friends or relatives and 14% (n = 8) had taken raspberry leaf after reading about it.

Safety issues

The safety aspect of raspberry leaf consumption in pregnancy was analysed using three parameters: maternal blood loss at birth, babies' Apgar score at 5 minutes, and maternal diastolic blood pressure pre labour. No clinically significant difference was demonstrated in any of these areas.

Gestation, labour and birth outcomes

The possible impact of raspberry leaf consumption was examined by comparing the raspberry leaf (RL) and control (C) groups for gestation period at birth, the incidence of medical augmentation and artificial rupture of membranes, the need for an epidural, the occurrence of meconium liquor, the need for babies' admission to Neonatal Intensive Care facilities following birth, the length of each stage of labour and the mode of delivery.

On average the gestation period (in days) for each group of mothers was the same. However, there was a marked difference in the standard deviations of this variable between the two, suggesting raspberry leaf mothers birthed closer to their expected date. The distribution of gestation periods was reasonably symmetric in both groups (Table 9.2.1).

There was no difference between the groups on the likelihood of medical augmentation of labour ($X^2(1)$ = 0, p = 1.0). There was, however, a greater likelihood of artificial rupture of membranes in the control group (52.9%, n = 51) compared with the raspberry leaf group (38.6%, n = 57) ($X^2(1)$ = 2.2, p = 13).

No difference was found between the two groups on the occurrence of meconium liquor ($X^2(1)$ = .07, p = .78) or the need for an epidural block ($X^2(1)$ = .02, p = .87) during labour and delivery. Basically there was no difference in the likelihood of babies being transferred to Neonatal Intensive Care facilities following birth ($X^2(2) = 1.25$, p = .53).

The analyses of time in first and third stages of labour excluded mothers who gave birth by Caesarean section. The analyses of time in second stage labour excluded mothers who were delivered by Caesarean section, forceps or ventouse extraction.

The timing of first stage labour differs markedly between the groups ($sd_{RL} = 212.5$, $sd_C = 349.8$, $F(42, 51) = 7.73$, p = .007). The unequal variance assumption was applied in the independent t-test of difference between means (Table 1). The mean time in first stage labour is substantially lower in the raspberry leaf group ($M_{RL} = 301.6$, $M_C = 387.3$, t = 1.41, df = 93, p = .165) than in the control group. As Table 9.2.2 shows, there were no statistically significant differences between the groups on measures of time in second and third stages of labour.

Compared to the control group (66.7%, n = 51), the raspberry leaf mothers (77.2%, n = 57) had a slightly larger percentage of normal deliveries ($X^2(1) = 1.48$, p = .22) (Table 9.2.3).

Discussion

In this retrospective study, the convenience sample in the raspberry leaf group was reasonably equivalent to the randomly selected control group for age, weight, and parity although primiparous women were more likely to ingest raspberry leaf than multiparous women. The use of retrospective convenience samples limits the generalisability of the findings. It was not possible to control the level of raspberry leaf ingestion by the treatment group, and the findings were confounded by the mix of multiparous and primiparous mothers in the two groups.

According to the data collected and the final analysis, the raspberry leaf herb appeared to be safe for pregnant women and their babies during pregnancy, labour and birth, and in the early postpartum period. Only one woman reported an incidence of diarrhoea after taking raspberry leaf for one week. Diarrhoea is a known side effect of raspberry leaf if taken in greater than therapeutic dose. Anecdotally women occasionally complain of strong Braxton-Hicks contractions (normal contractions of pregnancy) while taking raspberry leaf herbs and it was found in this study that one woman did stop taking raspberry leaf for this reason during her pregnancy. As pregnant women complain of strong Braxton-Hicks contractions even when not ingesting raspberry leaf products it is unknown if these contractions are strengthened by raspberry leaf or if they are normal for some women.

Despite the inconsistent consumption of this herb among the women in the treatment group the analysis suggested a shortening of the first stage of labour and reduction in spread of time in first stage of labour. It seems that raspberry leaf may not only shorten labour but may also lessen the likelihood of precipitate or prolonged labour. This obviously requires further investigation.

One unsubstantiated concern has been that raspberry leaf may cause preterm labour and birth. In this study only one woman in the control group birthed before 37 weeks gestation; there were no preterm labours or births in the raspberry leaf group.

The analysis also suggested that women who consumed the raspberry leaf herb during their pregnancy were more likely to give birth to their babies naturally and less likely to require artificial rupture of membranes, forceps, ventouse extraction or Caesarean section delivery compared with the control group. This supports the research expectations proposed by the investigators that raspberry leaf may have an effect on shortening the labour process and reduce the need for medical intervention, in this case the need for birth assistance.

To address the limitations in this study and further explore the research expectations, the controls of a double-blind, randomised, placebo-controlled trial are appropriate. Such a trial was commenced at Westmead Hospital in Sydney, Australia, in 1999.

REFERENCES

1 Beckett AH, Belthle FW, Fell KR, et al. Active constituents of raspberry leaves. Journal Pharmacy and Pharmacology 1954; 6:785–796.
2 Burn JH, Withell ER. A principle in raspberry leaves which relaxes uterine muscle. The Lancet 1941; July 5:1–3.
3 Whitehouse B. Fragarine: An inhibitor of uterine action. British Medical Journal 1941; Sept 13:370–1.
4 Bamford DS, Percival RC, Tothill AU. Raspberry leaf tea: A new aspect to an old problem. Proceedings of the British Pharmacological Society, 8th-10th July. British Journal of Pharmacology 1970; 40 (1):161–162.
5 Castleman M. The healing herbs. Melbourne: Schwartz; 1991.
6 Hoffinan D. The new holistic herbal. Dorset: Element; 1990.
7 Mills S. The A-Z of modern herbalism. London: Thorsons; 1989.
8 Pharmaceutical Society of Great Britain. Herbal medicines: A guide for healthcare professionals. London: The Pharmaceutical Press; 1996.

How did it feel to you?

An informal survey of massage techniques in labour

Linda Kimber

The 1970s were a time of increased technological intervention in maternity care, with induction of labour, epidural anaesthesia and operative delivery becoming commonplace.[1] Over the next 20 years attitudes began to change, giving more control to expectant parents.[2]

Touch, in the form of a positive massage during labour, was an area I wanted to explore to determine whether it is a useful way of shifting the focus of active support away from the midwife and towards the birthing partner.

The following report summarises a review I undertook of my practice of the massage techniques previously reported in *The Practising Midwife*.[3]

Background

Throughout the 17 years that I worked as a community midwife at the John Radcliffe Hospital, Oxford, I witnessed many changes in attitude and approach. During the 1970s it was common for doctors and midwives to take absolute control over childbearing women, leaving many women feeling disempowered and very dissatisfied with their experiences. Groups such as the NCT evolved in response and actively challenged this type of care,[4,5] emphasising the normality of childbirth.

During the 1990s alternative and complementary therapies began to gain popularity. Books and courses became available on such topics as massage, aromatherapy, reflexology, homeopathy and acupuncture.[6,7] There was a shift towards acceptance of complementary therapies, both by the users and the providers of health services.

Guidance on the use of complementary therapies is given in the *Midwife's Code of Practice*, and their use is to be based upon a sound knowledge and appropriate training.[8]

Massage is one such complementary therapy. It is a form of touch, and as such is an important form of communication. When performed in a positive and conscious way it can provide an active role for a support person. In investigating the physiological changes associated with touch, two small studies are of relevance. The first looked at the effects of massage on 11 preterm infants, and indicated that, while pain results in an increase of cortisol concentrations, the opposite occurs in response to massage.[9] The second study shows the effects of connective tissue massage and suggests that it results in a rise in beta endorphins.[10]

The needs of men

Women and their partners, during the 1980s, were encouraged to play a greater part in their 'birthing experience' and couples became better informed.[11] There has also been an emphasis on the importance of promoting options and choice for childbearing women and their partners.[12]

Despite this, many men still do not feel part of the labour process. Some fathers have expressed a need for more support to achieve an active role within the labour experience.

One commentator has written to men:

'You may be all too aware of the feeling of helplessness and frustration that you are not able to do enough to help your wife, especially with her pain in first stage.' [12]

In a survey of fathers' needs[13] the men considered themselves as essentially helpless in supporting their partner with the pain. Furthermore, two men out of the 30 in her survey:

'perceived health professionals as likely to increase the sense of powerlessness with which they viewed labour.'

Another important finding of this survey is that men want an active role during labour:

'because doing something seems more controlling than doing nothing.'

Questions

As a midwife, I used massage in labour, and the women found it both soothing and comforting. In addition, it gave me a positive, supportive role. I wanted to find out if I could pass this role on to the birthing partner; whether the partner could be more actively involved in the process of labour through the use of massage.

I therefore decided to undertake a review of the use of massage in my practice. This took place over a ten-month period. My purpose was to clarify:

- How best to implement massage for the woman, with her partner being the primary masseur
- How to help the couple become more reliant on each other and not focus entirely on the midwife for support
- How couples overall responded to this care option
- Whether any modifications of the specific massage techniques were called for
- Whether this programme would be of value in the future.

Participants

During my employment as a community midwife at the John Radcliffe Hospital, I offered massage to women whom I attended antenatally, others were referred to me by my colleagues, and some were women I met in early labour.

Altogether, 50 women and their partners were included in the review. All the couples were interested in learning the massage techniques and agreed to complete a questionnaire between two and five days after delivery.

The questionnaire included closed and open questions and sought to gain information on their views of their preparation for labour, on their perception of massage for pain relief, the outcome of labour, the couples' feelings about the labour and the effects of the massage. Both partners completed the questionnaire.

Women were not offered massage if they were 'high risk' (for example with hypertensive disorders), if they were anticipating a Caesarean section, or if they were planning a water birth.

Massage in action

At 36 weeks gestation onwards the participating women were asked if they wished to join the massage programme. The massage techniques taught were those described in a previous article.[3]

Of the 30 nulliparous and 20 multiparous women to whom I taught the techniques, two were booked for home delivery. Two of the nulliparous women declined massage in labour (one of whom subsequently had an elective Caesarean section). Overall, I was able to attend the labours of, and therefore observe the massage techniques of, 22 women – 12 of whom were nulliparous and ten of whom were multiparous.

The effects of rnassage on labour

The types of onset of labour, differentiated between the nulliparae and multiparae, are shown in Table 9.3.1. Augmentation of labour was noticeably higher in the nulliparous women.

The uptake of analgesia by women employing the massage techniques is shown in Table 9.3.2.

Nine nulliparae women (33%) did not require any analgesia, and nearly half used just Entonox. It is interesting to note that none of the women received pethidine. In those women who opted for an epidural, the massage was given to them up until the time of the epidural.

All the nulliparous women who did not receive any analgesia had a normal delivery. There was 100% spontaneous vaginal delivery in the multiparous women (Table 9.3.3).

Women's views of the effects of massage

Some of the comments which the women wrote on the questionnaire, on the effects of the massage techniques, were as follows (with the number of women who made the comments in brackets):

- Helped to cope with pain (21 nulliparae, 16 multiparae)
- Helped with breathing (5 nulliparae, 11 multiparae)
- Useful helpful in labour (23 nulliparae, 42 multiparae)
- Relaxing (1 nullipara, 1 multipara)
- Gave control (1 nullipara)
- Poor effect in advanced labour (2 nuiliparae, 1 multipara)
- Useful distraction (2 multiparae)
- Gave sense of wellbeing (1 nullipara, 1 multipara)
- A positive contact (20 nulliparae, 18 multiparae)
- Invaluable (1 nullipara)
- Reassuring (1 nullipara)
- I would recommend it (1 nullipara, 2 multiparae)

These comments suggest that the massage had positive effects, helping women to cope with pain and promoting a positive feeling of labour.

Coping with pain

Specific comments made by the women about how massage helped them to cope with labour included:

Table 9.3.1 Type of onset of labour

	Spontaneous	Induced	Augmented
Nullipara (n = 27)	18 (66.7%)	1 (3.7%)	8 (29.6%)
Multipara (n = 20)	18 (90%)	2 (10%)	0

Table 9.3.2 Type of analgesia used

	Pethidine	Epidural	Entonox	No analgesia
Nullipara (n = 27)	0	5 (18.5%)	13 (48.1%)	10 (33.3%)
Multipara (n = 20)	0	0	8 (40%)	12 (60%)

Table 9.3.3 Mode of delivery

	SVD	Forceps/Ventouse	Caesarean section
Nullipara (n = 27)	22 (81.4%)	4 (14.8%)	1 (3.7%)
Multipara (n = 20)	20 (100%)	0 (0%)	0 (0%)

'Very useful means of pain relief. Used for the first ten hours with breathing techniques as the sole means of relief. It proved very good. I feel it would have been possible to rely on massage, had I not failed to progress, for the entire labour' (nullipara).

'In some ways (and this is very difficult to describe in words), the massage focused my attention on the pain, but at the same time gave me a way of coping with it. Previous to starting the massage, I had been walking around, almost as though trying to walk away from the pain. The massage was a way of facing up to it' (multipara).

'Good for breathing, rhythm and a distraction from pain' (multipara).

The effects of massage techniques in combination with the breathing appear to provide a focus for women which was a distraction from the pain.

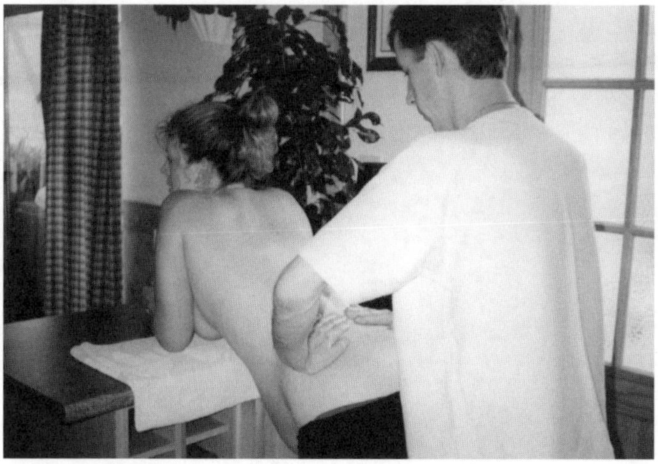

Figure 9.3.1 Pregnant woman being massaged by partner

Feeling in control and reducing anxiety

The relationship between feeling anxiety, feeling in control and pain relief is sometimes difficult to tease apart, but the following quotes indicate that massage assisted some women in feeling in control of the pain of their contractions:

'It helped me concentrate on the breathing, which helped me override the pain to the best of my ability, also made me feel in control to a certain degree' (nullipara).

'I felt that the massage helped me to have more control of the pain. It also seemed to provide pain relief, as I compare contractions I went through without massage with those with the massage. I had no pain relief during my first labour and I found the massage during the second one a much more pleasant way of getting through it' (multipara).

Partners' views on the use of massage techniques

A summary of the comments made by the partners in using the massage techniques is given below:

- Helped feeling of involvement (12 nulliparae, 7 multiparae)
- Helpful/useful (9 nulliparae, 10 multiparae)
- Practical/positive contribution (7 nulliparae, 1 multipara)
- Active role (7 nulliparae, 1 multipara)
- Togetherness (1 nullipara)
- Rewarding (1 nullipara)

Most partners found that using massage techniques assisted them in being involved and taking an active part in the process of labour. Some of the comments made include:

'A significant effect. During the very early stage I felt uninvolved and unable to help – a bit of a "spare part". When using massage, I felt very much more involved and glad that I was clearly having some impact in assisting pain relief' (partner of nullipara).

'It enabled me to get more involved in an active way and contribute positively, to help my partner get through the contractions. If not for the massage, I would have held her hand, wiped her face, etc., all very useful, but this way I was able to help her get through the contractions directly' (partner of multipara).

The partners appeared to find it beneficial to take an active role. For some this increased their sense of sharing and involvement at this time:

'The massage was a very positive aspect of my wife's labour. I felt that I was making a practical contribution to the labour and as a result of this feel that I would take a different approach to massage as a form of pain relief in future' (partner of nullipara).

'I felt usefully involved during labour, and looking back, feel that I had a part in the baby's delivery' (partner of multipara).

Partners who took an active role also felt a sense of taking part in the birth of the baby, and their positive contribution reduced their anxiety. The benefits of the partner undertaking the massage are not just the massage itself, but also the specific role they are provided with during labour.

Preparation for massage techniques

Effective teaching of this type of massage needs to be done on a one-to-one basis, either antenatally or in early labour. Group teaching does not work well, as the women become inhibited when taking their clothes off to learn the techniques. Although the massage techniques in themselves are simple, it is necessary for the couples to practise them for it to work well. An hour taken to teach the partner is very worthwhile.

I wanted to find out what women felt about their preparation for the massage. The majority of women appreciated the preparation antenatally and would have liked to have had the opportunity to learn massage techniques to use in pregnancy. Some responses to the preparation included:

'Invaluable – it would have been impossible and impracticable without it ' (nullipara).

'Yes, I would have jumped at the chance [to use massage during pregnancy], *to help with sleeping, relieving tension and general relaxation'* (nullipara).

'Yes – essential!! Particularly synchronising massage and breathing' (multipara).

'The more the better' (multipara).

Conclusion

This review of my practice of massage suggests that it has a value in achieving positive physical and psychological effects. It may also have a role in reducing the amount of analgesia and promoting women's ability to cope in labour.

The positive responses from the partners were centred on their feeling involved and helpful. Massage will not always be a viable care option for everyone and the wishes of the individual to opt out of massage need to be respected.

For those who are interested in massage, it is a positive way of giving the birthing partner an active role and therefore empowering the couple.

These massage techniques offer one way of overcoming the helplessness felt by many men when they are with women in labour.

REFERENCES

1 Tew M. Safer childbirth. London: Chapman and Hall; 1990.
2 DoH. Expert Maternity Group. Changing Childbirth (Cumberlege Report). London: HMSO; 1993.
3 Kimber L. Effective techniques for massage in labour. The Practising Midwife 1998; 1(4):3–9.
4 Inch S. Birthrights. London: Green Print; 1989.
5 Moorhead J. New generations: 40 years of birth in Britain. London: National Childbirth Trust; 1996.
6 Tisserand R. Aromatherapy today – part 1. The International Journal of Aromatherapy 1993; 5(3):26–29.
7 Thomas R. National occupational standards for alternative and complementary therapists. International Journal of Alternative and Complementary Medicine 1995; 13(11):23–26.

8 UKCC. The Midwife's Code of Practice. London: UKCC; 1994.
9 Acolet D, et al. Changes in plasma cortisol and catecholamine concentrations in response to massage in preterm infants. Archives of Disease in Childhood 1993; 68:29–31.
10 Kaada B, Torteinbo O. Increase of plasma endorphins in connective tissue massage. General Pharmacology 1989; 20(4):487–89.
11 Balaskas A, Balaskas J. Active birth manifesto. 1982.
12 Brant H. Childbirth for men. Oxford: Oxford University Press; 1985.
13 Nolan M. Caring for fathers in antenatal classes. Modern Midwife 1994, 4(2):25–28.

Piles

Ideas on how to reduce the pain from haemorrhoids

Jo Hartley

Participating practitioners

Anne Adamson
Independent midwife, SW London and Surrey

Mr J Eiles
Homeopathic pharmacist, Galen Homeopathics, Dorchester

Jo Hindley
Midwife, Birmingham

Lesley Hobbs
Independent midwife, Hampshire

Jo Hogan
Aromatherapist, Devon

Janie Price
Acupuncturist, Dorset

Cheryl Reynolds
Medical herbalist, Dorset

Jilly Rosser
Midwife, Bristol

Cynthia Walcott
Midwife, Dorset

Ros Weston
Midwife (independent and NHS), Powys and West Midlands

Pondering the difficulties of writing an article about pregnancy and haemorrhoids (possibly not the easiest subject with which to open a conversation), I noticed how pregnant and postnatal women tend to resign themselves to the condition. They are generally long-suffering in their acceptance of what is regarded as just another of those 'minor' problems of pregnancy. Their GP may prescribe them standard treatments such as Anusol or Sheriproct, or give Lactulose to guard against constipation, but on the whole they bear the discomfort, assuming it will eventually improve.

Ask specifically

Lesley Hobbs, midwife, suggested that women should be warned that they may well suffer from haemorrhoids while pregnant or after the birth. She has noticed that women with varicose veins in the legs seem to be more susceptible to haemorrhoids. All the midwives I spoke to thought that the pain caused by haemorrhoids in the postnatal period was drastically underestimated. Jilly Rosser, midwife, said that women are often reluctant to talk directly about the subject and midwives need to ask them specifically about the nature of any pain they report in the genital and peri-anal area – otherwise it is assumed that any pain from that area arises from perineal trauma.

It seems to be the case that midwives rarely ask specifically about haemorrhoids, concentrating much more on perineal pain and healing. Cheryl Reynolds, a medical herbalist, explained that it is necessary to be sure that the woman is actually suffering from haemorrhoids. For example if she complains of bleeding when opening her bowels it is important to exclude other, potentially more serious problems.

The practitioners I spoke to on this subject use of a variety of treatments, most of them coming under the heading of 'complementary therapies'. Only one midwife, Anne Adamson, recommended one of the more orthodox remedies: lignocaine cream 1% or 2%. This is perhaps a reflection on the limited effectiveness of some of the proprietary treatments.

Mr Eiles, a homeopathic pharmacist who recommends that treatment be commenced as early as possible, uses hamamelis and aesculus, particularly in oral preparations to reduce swelling of the veins. These preparations are safe during pregnancy and breastfeeding and tend to lead to an improvement relatively quickly.

Jo Hogan, an aromatherapist, treats haemorrhoids with a witch hazel compress and an ointment of geranium and cyprus oil. Although cyprus oil is contraindicated in pregnancy, it is safe when used topically and in small amounts. Acupuncture can also offer effective relief. Janie Prince, an acupuncturist who provides holistic care, first analyses the energy patterns of the woman and then chooses treatment points specific to her.

Hot or cold?

There was interesting disagreement about temperature of treatments. Janie Prince suggested using witch hazel that had been stored in the fridge and Anne Adamson recently treated a woman with haemorrhoids using sanitary towels soaked in witch hazel and stored in the freezer. The woman had obtained a very pure form of witch hazel and found this to be very effective. Jilly Rosser mentioned the time-honoured practice of using frozen peas (still in the packet!) for reducing the swelling. However, Cheryl Reynolds believes that the greatest pain is caused by the spasmodic nature of haemorrhoids and treating them with cold compresses or ointments causes them to go into spasm. Hence she would use an anti-spasmodic such as atropa belladonna taken orally although this is contraindicated in breastfeeding women. She would also advise the woman to sit on a bucket with an infusion of camomile in hot water and would prescribe a liver bitter (orally) such as gentian, milk thistle and dandelion to tone up the portal vein.

There was broad agreement on the importance of a healthy diet. Jo Hogan recommends eight to ten glasses of water a day. Ros Weston, a midwife, advocates increased fluid and fibre intake and Cheryl Reynolds offers a tea of camomile, fennel and senna to prevent constipation.

Several of the midwives were aware of treatments bought directly from health shops. Jilly Rosser had found a very effective haemorrhoid ointment made of witch hazel, pilewort, agrimony, calendula and elder. Jo Hindley, another midwife, has come across an aromatherapy preparation that contains magnetised essential oils of peppermint, tea tree and marigold that is applied to the painful area as well as being massaged into the abdomen. However, midwives should direct any woman seeking advice on complementary therapies to a qualified practitioner.

Compresses

Cynthia Walcott sometimes advises a woman to try and gently push the haemorrhoids back in place while in the bath, using a lubricant such as KY jelly. Jo Hindley offers similar advice, using olive oil to minimise the discomfort.

Jilly Rosser sometimes places a pad over the anal mouth during second stage to apply counter pressure. Ros Weston agrees that there is possibly a link between pushing and the appearance of haemorrhoids and will sometimes apply a warm compress or suggest the woman gently pushes them back in the postnatal period. She also said it was important to reassure the woman that they will eventually improve greatly as her body reverts to its pre-pregnancy state.

Anne Adamson recommends to women who are uncomfortable when breastfeeding that they lie on their side rather than sit up, thus reducing the pressure.

There appear to be many different treatments commonly used by experienced practitioners for haemorrhoids. It is reassuring to know that this very painful problem can be treated quickly and efficiently.

It behoves midwives to be sure that what the woman describes as perineal pain is not actually haemorrhoids, to acknowledge the level of discomfort that haemorrhoids can cause and to offer suggestions for treatment. By asking specific questions, midwives can make it easier for women to disclose their pain. This is not a condition which women have to suffer in silence.

The introduction of complementary therapies into a maternity service

Mandy Curry

The maternity service in Peterborough offers care to approximately 3,500 women each year. In October 1996 a group of midwives introduced a new complementary therapy service into the maternity unit. The service, which includes massage, aromatherapy and reflexology, provides for the training of staff and parents-to-be and for the use of therapies in the antenatal period, labour and the postnatal period.

Complementary therapies are gaining in popularity and in acceptance in many areas of social and healthcare.[1] In Peterborough we agree with others working in our field that providing complementary therapies gives women more choice and control in pregnancy.[2] The development of such a service within our unit fits well with our work towards meeting the indicators and philosophy of *Changing Childbirth*.[3] We believe that the holistic approach of complementary therapy – treating each client as an individual – enhances the development of a truly woman-centred service.

Legitimate concerns have been raised regarding the use of complementary medicines and therapies,[4] highlighting issues regarding training, evidence-based practice, resources and practitioner competence. The service in Peterborough addresses these concerns; training is provided for staff and for women and their partners; the oils and therapies used are only those which the evidence suggests are safe to use in pregnancy, and the therapies are offered within clear guidelines. The staff who provide the complementary therapies are all midwives, and as such are supervised in their practice by their supervisor of midwives. The service is resourced within the maternity budget.

Developing the service

The service was the brainchild of Sonia Gent, a senior midwife who works on the delivery suite in Peterborough and who holds diplomas in massage, reflexology and aromatherapy. She is now seconded for two days each week to develop the complementary therapy service. During these two days she develops training as well as providing therapies on an appointment basis to both service users and to staff.

Sonia was the key mover in getting the service established. This was no mean feat; it took a number of years for the proposal to gain the support of management and the clinicians and be taken forward. Sonia prepared a business case for the service which was presented to the manager, clinicians and to the trust. This covered staffing and financial costs as well as clinical and research issues.

The case had four key points:

1. Therapies would be offered within clear guidelines.
2. The service would be evidence based.
3. The practitioners would complete a certificated course of training.
4. Client satisfaction would be evaluated.

Initially, not all of the consultants agreed to women booked under their care being offered the service. However, as time has passed and confidence has been gained, this is no longer the case.

Our experience echoes that of others who suggest it is more difficult to gain acceptance for the introduction of complementary therapies than for other innovative activities in healthcare.[4]

The importance of the support of our obstetricians in enabling this service to progress cannot be overestimated. Their main concerns, prior to introducing the service, were around the safety of the therapies. Therefore the development of clear guidelines, detailing the parameters of the service, was of paramount concern.

The key to the success of introducing a new service lies in gaining the support of the entire multidisciplinary team.

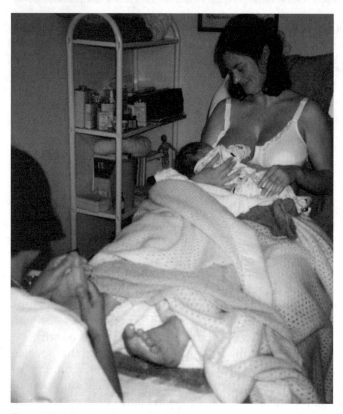

Figure 9.5.1 New mother receiving foot massage

Guidelines

The guidelines are designed to ensure the consistency and safety of the service offered. They include details of the oils to be used, which women are eligible for the therapy and the therapy process. Eligibility criteria require women to be 37 weeks pregnant, with a singleton pregnancy and cephalic presentation, not taking regular medication and with normal blood pressure. Babies for massage need to be four weeks old and have no medical problems. Guidelines also cover record-keeping and the storage of oils and equipment.

The guidelines take a cautious approach, reflecting the limits to current evidence regarding complementary therapies. They were drawn up by Sonia and negotiated with midwives and the consultant lead clinician prior to their implementation. They will be reviewed and amended as new evidence becomes available.

Only those midwives who have completed the training are recruited to offer complementary therapies. Sonia blends the essential oils and calculates dosage. Other midwives can refer women to the complementary therapy midwives if they wish to use aromatherapy during labour. In the antenatal period Sonia receives referrals for treatments from consultants, midwives and physiotherapists.

Pilot study

A pilot study began in October 1996. Initially planned to run for a year or to include 500 women (whichever the sooner), this period was extended to April 1998 due to difficulties in the early months in collecting data. These were resolved and the evaluation is now complete.

In preparation for the pilot study a group of eight midwives were trained to offer aromatherapy, reflexology and massage. Subsequently a further eight midwives completed the training and the complementary therapy group is now well established and meets regularly to maintain the service. Further training will be offered to staff on a modular basis. This modification is in response to an initial evaluation of the training course in which some midwives expressed a desire to learn only massage or aromatherapy or reflexology, rather than all three.

Accreditation has been obtained for two ENB study days entitled Baby Massage and Massage for Mothers, to be run in 1998.

The pilot study has two main aspects: training and direct care.

Training

Training consists of courses for staff and partners and parents in massage for labour and, postnatally, for babies.

Staff attend a basic complementary therapy course which equips them with the skills to offer therapies according to the unit policies. This course is run and assessed by Sonia and includes a rigorous examination. Further courses are planned, on a modular basis, to teach massage for pregnant women, baby massage, aromatherapy and reflexology.

Baby massage is also being taught to staff working in SCBU and to staff on our children's ward for children with special needs.

Partners are offered training in massage for their partner in labour and attend sessions at the maternity unit when their partner has reached 36 weeks' gestation. Parents are also offered a course in baby massage in the postnatal period. A charge is made for this course, which is used to fund the essential oils required and to support staff in training.

Direct care

Direct care is the application of therapies to the individual. It is offered to staff, mothers and babies.

Staff are offered reflexology and neck and shoulder massage by Sonia. This takes place in her therapy room, and appointments are made through a dedicated phone line with an answering facility. This is proving to be very popular amongst staff from all disciplines within the maternity unit. It is not yet available to staff throughout the trust, due to lack of time. A small charge is made.

Women are offered aromatherapy during labour and in the postnatal period, reflexology in the antenatal period from 36 weeks' gestation and in the puerperium, and massage from 36 weeks' gestation. Referrals for treatment come from midwives and members of the maternity unit team, using the unit guidelines. For women less than 36 weeks' gestation a referral is required by a consultant or named midwife (for women booked under midwife-led care). Treatment with massage and reflexology is offered for back pain, insomnia and other problems. This part of the service is well used and demand is increasing.

Evaluation

The service is currently being evaluated using a client survey. The results will be available later this year. The evaluation will assess the demand for the service, how well it is received by the women using it and its perceived effectiveness. Evaluation of the training takes place at the end of each course. Progress updates for staff within the unit have been circulated by Sonia at regular intervals and the views of staff are sought and received on an informal basis. Information sessions have been organised both within the unit and at the local health fair in the Town Hall on several occasions. These have been well supported by both staff and visitors.

Conclusion

Complementary therapies are used informally by many women and by midwives in practice. It is therefore important to ensure that the standards and practices of staff within a maternity service are maintained at a high and safe level. The best way to do this is to provide the therapies as an integrated part of the maternity services.

There is currently some scepticism amongst professionals about the value of such practices; this has been demonstrated in the response of midwives across the country to our recent article in *Changing Childbirth Update*.[5] Midwives have contacted us in writing and by telephone to find out more about our service. Midwives in several units have found intense resistance from professional colleagues to proposals to introduce complementary therapies into practice. This is despite the revised guidance within *The Midwife's Code of Practice*[6] which outlines the place of complementary therapies in the role of the midwife.

It is important to plan the introduction of a new service thoroughly and to acknowledge that the anticipated health gains need to be balanced by the costs of the service. The value of client satisfaction and qualitative gains are difficult to cost but should not be underestimated.

The investment in the wellbeing of our staff this service provides, both in supporting them physically and professionally, and through encouraging the development of their practice, is of prime interest to myself as the manager of the service.

REFERENCES

1 Raukin-Box. Complementary therapies – a guide for nurses and the caring profession. London: Croom-Helm; 1998.
2 Tiran D, Mack S (eds). Complementary therapies for pregnancy and childbirth. London: Baillière Tindall; 1995.
3 Department of Health. Changing Childbirth: Report of the Expert Maternity Group. London: HMSO; 1993.
4 The NHS Confederation. Complementary Therapy in the NHS: Managing the issues. Research Paper no 4. 1997.
5 Curry M. Complementary therapies in Peterborough. Changing Childbirth Update 1997; September: 10.
6 UKCC. The Midwife's Code of Practice. London: UKCC;20.

Osteopathy in pregnancy and childbirth

Jenny Green

Osteopathy is a non-invasive and holistically based profession, with much in common in terms of philosophy, with midwifery. Ordinarily, midwives are not exposed to osteopathy as osteopaths predominately do not form part of the multi-disciplinary team within the hospital maternity care services. These two interviews aim to explore the role of osteopathy in the care of pregnant women and newborn babies. The interviewees are leading experts in the field of osteopathy Stuart Korth (International lecturer in paediatric osteopathy and Consultant at the Osteopathic Centre for Children) and Stephen Sandler (International Consultant Osteopath at the Expectant Women's Clinic (EMC) in the British School of Osteopathy, Osteopath at the Portland Hospital). The format of the questions are similar as, in the writer's opinion, the two institutions associated appear to differ philosophically in that the Osteopathic Centre for Children (OCC) appears somewhat esoteric when compared to the more traditional British School of Osteopathy (BSO). The interviewer is an undergraduate student midwife. Unlike midwifery,[1] there are no international or nationally agreed definitions of osteopathy, and the Osteopaths Act 1993[2] is intriguingly devoid of any standard definition. It confers control of the osteopathy profession via the statutory formation of a General Osteopathics Council (GOsC), a body with power to register and regulate osteopaths and any person purporting to be an osteopath from the 1st May 2000. Unless osteopaths are registered (and approved) from this date, they will be acting illegally by virtue of the act. Thus the profession has recently undergone a certain amount of turbulence whilst acquiring a legal status.

Interview 1

Stephen Sandler is director and founder of the Expectant Mothers' Clinic (EMC) at the British School of Osteopathy (BSO) where he is also senior faculty member, clinic tutor, examiner, and senior lecturer in obstetrics, gynaecology and the gastrointestinal system. He works in private practice in Chingford and is also the Consultant Osteopath at the Portland Hospital for Women and Children. He guest lectures and speaks nationally at osteopathic schools and on postgraduate courses in physiotherapy.

What is osteopathy?

It is one of the 'so called' complementary medicines… we do not follow the same principles of practice as mainstream allopathic medicine, not that we reject them, we just use them in a slightly different way. Contemporary osteopaths are trained to a very high standard, completing a four year full time BSc (Hons) consisting of anatomy, physiology and pathology with an addition of a sense of palpation, a sense of touch, to aid us in diagnoses. We consider as a whole why people become sick. Allopathic medicine is concerned with the disease base, whereas osteopathic medicine is more concerned with the fault in the tissue. It is not necessarily the tissue at fault, but it's a fault within the tissue.

One of the fundamental precepts of osteopathy is that structure governs function, in other words if a thing is built properly, it will work. The sense of touch with palpation links to an orthodox medical training but we use it to evaluate what is happening within the patient and then we use our hands to physically treat the patient. That doesn't mean to say that I do not recognise the value of orthodox drugs. I work in conjunction with allopathic medicine, not in competition with it.

Why are osteopaths interested in pregnancy?

Pregnancy is a changing situation, there is a dynamic. This is why I have found it so exciting to work with pregnant ladies over the last twenty years. Women acquire excess weight (two stone plus) and posture has to change to accommodate it. Concurrently, (in nature this is the only time that it may go wrong), the ovaries are secreting relaxin so that the pelvis can widen and women can deliver their baby. But, when it comes to loosening the joints, where muscles are already trying (too) hard to accommodate, women get all sorts of problems. My research suggests that 85% of pregnant ladies get back pain. The big problem is, what do you do with that back pain? Medication, corsets, bed rest are contraindicated, thus physiotherapy is the only viable treatment, but few physiotherapy departments have people trained both in manipulative back pain care and obstetrics. I founded the EMC in 1980 because of that huge gap in patient care.

My personal research on the change in collagen that occurs in women's bodies has discovered that every woman's joints get progressively looser through the month as she approaches menstruation. It's probably caused by relaxin, progesterones and oestrogens because loosening occurs on days 14 and 25 of a 28 day cycle, when women are more likely to injure themselves. But in pregnancy, relaxin is an important hormone. There is differing opinion about when it is produced and my own experience is that women are looser at different times so I think relaxin is actually produced according to demand. A woman who is stiff will need relaxin early, but a 'looser' woman will probably produce it much later.

How can osteopaths help women: antenatally, intrapartum and postpartum?

Antenatally, examining women and predicting the changes that need to take place are important. The majority of women that have severe back pain have had a previous back injury such as trauma injury, disc injury, something related to a previous birth. These tend to be elderly patients… the women we tend to see in the EMC are primiparous aged 28+. Society of course will tell you that this is not surprising, women are leaving pregnancy later and later…

But physiologically it's harder?

There's a question mark about that, you don't menstruate at the age of twelve for no reason. When a woman presents initially, she often has pain, so my first ambition is to treat it. Sacro-iliac joint problems very commonly occur because the pelvis is open and one side will get 'hitched' while the other side will not. So I give treatment and then like to see her throughout her antepartum period at ever increasing intervals so that I can predict changes that occur. I treat prophylactically to facilitate them and reduce the incidence of pain.

I have been called to a few births… commonly, in the midst of labour a woman gets a sciatica – usually because there is compression of the piriformis muscle, or the nerve is pinched. If she asks for me I can very quickly do something, it takes less than a minute to manipulate a joint and release a spasm. I then leave because personally I don't think there's a major place for osteopathy in the delivery room – it's for the mother, her midwife and her child.

Postpartum I see women at six weeks after they have been discharged by their doctor and I usually check the baby's skull. Those 26 bones are nothing more than croutons floating in soup!

What do you do?

I apply osteopathy in the cranial field. It is not a different type of osteopathy, just a different technique. In this country we have 'created' structural osteopathy, visceral osteopathy, cranial osteopathy; everywhere else in the world you treat a patient with a multitude of techniques. I believe that as a practitioner, you're pretty poor if you only practice one technique. With babies it's the technique of choice because they are so small and young and responsive to it. What the osteopath and the doctor are looking for when they examine babies are completely different. I am interested in the functioning child and when the child takes its first breath, there is positive pressure from within that the cranial plates need to come back following delivery. They are designed to be so mobile to facilitate delivery, with moulding. Where there has been a ventouse delivery, I would advocate examining the baby. At the hospital where I work, The Portland, most of the obstetricians refer women and their babies to me automatically following a ventouse delivery.

Is there anything that osteopaths can recommend generally to women to help them in their pregnancy, intrapartum or postpartum?

Janet Balaskas' book, *Active Birth*, I like the yoga and I think she says some very sensible things about lifestyle.

Are there any specific problems or conditions pregnant women might encounter that an osteopath can help with?

Yes, things like pelvic torsion. My research has shown that 85% of women have problems with back pain and most have causes which are sacro-iliac or pelvic related.

Is this because the gravid uterus doesn't sit in the pelvis in a perfectly symmetrical way?

No, I did a posture survey years ago. Only 20/1000 people have straight backs, so it's not normal to have a straight back. Stick a gravid uterus in there with its gravitational forces and you're going to get problems. Pelvic torsion is the major problem that osteopaths can help with. Old adhesions can also be effectively dealt with. If there is any history of back pain, it's a good idea to get checked out by an osteopath, pre-pregnancy. One of the best things for some women is pregnancy because we can use the effect of relaxin to effectively treat chronic problems.

Is osteopathy safe?

In 1980 I spent the year before opening the EMC researching articles to find any evidence that miscarriage is produced by manipulation. I couldn't find any and offered a prize of £1000 to the first person that could provide me with any proof. I have said this in all countries over the world where I have taught and the money is still sitting on the table. What I do is restore normal physiology and function. However, if a woman miscarries shortly after a visit to an osteopath she and the osteopath will feel very guilty, despite what I say, that it just happened. We know that week 12 and week 16 are key periods for miscarriage, so I advise students not to treat women during these times, but only as a precaution. However, my own view is that I treat all the time.

The force used on a baby is less than a gram – really minuscule. If they didn't like what I do I would soon know about it! How they respond to treatment validates it. I am insured personally for £2,000,000 and the premium is very small. Insurance is a prerequisite to my registration with the General Osteopathic Council. I recommend all newborn babies be checked. If there is a problem it can be treated with one or two visits. The same problem in a five-year-old takes longer to treat.

Why is there so little osteopathy research?

I think osteopathic research must do its own thing. There are huge problems and I think they are going to be addressed in the next five years. There is no osteopathic research database.

Misunderstanding about what an osteopath does has contributed to a lack of inclusion of osteopathic research in conventional databases. Initially when I was asked to work at the Portland it was to treat back pain, now I am invited to deal with many more obstetric related cases. Over a thousand pieces of research a year are currently being produced at osteopathic schools throughout Europe yet where are they? It is a weirdness associated with osteopathy, not a question of funding.

We are addressing this at the BSO, developing a database and a website that links osteopathic research published in the UK. Once that is done, automatic links will come up with, say, a search for obstetrics and complementary therapies.

Has the work been evaluated at the BSO?

We did a pilot project at the EMC of 400 women treated specifically looking at each 100, comparing them to the next 100 to determine how effective their osteopathic treatment was. To date, we have researched over a thousand women. The results suggest that the majority of women show some improvement. We aim to publish in the next three months.

Interview 2

Stuart Korth is co-founder and director of the Osteopathic Centre for Children (OCC), where he works as a Consultant Paediatric Osteopath. He qualified from the British School of Osteopathy in 1964 and is currently an international lecturer in paediatric osteopathy. The OCC is a registered charity: its motto is Every child has a success story to live. Children up to the age of 19 and pregnant and post-partum women are treated at the Centre for a suggested minimum donation of £15. However, treatment is offered irrespective of ability to pay a donation.

Please explain osteopathy, for the benefit of midwives, in your own words.

Osteopathy is concerned with the arrangements of parts of the body. By definition, osteopathy employs manual means to make improvements in the body physiology, by working on its surface. To most people in the UK, osteopathy suggests somebody using manipulation in the broadest sense to aid those with painful disorders of the musculoskeletal system to be in better shape and less pain. This, in my view, is only a speciality within a much broader view. An American physician, Andrew Taylor Still, first formulated osteopathy in 1874. It is very interesting to note that in his writings he is one of the first practitioners to advocate gentleness and non-intervention in childbearing if possible.

Why are osteopaths interested in pregnancy?

Consider the postural adaptation of a pregnant woman. This adaptation is not just a matter of the body framework, it can also affect more specific parts, for example by causing an oesophageal reflux. I believe that I need to do everything I can to encourage health so that the baby is delivered with the least intervention, 'in the most natural way'. As pregnancy proceeds with the secretion of relaxin, osteopaths are better placed to make changes within the body framework to expedite the process of delivery. This is not simply a matter of ensuring the pelvic girdle is free, that there is proper sacroiliac motion and correct relationship of parts of the pelvis. All of the bodily changes have an interaction with the changing hormonal state and the readiness for parturition itself... in the relative tensity of the tissues of the pelvic floor and the ability of the uterus to contract for long enough. They all interact through the nervous and the endocrine systems. The body framework is not simply there to stop the guts falling out, it is the primary machinery of life. It is through this neuromuscular system that we experience everything, that we give vent to emotions and express ourselves. Such experiences are dependent upon the health of that system. Their effects upon it feed back into other organ systems and especially the endocrine system.

How can osteopaths help women: antenatally, intrapartum and postpartum?

My own feeling is that in an ideal world an osteopath would assess all women early on in pregnancy. Those who are well could perhaps be assessed at six months and just prior to the expected date of parturition. There may be many women who would require more treatment for a variety of reasons. In particular, osteopaths can help to prepare the pelvis mechanically for parturition. Ideally I would like to see an osteopath as part of the obstetric team so that the woman also has the option to be treated by an osteopath during labour. There are many instances of uterine inertia, and delayed parturition being expedited by specific work particularly on the spine. It is also important to examine, and where appropriate adjust parts of the body that have been strained through parturition. Particular attention to the relationship between the sacrum and the pelvis is essential in view of its relationship to competence of the pelvic floor. Stress incontinence would be reduced very markedly if this were done.

Osteopathy is often helpful with reflux oesophagitis and hiatus hernia, where posture affects these conditions. The autonomic nervous system can also feature in hyperemesis and morning sickness. In particular, where the vagus nerve is involved, osteopathic treatment in the neck may improve symptoms. It would be wrong for me to state that we have an answer for all women with sickness, but we can help a significant number.

Is there anything that osteopaths can recommend generally to women to help them in their pregnancy?

Nutritional status is always important. Perhaps the biggest difficulty facing most pregnant women is that they have other children and a job. People suffer as a result of too much stress. Osteopathic treatment frequently involves de-stressing at a mechanical level, which helps people to cope again. This enhances the

functioning of the body by facilitating a release from its sympathetic tone – its hyped up state of action – and getting it down to a state of repose from which more stress may be adequately dealt with.

I understand that you have a particular interest in cranial osteopathy and newborn babies and children. What is cranial osteopathy?

Cranial osteopathy is a misnomer. The principles of osteopathy can be applied to the cranium as they can to any other part of the body. The way that cranial osteopathy has become termed comes from usage that is political. It implies a speciality that doesn't exist, so I prefer not to use the term. I will say that osteopathy in the cranial field is a phrase that describes application of osteopathy to a particular part of the body, whereas the osteopath is always looking at the whole.

It is my perception that people fear that osteopathic treatment applied to children/babies may be dangerous. What are your thoughts on this issue?

In actuarial terms we are safe because professional indemnity insurance for osteopaths is around £100 per annum. However, manipulating the head of a newborn baby is a very skilled procedure and in the wrong hands it is dangerous. Provided the operator is a suitably qualified practitioner (a paediatric osteopath), and has the specialist knowledge necessary to treat babies, it is a safe procedure. This is evidenced by the fact that we are invited to participate on the Starlight Unit (SCBU) at Barnet General Hospital.

Is there anything you recommend for newborn babies?

A paediatric osteopath should examine all newborn babies: in most cases there is some degree of mechanical stress that remains unresolved... when there isn't, I rejoice. I once said (at considerable risk!) in a lecture to group of midwives, that when labour proceeds normally there is no need for a midwife or an osteopath. Unfortunately, for most labours women need a midwife and some intervention. Osteopathically, this may be a very fine adjustment on a predominantly healthy baby, or extensive work on someone with prenatal hypoxic damage. I view paediatric osteopathy as the cheapest, most effective form of prophylactic medicine as yet not being used in the care of pregnant women and babies.

Could you explain your work at Barnet Hospital?

The parents of children in special care and intensive care are offered the opportunity to be examined and treated by an osteopath from the OCC. The hospital makes it known to the parents that this service is available, but is not in a position to recommend it. In effect, we have a collaborative venture with the Consultant Paediatrician, Simon Roth, being very fair minded and satisfied that his patients are safely cared for. We are both keen to enter into collaborative research on the treatment given because the anecdotal evidence to date is favourable and we are actually in the process of examining mutually suitable protocols for the research.

Can you describe what you do?

We visit once a week and have done so for the past six years. Basically, neonatal staff help the patients survive and we contribute to the improvement of their quality of life. In practical terms, we save them money… it appears that we help to get the patients out of intensive care more quickly.

Hospital staff now accept us and we have developed cooperation in certain other circumstances, for example, where we believe that older children have perhaps been overmedicated for asthma. We can often treat these children in communication with the hospital and significantly reduce or eradicate their medication.

Do you have any advice for midwives, in terms of what does and does not facilitate the physiological mechanisms of birth?

Well, this could be controversial! I would ask those midwives with perhaps a feel for this, to use their hands on the mothers as much as possible, although I'm sure a lot of them already massage the right parts. In terms of what influence professionals can have upon a birth, much depends upon existing family factors yet the influence is still enough to make a difference, but only if the mother and baby want you to.

Can you see any parallels in terms of midwifery philosophy, with the osteopathic approach to care?

Yes, both professions deal with people and their feelings – that is as important to us as the medical condition.

Osteopaths never seem to be consulted for input in, for example, the Cochrane reviews/research. Does this bother you, or are you not interested in the allopathic models of medicine?

If you ask me whether my profession is interested in the allopathic model the answer would be a categorical yes. If you asked me personally, the answer would be a qualified no. I think that if we try to make our practice and research acceptable to the medical profession… if that is our starting point… we are in great danger of denying the very distinctness that we represent. I believe that the shift in acceptance will come because the Government and public will move more and more towards qualitative assessment. Through concepts such as consumer satisfaction, sociological measures are already beginning to make their way into medical practice. That to me is valid because it is actually measuring people's experiences.

Conclusion

Research based evidence into the benefits of osteopathy for treatment of back pain is established[3-6] as is treatment of lumbar pain during labour. Effectiveness of osteopathic care of pregnant women in relation to alleviating mechanical stress and associated pain also exists.[7] The cost effectiveness of general osteopathic treatment when combined with services offered in the NHS is also demonstrated.[8,9] Sandler's contemporary research into pregnant women is promising although not yet complete. Some evidence suggests that osteopathy in the cranial field may be effective in treating infants with poor feeding/sucking, vomiting, irritability, crying, recurrent ear infections, asthma, neurological dysfunction (including cerebral palsy), learning difficulties and sleep disorders[10-15] – this is certainly endorsed by the experience of the OCC. It is hoped that the proposed research plans for the work at Barnet General Hospital and the OCC will yield more tangible results.

The lack of published research available on the effectiveness of osteopathy in the care of pregnant women and their babies is a major weakness when attempting to critically assess its value. The proposed research of the BSO and OCC is awaited with great interest. Despite occasional disparity of opinion between the two interviewees, their testimonial evidence is compelling and the expanding success of the respective clinics devoted solely to this care is strong evidence to support it. However, the writer was motivated to challenge the osteopathic view of prophylaxis as an essentially medical model perspective and not in harmony with the philosophy of either midwifery or osteopathy. The replies centred upon the effect of modern lifestyle and relative safety of 'osteopathic type of intervention'. On balance, there is a value of osteopathic care in the maternity services and further research into the feasibility of osteopaths becoming part of the multidisciplinary obstetric team could be of benefit to midwives.

REFERENCES

1 World Health Organisation 1992, European Union, International Federation of Obstetricians and Gynaecologists 1991.
2 Chapter 21.
3 Kane M, Costello M, Sandler S, et al. Low back and pelvic pain. Journal of Bodywork and Movement Therapies 1998; 2(2):66–67.
4 Koes BW. Randomised clinical trial of manipulative therapy and physiotherapy for persistent back and neck complaints. British Medical Journal 1992; 304:601–605.
5 Ongley MJ. A new approach to the treatment of chronic low back pain. Lancet 1987; 2:143–146.
6 Pringle M, Tyreman S. Study of 500 patients attending an osteopathic practice. British Journal of General Practice 1993; January: 15–18.
7 Guthrie RA, Martin RH. Effect of pressure applied to the upper thoracic (placebo) versus lumbar areas (osteopathic manipulative treatment) for inhibition of lumbar myalgia during labour. Journal of American Osteopathic Association 1987; 82(4):247–251.
8 Aswani K. Fund GP reveals benefits of osteopathy. Fundholder 1994: 18–21.
9 Budd C, Fisher B, Parrinder D, et al. A model of co-operation between complementary and allopathic medicine in a primary care setting. British Journal of General Practice 1990; September (40):376–378.
10 Coppinger JC. Osteopathy in the cranial field. New England Journal of Homeopathy 1998; 7(2):127–129.
11 Coppinger JC. Fryman effect of osteopathic medical management on neurologic development in children. Journal of American Osteopathic Association 1992; 92(1):20–23.
12 Holmes P. Cranial osteopathy. Nursing Times 1991; 29(87):36–38.
13 Pearson D. The therapy every baby needs. Here's Health 1997; August:30–32.
14 Sandler S. New ways to health: A guide to osteopathy. London: Hamlyn; 1989.
15 Sullivan C. Introducing the cranial approach in osteopathy and the treatment of infants and mothers. Complementary Therapies in Nursing and Midwifery 1997; 3:72–76.

Baby massage classes

Joyce Reid

In a warm, quiet room, with the faint aroma of lavender, six contented babies are lying out naked on towels with their mothers kneeling in front of them. These lucky infants are about to have a massage.

Health visitor, May Crerar, makes sure that everyone is ready to begin. 'Take off any jewellery,' she says, 'and make sure you have no rag nails. I have a nail file if you need it.' She then checks that everyone has enough sweet almond oil before beginning the baby massage class. The oil, which May provides, is all that is needed for the massage, other than a soft towel on which the baby lies.

May has been running these classes at Whitehills Maternity Unit in Forfar for three years, having received her Baby Massage Instructors' Course certificate following a weekend training session in Edinburgh in 1996. Her training was partly funded by the health board – the trust paid for the course, while May paid for her own accommodation and travel. She is enthusiastic about the benefits to both the babies and the mothers. 'It can be difficult coping with a new baby', she acknowledges, 'and these classes will give you special protected time with your baby. It is definitely a getting-to-know-you session for both mum and baby.'

May likes to have around eight to ten babies in each class, and for each baby and mother to attend six sessions. The babies can come when they are three weeks old. May points out that massage is done in special care baby units, so there is no reason to wait until the baby is any older.

Baby massage is not new. It is believed to have originated in India over 2,000 years ago and still today many women in other parts of the world do it automatically. Massage helps young babies in many ways. First and foremost it is a form of communication, which can help to form a strong bond between the mother and the infant. May believes that it can also be beneficial to a baby's physical health and wellbeing by helping to eliminate toxins, encouraging good muscle

tone, soothing the baby and helping him to sleep.

Another aspect of the class, which is very important to May, is that it gives new mothers the chance to meet one another. She says 'Mums are so relaxed at the end of a massage that they like to sit and chat.' It also provides an opportunity for May to give them advice about diet or immunisations – about anything, in fact, which you would contact a health visitor for. May says 'It doesn't matter that I am not their own health visitor. They can ask me about anything that they are unsure of.'

Other health visitors have taken a keen interest in May's classes and several have requested training. Of course, this would inevitably require funding. May would certainly like to see training for health visitors in the area, so that every practice had at least one health visitor who did massage.

During the class, May 'massages' a life-sized doll, always showing the mothers exactly what to do, explaining the importance of certain parts of the massage. She starts off by saying to the mothers 'Ask your baby's permission to start.' She then explains that the babies can smell the oil and know what is coming. She feels it is important to keep talking to the baby – 'Your face in front of them, your voice – that is the best toy they can have' – and to look out for visual signs that the baby is getting fed up or does not like what is being done at any time. 'If the baby is not enjoying it, he will twist about,' she says. 'If this happens draw your face into focus and reassure your little one.'

Certainly, all the babies seemed to be thoroughly enjoying their massage. Arlene Kerrigan, who was attending the class with her 14-week-old son, Ryan, says 'My health visitor suggested the course. I really enjoy doing the massage and Ryan enjoys it too. I have been trying to do it at home.'

May explains that this massage can be done until the baby is around five months old, by which time he will be rolling over and the massage can progress to something more boisterous. She suggests that by then the mothers should be saying nursery rhymes to their babies, such as 'This Little Piggy', while doing the actions. 'Your Mum probably said these rhymes to you', she says. 'We don't want to lose them.'

If a mother already has a toddler and wants to learn how to massage her new baby, May will visit her at home for a couple of sessions. It is all part of the juggling act. She says 'I have to juggle my caseload with the classes, but it is worth it.'

Reflecting on alternative therapies

- Bearing in mind the professional constraints on midwives who are not separately qualified in an alternative therapy, how can midwives appropriately give information about different alternative therapies to women who are interested in this? Which alternative therapies are within the scope of the midwife's role, and which are not?
- How are alternative therapies best evaluated? Should they be subjected to quantitative research studies, in the same way that drugs and other interventions are (or should be)? Or should we be developing tools which are more in line with the original philosophy of the therapy?
- Are alternative therapies interventions? Why do some midwives feel more comfortable with offering an alternative therapy that has not been fully evaluated in midwifery practice than with offering a drug or other intervention that has been evaluated? How does this impact our own philosophies?
- Do women have access to a list of alternative therapists locally? Would this be a useful and appropriate thing to offer women who were interested in this? Bearing in mind that it is always better to refer women to any other professional by personal experience, could such a tool be collated from the experience of local midwives and their families?

- How can midwives gather evidence on the efficacy and effectiveness of therapies which have been researched? Can this information be used to inform local initiatives and the range of services on offer to women?

Group exercise

One of the best ways of gaining the knowledge needed to talk to women about alternative therapies is for midwives to experience the therapy themselves. However, it is not always practical or possible to experience every available therapy firsthand; a good alternative to this is to discuss someone else's experience with them and to be able to ask questions about this. If you are interested in finding out more about the different alternative therapies on offer, a group of midwives can undertake to experience one new therapy each, and then feed back to the group about their experience.

This can also enable midwives to gather local contacts and talk to therapists about what they might be able to offer women during the childbearing year. Most therapists offer information leaflets and details of other resources; collating these for the group builds up quickly into a small library of information which may be useful for women wanting to find out more.

Stories and reflection

Midwives have always learned from stories. Traditionally, midwives learned their art at the feet of an older and more experienced woman. Both before and after development of the written word, stories were a tool to teach students and colleagues important lessons in a way that was both accessible and easily recalled. Women and midwives love hearing and telling stories, especially birth stories. Every midwife has sat next to an eighty-year-old woman who, upon finding out what she does, delightedly recounts her birth stories as if they happened yesterday.

I have spoken to lots of different groups of students and midwives, and in almost every group people will sometimes turn to whisper to their neighbour while I am speaking. I have learned to not mind this, since I discovered that this is often because they have a story or anecdote relating to the topic that they need to share. But I also discovered that, when I take a break from discussing the evidence, or the ethics, or the politics of an issue, and tell a story, nobody whispers anymore. Other midwife teachers agree that, if you want to get a group's attention, you only need to tell a birth story or two! Stories speak to women; they are an important – and universal – way of knowing for women. They are also an important form of the evidence which informs midwifery practice.

The following stories and reflective pieces speak for themselves. Some are funny, some are sad; some contain great and timeless wisdom. It seems only fair to give the last word in this book to Jilly Rosser; it was under her and Tricia Anderson's vision and direction that *The Practising Midwife* took shape as the journal which openly celebrated stories and other ways of knowing and became a resource for best practice in midwifery.

Pictures at a birth

Caroline Flint

Photographs can be such a comfort. My mother, widowed for ten years, always brings a photo of my father with her when she comes to stay. He stands on her bedside table, beaming at the world from his photograph.

For me, perhaps one of the most moving aspects of a labour and birth are the photos that women bring with them – pictures of those they love who watch over them and give them strength. I was moved to tears when a woman whose first child had been killed in a car crash at the age of two kept talking to her daughter's photo, convinced that the reason that she was coping so well was due to the benign influence of the little angel looking down on her. But the particular labour I am thinking about now was graced with the photo of a beloved mother who had died a year previously.

For women whose mothers are dead, having a baby is especially hard. At the time of becoming a mother, many women find an empathy with their own mother which brings them closer – for many mothers and daughters it is the reawakening of a relationship which brings great joy to both of them.

However, it isn't mother-daughter relationships that are the point of this story – it is underpants.

A young couple had decided to have their first baby in our Birth Centre. She (we will call her Joanna) called me at 10am on a Friday morning last summer when she was eight days overdue. Joanna had been having period type pains occasionally all through the night, she had also had a show. I examined her abdomen, the fundus was compatible with dates, presentation was cephalic, head engaged, LOA and FHHR 132-144. I did not do a vaginal examination because Joanna was so chatty and full of beans that it made me think that this was not yet established labour. The couple were planning to go on a forty-mile journey in the car and they would be back at about 5-6pm. I thought this was a good idea; it would keep Joanna occupied and they had a mobile phone to keep in touch with me if they needed to. Joanna and Martin sped off and I went about my business.

At 6.30pm I telephoned them. Joanna sounded as bright as a button. She was leaking small spurts of clear fluid and the baby had been moving. I wished them well and told them that I expected that they would ring me during the night.

Just as I lay my head on the pillow at 11pm, my bleep went off. When I arrived at their house Joanna was having contractions every four minutes. The abdominal palpation was the same as in the morning, but this time I did a vaginal examination – cervix completely effaced and thin, posterior and 2cm dilated.

The membranes were intact and the FHHR 150-156. We decided to go to the Birth Centre – I went first to warm up the room and run water into the birth pool and Joanna and Martin followed. They arrived at 00.45 and Joanna put the photo of her mother on the side of the pool and then got into the water with a sigh of relief.

Then the underpants discussion started. Martin had already decided that he would also get into the pool, but should he wear his underpants? Joanna thought no, I said I didn't mind one way or the other. The labour was obviously hotting up and I went into the office and called Val, my midwife colleague, to join me – I told her about the underpants discussion.

I went back inside the room – the underpants discussion was still in full flow, Joanna voicing her thoughts between contractions and Martin voicing his during contractions. Well, this is one way of passing the time, I thought. Joanna's cries were increasing, she was taking entonox, it seemed to me that labour was progressing rapidly. The condition of both mother and baby was fine, but still the discussion raged. I said to Martin that if he didn't hurry up and decide, the baby would be out first.

Joanna was beginning to grunt. I pointed this out to Martin, at which point Joanna's mother made the decision; he looked at her photo and said 'Well, she wouldn't want to see me naked'. And with that he jumped into the pool in his underpants and cradled Joanna in his arms. Baby Leo emerged from his mother while she lay on her husband. The baby looked around and then settled down on his mother's chest to breath efficiently and quietly.

After the birth, when Joanna was sitting on the birth stool to deliver the placenta, the underpants discussion started again! Would Martin wear wet underpants under his trousers, or would he wear no underpants under his trousers? The placenta plopped out and Joanna snuggled into bed.

But I can't tell you what Martin decided to do; I went off to make a cup of tea and scrambled eggs on toast – much more important!

Caring for Ann
A reflective case study

Jenny Fraser

I first met Ann when she was 12 weeks pregnant. She came to see me at her GP's surgery for her first antenatal appointment. Ann had obvious physical disabilities. She was short in stature with a visibly curved spine and deformities of both legs. She was late for the appointment and explained that she found the narrow toilet in the surgery difficult to squeeze into, and that she needed to empty her bladder regularly.

As Ann apologised, I noticed that she had a speech impediment. She told me that she had been profoundly deaf since birth, hence her speech difficulty. It was obvious that Ann was going to need extra time to communicate during this first antenatal, and addressing the most suitable means of interaction was a priority. She could lip-read and could also sign, but she did not want a sign interpreter with her during antenatal visits as she liked her privacy and only wanted to share these intimate moments with the relevant health professionals.

I was very conscious of a busy afternoon's antenatal clinic, and I knew that I would inevitably keep other women waiting if I focused my attention on Ann. However, I felt that Ann was in great need of support and that it was vital to begin to establish some mutual trust and confidence.

A difficult life

Once comfortable, Ann continued with some more of her background. She was rubella damaged whilst in her mother's womb. As well as being deaf she had a closed spina bifida and talipes of both feet. Daily activities were difficult; because of her curved fused spine she was just 4'10" tall and could only walk slowly. She was 25, single and lived alone in a specially adapted ground floor flat with low surfaces and handrails. Her doorbell and telephone were fitted with flashing lights, and she had a minicom system using typetalk to enable telephone conversations.

Ann was very much on her own, with no particular close friends. She did not mention the baby's father, and I did not pursue the issue. Her mother deserted her as a baby when it became clear that profound disabilities were present. She had no brothers or sisters and lived with her father until she was 17. He subsequently moved to London, remarried and kept minimal contact with his daughter.

Despite this, it was obvious from this first meeting that Ann was intelligent, with a noteworthy sense of humour. She valued her independence and did not want to share her life with someone who would tell her what to do.

Special needs

This first meeting took up a great deal of time. I offered Ann home antenatal visits, because in addition to everything else, she found it difficult to clamber onto the couch for examination. She declined this offer as she was determined to be independent and preferred to travel to the surgery. We made a double appointment for Ann's next visit, to allow more time for her special circumstances.

Ann told me several times that she would like to give birth at home, where she would be in familiar surroundings and could maintain some feelings of control. However, she needed consultant-led care because of her condition. I accompanied Ann to her consultant antenatal appointments at her request. She hated having to go to the hospital, because although she was treated kindly and warmly, it brought back distressing memories of many hospital visits in her life.

During the first consultation the possibility of a Caesarean section was discussed because of Ann's misshapen pelvis. Her consultant stated that a decision would be made later, once the size of the baby and the lie were determined. As the pregnancy progressed it became clear that a Caesarean would be necessary, and that Ann would need a general anaesthetic for the operation because of her curved fused spine. Ann was very frightened by this prospect and talked through the procedure with me over and over again. She felt that it was vital to have a familiar face in theatre and to have support from someone who knew her during her recovery. I made arrangements with my colleagues and managers so that I would be free to be with Ann.

The best laid plans...

Unfortunately the premature rupture of her membranes three days before Ann's elective Caesarean section made an emergency Caesarean section necessary. I was on annual leave, and I did not find out that Ann had had her baby until my first day back at work, which was the day of the initial planned Caesarean. By then her baby was three days old.

I went to see Ann immediately. She was very upset and distressed that I had not been with her for her Caesarean. She had felt very let down by not having a familiar face in theatre. She said that although the midwife who had been with her was kind and caring, she did not know her and had felt unable to communicate freely.

Postnatal stay

Ann spent ten full days in hospital on the postnatal ward. She had very few visitors. Her physical disability was obvious and this provoked adequate practical responses from staff; a stool was found to enable her to climb onto the bed, and the cot was adjusted to aid her. However, her transition to parenthood, which should have been enabling and empowering, was hampered by paternalism. Her short stature and speech difficulties led to the staff and the other women on the ward viewing her more as a young girl than as an adult who had overcome enormous challenges in her life. Many midwives became 'motherly' with her and kindly took over the care of her baby, instead of supporting Ann and allowing her to learn to care for the baby competently herself.

During her hospital stay, Ann was rarely asked to make any decisions – assumptions about her care were made on her behalf. Staff would often lift her onto the bed in order to 'help', resulting in her feeling particularly undermined and incapable. However, Ann's deafness, which was not immediately visible, was the disability that caused her the most distress. Several times she told me that she just nodded and smiled at staff if it was too difficult to try to communicate. She was worried that if she asked too many times for words to be repeated, staff would think that she was mentally as well as physically impaired. During this time Ann also received some negative reactions about her ability to parent her child, mainly from the other mothers on the ward.

Problems at home

Ann had help available night and day during her stay in hospital. When she finally returned home with her baby, she felt desperately alone and isolated. I visited her on the first morning and found her in acute distress, crying inconsolably and feeling unable to cope. These feelings were unusual for Ann as she had coped with immense adversity in her life and has always preferred to be independent. Although she was used to dealing with her disabilities she found that the new baby added a further impairment to her life, and a confusing one at that.

Several days later Ann was still not coping with the demands of the baby. She became depressed and I felt that she was slipping into a situation in which she would be unable to cope at all, a position which she would have hated. Having to manage the baby all day meant that she had no reserves to cope at night, so she was extraordinarily tired. A visual sound activator was in place, to indicate whether the baby was crying, but Ann spent a lot of the night awake, watching the light because she felt that if she was asleep she would not see it flashing. Confusingly for Ann the light flashed indiscriminately with any sound – even the baby wriggling and murmuring would trigger it. She rang the 'on call' midwife every night. For Ann to summon assistance in such a way was a very genuine cry for help.

Support at last

I realised that something had to be done to help Ann immediately, and I set about organising some support for her. Through the social services, I eventually found a carer to help with the day-to-day care of the baby, allowing Ann to rest so that she was fresh for the night. We also found a 'befriender', to get to know Ann and take her out sometimes. Even though the situation was urgent, these support mechanisms took a while to get through the system and they were not in place until the baby was four weeks old. By this time Ann had begun to neglect her baby as a survival technique for herself. However, the supporters were very successful and Ann started to live her life again and be happy.

Ann's baby has subsequently flourished in her care and is now a happy and contented toddler; they have a confident and secure bond between them.

Reflection

I regularly see Ann out walking with her toddler. She looks brave and in control again. Every time I see her I reflect ruefully on the fact that much more could have been done to pave her way for a smoother transition to parenthood.

- If we had made contact with some support groups antenatally, Ann would have felt less isolated and lonely in the postnatal period. Time would not have been wasted getting Ann into the 'system' postnatally when the situation was grave. Midwives are in a unique position to foster coordination between agencies; for example, the daily carer and the befriender could have been in place in the antenatal period. It only took a few telephone calls to social services to discover the way of accessing the help. The delay postnatally was not their fault – they gave their attention to Ann as soon as was practically possible.

- In hindsight I had a responsibility not only to originate the provision of maternity care but also to provide Ann with information about the maternity services, thus promoting her self-reliance, independence and confidence. There are some excellent books available which enable the disabled mother to be better prepared for parenthood by presenting an insight into our world. For example, *The Baby Challenge*[1] speaks directly and effectively to parents-to-be in a non-judgemental, honest and easy-to-understand way.

- One-to-one learning about birth seemed to be the most appropriate way of helping Ann during the antenatal period. She would make out a list of questions, which we would painstakingly plough our way through. In hindsight I realise that I fell into the trap of thinking that I knew what was best for Ann. Choices should have been available to her, rather than a decision made for her. In fact, Ann was in desperate need of contact with other women at the same stage of pregnancy as herself, to generate some friendship and support. Antenatal classes are not just a forum for imparting information. When Ann was feeling 'low' postnatally, she found it impossible even to try to communicate with other women with new babies, whereas she may have been able to do so if she had formed a relationship earlier. The social benefit could well have staved off some of the awful feelings of gloom and desolation.

- A support mechanism should have been in place for the birth, to take into account any untoward circumstances, such as the situation that actually arose. Ann would not then have felt abandoned in the way that she did. It would have been straightforward for all of the midwives working within our small team to have been made aware of Ann's special needs, and she could have met some of the other midwives. She would then have had a familiar face with her in theatre, even though it may not have been the most familiar.

- Kelsall's pioneering work[2,3] on the care of a deaf woman during pregnancy was invaluable for enabling quality two-way interaction between myself and Ann. She had no hesitation in letting me know if something could be done to enhance her understanding of what was being said, such as moving me into a particular position so that she could lip-read more easily. I developed a better understanding of the wider issues relevant to Ann and of the difficulties faced by disabled mothers. But whilst it has been a truly learning and reflective experience for me, how much better it would have been to have had a wider knowledge in advance. There are excellent national self-help groups which can be tapped into, as well as any local help. Women who are connected to a network of disabled mothers in the community are better prepared to tackle the challenges of pregnancy, birth and parenting.[4]

- In retrospect it would have been better for Ann to have gone home earlier from the postnatal ward with community support as described, had it been in place early enough. Ten days in hospital were disorientating and it took a long time for Ann to pick up the threads of her life again.

I hope that others will reflect and learn from my experience. Let's make sure that we liaise with our professional and lay colleagues. By sharing specialist information we can deliver a high quality service that is truly appropriate for the women in our collective care.

REFERENCES

1 Campion M. The baby challenge: A handbook on pregnancy for women with a physical disability. London: Routledge; 1990.
2 Kelsall J. Giving midwifery care for the deaf in the 1990s. Midwives Chronicle 1993; 106(1262):80–83.
3 Kelsall J. Hearing impairment and midwifery care. In: Kargar I, Hunt S (eds). Challenges in midwifery care. London: Macmillan; 1997.

4 McEwan Carty E, Conine T, Hall L. Comprehensive health promotion for the pregnant woman who is disabled. Journal of Nurse Midwifery 1990; 35(3):134–136.

A mother's experience of Edgware Birth Centre

Krystina Kweik

A dimmed bedside lamp; peace and quiet; a lovely decorated bedroom with en suite bathroom; carpet underfoot; all colour coordinated. Everything is spotlessly clean without seeming clinical, a radio is playing music softly and the smell of lavender is coming from an oil burner. Am I in an expensive hotel? No. A yellow crib with ducks painted on it is in the corner. I'm in Edgware Birth Centre. It's twelve thirty on a Friday night and I've got two casually dressed women to help me – one is the midwife, the other her assistant. Not a clinical white coat in sight, no uniforms, no monitoring machines.

There's no stress. The birth pool, stool, chair and beanbag are there if I want them. If I want to give birth standing in the shower I could. I am encouraged to do what I want. If I feel the urge to run round the staff car park I am 100% sure my midwife will jog with me.

I'm not expected to lie on the bed – unless, of course, I want to… I'm certainly not made to… pinch me and wake me up, I'm dreaming… it can't be true, I've had two children in hospital… it doesn't happen this way.

My 9lb 3½oz daughter is born half an hour later without me using anything but a couple of puffs of gas and air. The midwives ask if they can bath Leila – of course, I say. They coo and fuss over both me and my baby, as if they are members of my family. Why is Leila so special? They must have delivered dozens of babies. The answer is them; they are special, the environment of the birth centre is special… it's job satisfaction… they care… they want to be working here.

It was a pleasure to deliver Leila… honestly.

I still physically and mentally cringe when I think of the births of my two older children. I was in hospital, not in control, I lay on a bed being monitored. Why? I wasn't ill, I was pregnant.

I made an informed choice as to how I was going to have my baby this time round and it was a great experience. My GP was against me coming to the Birth Centre and refused to refer me. But I came anyway and I'm glad I did.

Taken to the limit

Kate Olsen

I'm a great believer in informed choice. Waterbirth, homebirth, up-a-chimney birth – you name it, if that's what women want, I'll support it. Or so I thought. Yet recently I was pushed to the limits and found myself out at the grey edges of midwifery practice, which is, I can now report back, an uncomfortable and lonely place to be.

Sometimes women make choices that we do not feel comfortable with, and yet we cannot withdraw our support. Often there is little or no 'hard' information on which they can base their choices, or on which we can base our advice. Out at the edges there are few hard facts or solid statistics to rely on, and the familiar shape of the medical model suddenly becomes very reassuring.

Julia's choice

Julia, a woman on my caseload, was expecting her third baby, and her dates were certain. She made it clear during her pregnancy that she would not consider a 'routine' induction in the absence of any indication of fetal compromise. After a long and deliberate consideration of the evidence, she decided that the risk of intervening in a natural process by inducing labour was greater than any potential risk of not inducing her labour.

41 weeks passed. 42 weeks passed. No signs of labour. The head of the baby would sometimes be engaged, and sometimes not. At 42 weeks Julia had a CTG (which was fine), a visit to the consultant, and decided to 'wait it out'. She tried all the 'natural' things to get labour started – sex, homeopathy and so on. The baby seemed healthy and active.

Oligohydramnios

Then, at 42½ weeks, Julia had an ultrasound scan which was not fine. There was an almost total absence of liquor. All we could see was a tiny spit under the baby's chin, not even enough to measure. The ultrasonographers were marvellous; together, we pored over their charts to see just what the normal liquor volume range might be at 42½ weeks, but the charts just didn't go beyond 42 weeks. How much liquor could you expect at this late gestation, and what was the significance, if any, of having so little? The textbooks, one after the other, confirmed what I knew: that oligohydramnios was a risk factor for cord compression and fetal compromise. I showed the books to Julia; we discussed the risks in detail, but it was impossible to quantify them. I searched the literature, discussed it with my colleagues and asked the advice of several well-respected midwifery consultants, all of whom confirmed that oligohydramnios was a risk factor to be taken seriously.

Yet several subsequent CTGs were fine and the baby was active. Julia still believed that the risks of induction outweighed the risks of oligohydramnios, and felt intuitively that the baby was fine.

Desperate

The next few days were filled with my anxiety. In my mind's eye, there was no fluid left to cushion the cord or give it a slippery surface. One colleague had said: 'If that baby sticks out an elbow in the wrong place, or that woman stands up suddenly…' Every day I visited Julia I was afraid that today might be the day that there was no fetal heart to be heard. Every day I hoped that she might want to have labour induced. I was desperate for her to go into labour.

At night I would lie awake, trying to discriminate between needless anxiety – a result of working in maternity units where induction at term +10 days is routine – and valid concerns. I was haunted by that well-known graph showing the rate of unexplained stillbirths rising as gestation progresses, and tried to grapple with how that graph of statistics could be applied to Julia's individual situation. Yet whilst being totally, unblinkingly honest with Julia about my concerns (as was her consultant), I didn't want my fear to invade her.

I never thought I'd live to hear myself say this, but how I love supervisors of midwives! The support I received during this time was superb. They truly understood the meaning of the word 'responsibility': listening and responding to my needs without needing to take over or intervene.

Induced at last

Finally, at 43½ weeks, it was Julia who made the decision that she was now ready for labour to be induced. In her own time and her own way, she felt she had given 'nature' long enough to work. The induction was simple enough – a syntocinon infusion quickly put Julia into a short, straightforward labour. The baby was born easily with a meconium all-over body-pack! The placenta was calcified, the Wharton's jelly on the cord was shrivelled and dry, but the baby was absolutely fine.

Was Julia a foolish woman, and lucky to 'get away with it'? Or was I an overly-anxious midwife? What would the outcome have been if Julia had not opted for induction? I'm still puzzling and reflecting.

Sometimes, being a midwife who supports informed choice is very hard.

The 'D' word

Hannah Hulme Hunter

Don't tell anyone, but I pay a young woman (her name is Judy) to do my ironing. I know I should feel bad about this, but Judy does wonders for my husband's appearance, and she is incredibly good for my ego. In a nutshell, Judy thinks I am Wonderful. I think she has even used the word Cool. She spends quite a long time telling me so each week. And why? Because I am a midwife.

The conversation generally goes something like this;

Judy: Do you really deliver babies?

Me (nonchalantly): Oh, yes.

Judy: Every day?

Me (reluctantly): Well, just some of the time.

Judy: On your own, then? No doctors?

Me (casually, loving every moment): Goodness, no! Midwives work quite independently of doctors – so long as everything's okay.

Judy: Wow. That's brilliant. I wish you could have delivered my baby.

Deliver: rescue, save, set free from, disburden (women in parturition) of child (usu. passive)…
(Concise Oxford Dictionary)

Okay, you know where I'm heading and you've heard this before, and from writers far more eloquent and learned than myself; how words used carelessly in our daily work may inadvertently harm the women in our care. Words that patronise: 'all my ladies…', 'I usually allow…', 'we're having good contractions…'. And words that diminish: 'incompetent cervix', 'failure to progress', 'trial of labour', 'deliver'.

This (I hope) is familiar stuff and, as midwives, we try to chose our words carefully – but so often time is short, and confidence is low, and we think the medics won't respect us unless we talk like Dr Corday on ER, (it probably wouldn't hurt to look like her, either), and so I'm going to suggest just one very small, but incredibly powerful, change – we stop using the word 'deliver'.

'Don't worry, Mrs B, I will deliver your baby.'

Meaning? All you have to do is cope, Mrs B, exhausted, starving and frightened, for twelve hours with the worst pain you've ever experienced, before pushing with all your might for an hour (maybe more), straining, leaking and defecating in front of strangers, at the end of which I will – for a few brief moments – place my hands (almost entirely superfluously) on your baby as you push him out, yet it will be my name that is entered in the column marked 'Delivered By' in the Birth Register for all time (or for 25 years – whichever comes first). Surely what we really want Mrs B to hear is this:

'I will care for you, whilst you give birth to your baby.'

In other words: A first labour can be long and hard, but the female body is a wonderful thing. I know you can do it. I will be there for you when things get tough, I will protect you from unnecessary interference and unwanted distraction, and I will use my professional skills and knowledge to keep you and your baby safe and well, as you labour to bring him forth into this world.

Saying what we mean

So why not say what we mean? Why use sloppy and out-dated words?

Not saying the word 'delivery' isn't really that hard. Think about it. There are very, very few instances when the word 'birth', or something similar, cannot be substituted. It's really just a matter of practice:

'Mrs B gave birth last night. It was lovely. She was so strong and calm.'
(How much more empowering – and accurate – than the ubiquitous 'I had a lovely delivery last night.')

'I guide the mother as she breathes her baby's head out.'
('I aim to deliver the head slowly.')

'I attended Mrs B when she had her baby.'
('I delivered Mrs B.')

'I have to care for ten more women as they give birth.'
('I need ten more deliveries.')

Avoiding the D word isn't so hard, is it? The chances are that your colleagues won't notice anything different. But the women for whom you care will. Guaranteed!

Multiple sclerosis and homebirths

Susan Burvill

Multiple sclerosis is the most prevalent central nervous system disorder in the UK.[1] It involves a degeneration of the fatty sheath that protects nerves. This myelin sheath insulates and ensures proper conductivity of nervous impulses. 'Sclerosis' refers to hardened patches, which cover demyelinated nerves, and 'multiple' implies many areas affected in the same way. MS is very unpredictable and idiosyncratic, presenting with a variety of symptoms, some of which are mild while others can be very severe and debilitating for the sufferer. Individual impairment from person to person varies considerably, as does the course of the disease.

The majority of MS diagnosed people are women (ratio of 2:1) in their childbearing years and the disease is therefore of importance to midwives. The unpredictability of both the MS condition and childbearing can put stress on women who require sensitive and individualised care. This is the story of Virginia and her two births at home. The story illustrates clearly that MS, like childbirth, should not be treated as an illness, but as highly unique to each woman's personal experience. Also, MS, like childbirth, cannot be seen as purely physiological; there are powerful emotional and social elements that interact with one another influencing the course of the condition.[2]

The first time I met Virginia I was incredibly impressed by her strength and by her response to the diagnosis of MS that she had received four years before I first met her. Virginia called me in her first pregnancy at 27 weeks gestation. She was booked in at her local hospital for maternity care but had become increasingly concerned that her wishes and concerns had not been heard. Virginia had been a professional dancer before her MS had slowly taken away her sense of balance, mobility and ability to endure tiring workouts and rehearsals. She continued to be a singer but had obviously had to surrender her dancing ambitions since her diagnosis and the onset of various symptoms related to her MS.

Virginia was very clear at our first meeting what she was looking for. She had read Judy Graham's book about MS[3] and had spoken with the author directly. She didn't want to feel medicalised and have unnecessary interventions due to her MS diagnosis. She had decided to inform herself about the options and was very proactive in self-help approaches, using nutrition and homeopathy. She had resisted pharmacological prescriptions from her medical advisers as she felt this would only serve to weaken her already compromised immune system. For the same reasons she felt strongly that drugs in pregnancy and labour were to be avoided as much as possible. Weighing all the options available to her, she opted for a homebirth with an independent midwife who could spend time discussing her concerns about the whole process of childbearing in detail. The emphasis was put on ways to minimise fatigue, stress and need for medication while promoting a sense of the positive in the whole process. Virginia had found that the local hospital lacked the time to respond to her anxieties and were unable to provide the kind of sensitivity she required to face her journey to motherhood with MS and all its uncertainty. She told me that the staff at the hospital were all courteous but extremely busy and only concerned about her 'condition with MS' and not the fact that she was a woman behind the MS who was having a baby.

On my first meeting with Virginia, it was evident that there was grief and regret about loosing the life she had originally planned for. Virginia was very much in touch with her emotions and mental state. She understood clearly from experience with MS that her psychological and emotional wellbeing was imperative if she was to stay well. She had been seeing a psychotherapist since her MS diagnosis in an attempt to change her behaviour to a more positive one in order to stay healthy. Excluding the psychosocial aspects of her care would have been detrimental to her and I feel would have adversely interfered with her capacity to adapt to motherhood.

Although Virginia's physical symptoms were not totally debilitating, they were disturbing and distressing. She experienced much anxiety about what may eventually happen to her and each and every symptom of her pregnancy was addressed. For example, before the pregnancy she had endured frequency of micturition, mild incontinence and urgency. She had a degree of back numbness, a left-sided dull ache into the hips and bad occasional migraines that increased with fatigue and stress. These symptoms and other symptoms became exacerbated as the pregnancy advanced. Many studies show pregnancy to be a stabilising factor in MS[4,5,6] but it was difficult to know at times whether the MS was worsening, or whether Virginia was experiencing common pregnancy symptoms.

In order not to devalue her concerns we discussed the reasons for her symptoms and how they may be symptoms of pregnancy even without MS. Frequent MSUs were sent and occasional vaginal swabs for possible thrush to help allay her concerns for infections, which in themselves can accelerate MS pathology. Each symptom was examined and discussed at each antenatal visit. Improvements were celebrated and worsening symptoms carefully discussed, noted and monitored. I encouraged Virginia to understand her female body and its amazing adaptation to pregnancy and what a healthy, natural and dynamic process it was. I attempted to empathise with Virginia's situation by ensuring that she did not feel judged or labelled as being 'unduly anxious'. Most women experience emotional turmoil in pregnancy as they adapt and come to terms with a major life change, it was important with Virginia to maintain perspective while remaining alert and sensitive to potentially irrational concerns.

The main problems Virginia encountered during her first pregnancy were recurrent bouts of Candida. Many natural remedies and diet adjustment appeared to help and Canistan was eventually used. Towards the end, fatigue due to sleeping problems was a major problem for Virginia. Fatigue is generally difficult to control and unpredictable for people with MS, and it caused a lot of concern to the couple. We discussed help postnatally and contacted the local social services to find a home help, but to no avail. Luckily, Virginia's mother was able to provide a lot of support despite living far away. I was concerned for Virginia postnatally as MS has been shown in various studies to worsen 0-6 months post delivery.[5,6,7] We discussed broken sleep due to childcare and breastfeeding, and ways of dealing with this. Virginia was also worried that her fatigue would inhibit milk supply. She was very positive about breastfeeding for many reasons common to all mothers but in addition, she felt that due to the high levels of essential fatty acids in breastmilk her child would potentially receive a protective effect against MS.

Weight increases and body shape changes created problems with Virginia's balance and mobility. Her nervous system was constantly adapting to areas of numbness brought on by fatigue and the extra stresses of pregnancy caused her added problems. The fetal head on the bladder later in the pregnancy increased urgency and incontinence, making it more and more difficult to travel far from home. Heat regulation was difficult for Virginia. She had had increased sensitivity to heat that immediately exhausted her for some time. The increased blood volume only added to the heat problem, as well as the fact that she was heavily pregnant in July. We had discussed the use of water in labour and she felt warm water would be harmful to her energy levels and was not really a viable option. Postnatally it was imperative that Virginia didn't suffer unnecessary milk engorgement and its related pyrexia due to the fatigue issue, equally infection risks had to be kept to a minimum. Overall it was our plan to interfere as little as possible with the natural process, avoid infections and ensure adequate rest.

The first homebirth

Virginia called me in the night to say she was losing some pink discharge, she was feeling occasional contractions down her legs with some backache. She had felt uncomfortable and not slept all night, she could 'feel nothing' in her pelvis and her numbness was a little worse. She requested that I examine her to see if anything was happening. Abdominally the baby was lying LOA and was well engaged. Internally Virginia's cervix was 3 centimetres dilated with the vertex still above the ischial spines and bulging membranes. The plan now was to eat, drink and sleep, or at least rest. I went home to sleep more myself, returning later that day. Contractions were now more regular but not 'felt' as painful. Virginia was a bit fed up so we went for a walk in the local park but the contractions remained the same. I again left Virginia and asked her to call me when contractions became more uncomfortable and regular. Six hours later I returned. Contractions were now frequent, and Virginia was tired but not in a lot of pain. She asked to be examined; her cervix was now 5 centimetres with bulging membranes. She was passing urine at least half hourly. Shortly after the examination the membranes ruptured and within a few hours contractions became strong and regular. Virginia was now quite tired but positive and began complaining of rectal pressure. There was lots of clear liquor draining accompanied by a strong reactive fetal heart. I advised Virginia to eat and drink something and her husband gave her back massage. By the early hours of the morning Virginia was very tired, contractions slowed and there were no urges to push. Virginia was helped to bed to rest in left lateral position. A fan was used to keep her cool along with cold drinks. A few hours later she had an urge to push. Virginia wanted to try upright positions to allow gravity to help, but an hour later the urge to push had not developed into spontaneous pushing. We discussed an examination and agreed it would be good to know. An anterior lip was found, with a baby in an OA position, flexed, below the spines with no caput or moulding.

The contractions again slowed to 2 in 10 minutes. Virginia returned to left lateral and we encouraged her to rest. All maternal and baby observations remained healthy. By now Virginia was fatigued and her MS symptoms started to increase, especially the numbness in the pelvis and back. Two hours later anal dilatation was noted with only a very slight urge to push. There was a clear defined red line between her buttocks extending now to the top. Virginia got up and wanted to try and push in a squat and on a bucket alternately. She reported not being able to feel anything to push, the MS had taken the feeling away.

Two hours later the vertex could be seen. Virginia could not feel much but was very determined. Her legs could no longer support her so she continued left lateral. With lots of encouragement from her husband and her personal strength she birthed her 7lb 7oz baby boy and his placenta without being medicalised. There was no 'fetal ejection reflex' or 'Fergusson reflex'. In the final hours of her labour it was like caring for a woman with a dense epidural block as all sensation vanished in the second stage. The baby was born a bit shocked but responded to his mother's voice instantly and took straight to the breast. It was a long arduous labour, but the look of triumph and empowerment on Virginia's face was amazing. The only problem was when her husband and I attempted to bath the baby and managed to pour the contents of the baby bath onto the living room carpet, needless to say we were also exhausted.

The postnatal period saw an increase in Virginia's frequency and urgency. Due to the constant moisture and irritation her perineum felt sore and she complained of dysuria. MSU and swabs were taken, these were clear. I encouraged her to start pelvic floor exercises even if she could not feel everything. She had a small perineal tear that healed wonderfully with a herbal pack and good hygiene. Tiredness was an ongoing issue, which was difficult to resolve. At the end of the first week Virginia expressed milk so that her husband could feed the baby at night to give her some unbroken sleep. Her mobility quickly returned and the numbness slowly abated as the days passed. By day 17 she went out for a short walk. Liaison with the local health visitor and social services for support was again made. The postnatal period until

28 days passed well. Virginia was obviously worried about the future and we talked about this at length. We discussed family planning but Virginia phoned me 10 months later and said 'Guess what?'

The second homebirth

The MS had not progressed since before the last birth. The major problem this time on booking was her BMI, which was only 18. Virginia was visibly thin, nauseous and without appetite. We discussed nutrition and homeopathy as ways of helping. I decided to keep an eye on her weight at each visit. Her weight steadily increased, as did the size of her baby. She started on Floradix as a tonic from 10 weeks onwards. The thrush was again a problem and this was treated. Colin, the first baby, was vibrant and a real handful, still breastfeeding. During the pregnancy he had chickenpox, glue ear and was teething. This was a very different pregnancy for Virginia; she had less time to worry about a good diet, exercise or yoga as with the first. The advantage was that they had moved nearer to Virginia's mother who provided fantastic support on a daily basis.

Virginia's emotional state was far more affected this time. She often felt quite low and unable to cope. She felt she no longer had the ability to give birth, as she was constantly tired. After an episode of syncope at 34 weeks she took my advice and began afternoon siestas. We had many conversations about the labour and birthing positions. At 39 weeks labour began, after she took castor oil for constipation (not my prescription). The constipation was not resolved but contractions were induced. This labour was much quicker and did not deplete Virginia's energy. The waters ruptured 6 hours after contractions began. Virginia coped very well and adopted an all-fours position. The contractions were rapid and intense. She ate some lasagne and said 'I want to push, but it's probably the constipation', and continued to eat. Twenty minutes into her meal I advised her to focus on what she was doing as I could see the vertex! She was totally shocked by this and taking another mouthful of food put her fork down. Ten minutes later she birthed her second baby boy, this time 8lb 12oz. We all laughed and embraced each other. It was wonderful to see Virginia's triumphant face again. The placenta followed physiologically and the new baby fed brilliantly. The postnatal period passed quickly with no abnormal events. Fatigue continued to be a concern, especially to her husband who was concerned for Virginia's wellbeing. We discussed strategies for ensuring Virginia got enough rest.

Virginia's story is one of triumph for all women who face a life with MS. Virginia is a strong woman who has taken control of her life since her diagnosis. She said to me on discharge:

'You know... if I didn't have MS I would have done what all my friends do, go to hospital and hand it all over and have an epidural.'

The MS, although a devastating diagnosis, had provided Virginia with much personal growth and insight to life. Her changed outlook and questioning approach to all the options was an inspiration to me. I feel my role as midwife was truly exercised with this new family. 'Being with' Virginia was an honour, she taught me much about the power of the human spirit and positive thinking.

REFERENCES

1 Campion M J. The baby challenge. London: Routledge; 1990.

2 Taylor M. Multiple sclerosis and midwifery care. In: Kargar I, Hunt SC (eds). Challenges in midwifery care. London: Macmillan; 1997.

3 Graham J. Multiple sclerosis, pregnancy and parenthood. Stanstead: The MS Resource Centre; 1996.

4 Duquette P, Girard M. Hormonal factors in susceptibility to multiple sclerosis. Current Opinion in Neurology and Neurosurgery 1993; 6:195–201.

5 Birk K, Rudick A. The clinical course of multiple sclerosis during pregnancy and the puerperium. Archives of Neurology 1990; 3:7–19.

6 Runmaker B, Anderson O. Pregnancy is associated with a lower risk of onset and a better prognosis in multiple sclerosis. Brain 1995; 118:253–261.

7 Roullet E, Verdier-Taillefer MH, Amarenco P, et al. Pregnancy and multiple sclerosis: A longitudinal study of 125 remittent patients. Journal of Neurology, Neurosurgery and Psychiatry 1993; 56:1062–1065.

8 Birk K, Rudick R. Pregnancy and multiple sclerosis. Archives of Neurology 1986; 43:719–726.

Born before arrival

Becky Reed

Yesterday, in the space of six hours, two women in our practice had a BBA. My mind turns to Oscar Wilde (with apologies): 'To miss one birth … may be regarded as a misfortune; to miss two looks like carelessness'! Clearly carelessness is what it is not; the last thing either of the midwives would have wanted would be to miss the births. And yet BBAs happen, either because women wait too long before calling, or because they simply don't realise how close the birth is (we have been told more than once 'I was waiting for the pain to get worse'!), or – and this feels like the most common reason – because the labour changes dramatically into a different gear, from something that feels easy to cope with, to a roller-coaster of contractions culminating in a sudden and surprising birth.

How do we midwives feel when this happens? Anxious, certainly, as we speed towards a woman's home where we know she is probably giving birth alone or with a worried partner, friend or even children in attendence. Cheated, maybe? – we would genuinely have liked to be there to see this little person coming into the world, and, after all, that is part of our job description. Guilty, even – should we have been able to get there in time? Are we 'bad' midwives because we didn't?

And how do the women themselves feel? A mixture of emotions I'm sure, ranging from surprise, shock and possibly fear through to pride in themselves after the event. And there is always the exciting tale to be told over and over for years to come…

Elena was having her second baby; her little boy Kier had been born at home after an efficient six-hour labour, with the midwives finally arriving at the onset of the second stage. Because we were aware of this, we included in our customary 36-week 'birth talk' a discussion about fast labour, with guidelines on what to do if Elena and her partner Anton thought labour was progressing rapidly. This includes calling the midwives and any other help, leaving the front door on the latch, turning the heating on/up if there's time, making a nest

with towels and getting into a knee-chest position to slow things down as much as possible, blowing as the baby's head is born (to prevent tearing) and keeping the baby warm, preferably skin-to-skin with its mother. It also includes trying to keep calm if possible and remembering that the midwife is on her way! Elena said afterwards that she had felt very reassured by this discussion.

Elena's pregnancy began smoothly, but at a 23-week scan the baby, a little girl, was seen to have a kidney problem. By 30 weeks this had been diagnosed as a bilateral duplex renal system with hydronephrosis on one side associated with a ureterocele. An anxious few weeks followed, but finally, at 35 weeks, Elena felt that she had a clear idea of what to expect, and a plan was agreed for the care of her baby postnatally. Importantly for Elena and Anton, there appeared to be no contraindication to the home birth they very much wanted. Elena was able at last to relax and prepare for her baby.

Mild contractions

One morning, just under a week before her due date, Elena bleeped me to let me know that things were starting to happen: she had had a 'show' and was feeling very mild, irregular contractions. We agreed to stay in touch and spoke again in the afternoon and in the evening; there was no change. I went to bed, fully expecting to be called in the night. My pager message came at 8.17am: 'waters have broken, regular every 6 minutes'. I phoned and spoke to Anton, who wasn't sure if Elena wanted me to come. Elena, however, couldn't speak to me, and I heard her in the background saying 'It feels like one continuous contraction'. I told Anton I was on my way and quickly phoned Cathy (Elena's other midwife) to let her know. It was now 8.20am.

Elena and Anton live in a small cul-de-sac of terraced houses, very close and neighbourly. At 8.40am I arrived at the end of the road. Anton was leaning out of the bedroom window shouting loudly enough for all the street to hear, 'You're useless – she's had it!'

Elena was kneeling up in her 'nest', cuddling her baby. Flossie, her friend and neighbour, was sitting next to Elena with a big grin on her face. She had come to collect Kier and stayed to help Anton catch his daughter. Baby Freya had shot into the world at 8.30am – only ten minutes after I had spoken to Anton. All was well with both mother and baby, and the two honorary midwives were both looking very pleased with themselves!

These days, when a woman has a BBA, we are required to fill out a form detailing the sequence of events leading up to the birth, and answering the question 'Could the BBA have been avoided?' My answer was: 'Only if I had lived next door!'

The coffee break epidural

Hannah Hulme Hunter

Has this ever happened to you? You've been supporting a woman in nice, normal, established labour. Let's call her Jane. It's all going really well. You've established a good rapport, drawn the curtains, dimmed the lights, and Jane is kneeling on a pile of pillows. During contractions she kneels up, swaying and moaning. Between contractions, she dozes, head in her partner's lap. You can almost *smell* the endorphins. You check her pulse, listen to her baby's heart, whisper encouragement – and go for a cup of coffee.

Fifteen minutes later, you return – to be met at the door by Sister X. She smiles. 'Your lady's decided to have an epidural now. I think it's for the best. She's wearing herself out, poor girl. I've bleeped the anaesthetist.'

What can you say? What can you *do*? Jane's agreed to have an epidural. Maybe it was even at her request. It's her decision: to try and talk her out of it now may only cause upset. Besides, there's a tiny seed of doubt already sprouting in your mind. *Maybe I've misjudged how well she's been coping. Maybe this is what she's wanted all along.*

It certainly seems like it. Half an hour later, Jane is sitting up in bed, alert and smiling, and flirting with the anaesthetist. It doesn't feel like labour any longer. It doesn't even *smell* like labour. That warm, sweet woman-smell has gone, replaced by something sharp and antiseptic. The lights are bright, the monitor bleeps happily, the Dynamap hums reassuringly. It's labour, Jim, but not as we know it.

Have you noticed how, when we midwives talk about pain relief to women, we rarely mention the one method that is completely safe, amazingly effective, completely free and requires no special equipment or advanced training to implement? We give lots of good, balanced information about epidurals and pethidine, and there's plenty of right-on talk about water and complementary therapies – but rarely a mention of the body's own, ready-loaded, plug-and-go pain relief system: endorphins.

Maybe this is because the trouble with endorphins is that seeing really is believing. Unless you have witnessed (or experienced yourself) a labour flowing under the influence of these morphine-like hormones, it is hard to appreciate their power. Hardest of all, endorphins – like fairies at the bottom of the garden – tend to slip away at the first sight of an unbeliever. It can be so disheartening.

Maybe it's time we got a bit more bullish about endorphins. How about lapel badges – 'Endorphins Rule Okay (if you let 'em)', copies of Andrea Robertson's *The Midwife Companion*[1] in every staff room, quotes from Michel Odent[2] on every noticeboard? What about a *policy*, for goodness sake? Labour wards are full of protocols and policies about epidurals and waterbirths – but have you ever seen one about endorphins? Why on earth not? There's a jolly sight more evidence concerning the endocrinology of labour than there is about, say, lavender oil in labour. (Not that I'm knocking lavender. Love it.)

And if anybody even *dares* to question the research base for 10,000 generations of human physiology, perhaps we should suggest that next time they feel like making love, they and their partner leave their cosy bed, drive through the cold night to a strange building and then try to carry on where they left off in a brightly-lit room with strangers walking in and out. (If that doesn't faze them, maybe they would be better off making educational films for adults.)

In the meantime, don't take too long with that coffee.

REFERENCES

1 Robertson A. The midwife companion. ACE Graphics; 1997.

2 Odent M. Knitting needles, cameras and electronic fetal monitors. Reprinted in: MIDIRS Midwifery Digest 1996; September: 304–306.

Waterbirth and song

Sheila Kitzinger

The earliest birth in water recorded in Western Europe occurred in Pithiviers, France, some time in the 1970s. Dr Michel Odent had introduced a children's paddling pool into the birth room at the little hospital there, so that a woman having a painful labour might have the benefits of submersion in water.

The first waterbirth took him by surprise; he stepped into the pool still wearing his socks to catch the baby.

In fact, the pool was so successful in easing pain, enabling women to act instinctively, and facilitating the progress of labour, that he then installed a specially designed pool. The birth pool became the hallmark of this hospital and a symbol of his philosophy of birth.

Michel and I met at a conference on psychoprophylaxis in obstetrics, which was held in Rome, at a time when I was living near Pithiviers, and he invited me to come and see what he was doing there.

In 1977 I visited the hospital. It was not with the aim of seeing a waterbirth. Rather, it was to explore the non-obstetric milieu for birth which he had created with a group of dedicated midwives.

Pithiviers was essentially women's space, though fathers, other children and all members of the family were made welcome. As in traditional environments all over the world, birth was shaped and conducted by women. It was the same with pregnancy.

An enthusiastic older woman who had been an opera singer gathered pregnant women, and whole families, round her piano in the antenatal clinic, and they and any members of staff who could drop in sang together unselfconsciously, rousingly and jubilantly. It was a powerful bonding experience. Singing was an important element in antenatal clinic visits.

Song in other cultures

Singing in pregnancy and birth is a well established practice with a long history in many different cultures.

Women form choirs to welcome a pregnancy, to guide a woman through it with counsel and hope, to support her and join in the sounds she makes during labour, to praise her and greet the baby at the birth, and to announce the birth to the village.

Among the Galla of Ethiopia, for example, when the expectant mother returns to her mother's home to give birth she takes with her two, four or six women to be her companions, at least one of whom must be an accomplished singer.[1] Birth takes place in the back room of the house, and the mother kneels on freshly strewn grass, supported by her women friends.

The male anthropologist who wrote about this did not describe what they sang during labour, presumably because he was not allowed to be present. But as soon as the baby is born the women ululate, four times for a girl, five for a boy. Then they break into songs which proclaim the mother's gallantry in giving birth and her happiness, and give thanks to Maram, the goddess of childbirth. They compare the mother's achievement with that of the brave hunter who returns victorious to the village.

In New Zealand, when a Maori woman is pregnant a female choir traditionally sings to her about the progress of the pregnancy. If all is not well, they sing about this, too, preparing her for problems ahead. Pregnancy links women together in shared pleasure and concern which is expressed through song.

Water and birth

It is sometimes claimed that waterbirth has a long ancestry and that labour in water occurs in a variety of cultures. There is little anthropological evidence for this. Mostly women have sought out, or had built for them, a secluded, dark place, a room by the stove in temperate climates, a fern-cushioned space in the bush, a mossy enclosure, or a sand or fur carpeted tent.

There is a Maori mountain tribe in which women gave birth in a sacred river. Some Polynesian islanders went down to the beach to give birth where they could have a dip and freshen up immediately afterwards. But in general water has been in short supply and too precious to be used in a tub for birth. Like eating the placenta, waterbirth is more likely to be encountered in California, or, for that matter, in Kensington, than in traditional cultures. Waterbirth is part of a new birth culture that challenges the dominant medical system of birth. It does not need to be validated by tradition.

Women who are immersed in water in labour often insist on staying in the pool for the birth. Sometimes this is an ordinary household bath. But the problem with a bath is that the sides are often narrow so that the mother cannot move easily. It may also be difficult to have the water deep enough to cover her lower torso. Instead, she is sitting in a puddle. Once birth pools were on the market there were new possibilities, above all of movement in water.

When floating in a pool, a woman in labour can move unencumbered. The water bears some of her weight and she has the sense of being in her own private world within the margins of her pool. Immersion in water also enables her to move spontaneously. She squats, kneels, lies on her side, goes onto all-fours, or crouches forward holding onto the side of the pool.

She may explore gliding movements, using her arms to glide forwards and backwards during contractions or to turn from her back to one side, or from one side to the other, rolling her pelvis over as she does so. She lunges, bending one or both knees and pushing away from the side of the pool. She rolls her knees from side to side so that she is also rolling her pelvis. She rediscovers birth postures and movements that are common to traditional birth cultures all over the world.

Safety

Through the 1980s and 1990s increasing numbers of midwives in North America and Western Europe assisted at births in which women laboured, and sometimes delivered, in a birth pool.

A survey into the use of water in labour and birth in England and Wales commissioned by the Department of Health[2] revealed that in 1993 43% of maternity units offered a birth pool or allowed women to take in a hired pool, and all units reported that they had ordinary baths that women could use in labour.

In 1993 2,885 babies were born under water. In many units where there were pools, however, they were little used. Midwives lacked the confidence in assisting at waterbirths and could not develop their skills. This remains the case.

Following concerns about safety, a landmark study of 4,032 babies born under water in England and Wales between April 1994 and March 1996 was undertaken, involving all consultant paediatricians in the British Isles.[3] It revealed that the perinatal mortality rate for babies born under water was 1.2/1000. This is comparable to that for low risk babies born in air. No deaths occurred as a consequence of waterbirth. Thirty four babies were admitted to special care baby units, a rate of 8.4/1000. This is significantly lower than the rate for babies born to low risk primigravidae.

Why water? Why not song?

It intrigues me that waterbirth has become an alternative birth option for increasing numbers of women, and that many hospitals have installed birth pools, while singing, the other important element in the Pithiviers birth style, and a much more common practice in diverse cultures, has never caught on in Britain or North America.

The problem cannot be cost. A piano is no more expensive than a birth pool. Singing is unlikely to be considered an unevaluated risk factor.

One possible answer is that the social system of the modern hospital dictates the relative status of the behaviour of everyone in it. Singing in groups would blur the boundaries between staff, and between staff and patients. It might be disturbing for those who relied on a rigid social system to define their position and role and to maintain order in a hierarchically based institution. It is difficult to imagine informal singing groups consisting of consultants, midwives, cleaners, pregnant women, children, fathers and senior managers, or a choir singing while a woman was in labour in any NHS hospital.

On the other hand, singing can be formalised, as it is in church services and temples, where chanting conforms to a strict pattern. The priest intones the collect and, with careful timing and in unison, the congregation responds. There is no doubt about who is in charge, and the worshippers must not usurp the priestly role. It is conceivable that singing might be introduced into hospitals in a similarly regulated way, and that it would then reinforce, rather than blur, the hierarchical system. So this is an unsatisfactory, or at least incomplete, explanation as to why singing does not find a place in birth today.

Water has a powerful cultural symbolism that makes it particularly attractive and there is a long tradition of using water for healing: sacred springs, spas and 'taking the waters'. It is an essential element in the Christian baptism. In revivalist sects the faithful are 'born again' by submersion in water. Waterbirth draws on this traditional symbolism, bestowing the birth pool with esoteric meaning.

Yet communal singing is also rooted in northern cultures. It often marks major life transitions – wedding and funeral hymns in the rites around marriage and death, for example. It has a unifying function. When people join together in a national anthem, sing *Jerusalem* on the last night of the Proms, or football crowds roar out songs in support of their team, or traditionally when workers have toiled in the fields, singing has cohesive power.

Consumer choice

The dominant model of birth in northern industrial cultures today is both technocratic and individualistic. Birth is technologically managed with electronic fetal monitor, intravenous drip and epidural cannula – all regulated by the clock, the oldest technology of all, on which all the other technology is based. The object of attention is the fetus in the pelvis and the patient in which the fetus is contained.

When a woman presents in an antenatal clinic, or is admitted in labour, she is 'managed' as an isolated reproductive organism, separate from her family and community. The web of relationships in her life outside the hospital doors is seen as irrelevant, or, if it intrudes, as an inconvenience to be dealt with by teaching midwives about ethnic minorities and the communication and management skills required to achieve patient compliance.

Over the last 25 years women have begun to resist being treated as ambulant pelvises and contracting uteruses. The result is that the focus is shifting, slowly but inexorably, to 'the whole woman'. But that is as far as it goes.

A patient is seen as a consumer who must be given the information to make choices between alternatives. These are ranged in front of her: induction of labour, pethidine, breathing exercises, an epidural, a 'walking' epidural, an elective Caesarean section, or waterbirth. The pregnant woman selects what she wants, much as she would a breakfast cereal on the supermarket shelf.

Song, in contrast, is part of a communal experience.

Traditionally, in cultures throughout the world, birth is an activity shared by a group of women who come together to support the woman in labour and thereby reinforce the bonds between them.

Though in some cultures the ideal is for a woman to go off into the bush alone and come back with a baby, these societies are few and far between, and even there, a woman having her first baby is usually attended by several female friends. The norm in most cultures is for birth to draw together a group of women, all of whom already know each other well. It takes place in women's space, and is choreographed by them. Prayer and invocation, embraces, joking, the telling of stories and sharing of news in the community, sounds of encouragement, massage, movement, dance and song all have a place in the unfolding birth drama.

Groups of women singing are foreign to birth today in northern cultures. This is so because the experience of birth has been medicalised and socially fragmented. A woman nearing the end of her pregnancy may not even know who will be attending her during labour. A group of female friends, especially if they were singing and in festive mood, would be unlikely to gain admission to the birth room. She is lucky if she has even one individual who stays with her through labour and till after the birth. If this happens, it is likely to be a male partner, perhaps with no previous experience of birth.

Childbirth is no longer an act shared between women who are well known to each other, in which the bonds between them are reinforced and celebrated. It is an isolated process which is seen increasingly as a matter of individual consumer choice.

A consumer may be permitted, with careful negotiation, to opt for the use of a birth pool. If one is available it can be offered as another 'method' and incorporated into the hospital system.

Singing, in contrast, does not fit the paradigm of birth 'methods' and techniques that can be regulated by agreed protocols. Perhaps this is why the other element in the birth experience at Pithiviers has still to be explored.

REFERENCES

1 Bartels Lambert. Birth songs of the Macha Galla. Ethnology 1969; 8: 406–422.
2 Allerdice F, Renfrew M, Marchant S, et al. Labour and birth in water in England and Wales. BMJ 1995; 310:837.
3 Gilbert RE, Tookey PA. Perinatal mortality and morbidity among babies delivered in water: Surveillance study and postal survey. BMJ 1999; 319:483–487.

In praise of an unusual midwife

Sandy Kirkman

I enjoy being old. I particularly enjoy telling my students that I trained halfway through the last century and that I can remember the physiological management of the third stage, first time around.

I was reflecting recently on my community midwife all those years ago. Mrs Silver (I shall call her) was a married woman who lived at home with her husband, daughters and cat. She had been a community midwife in a poor area of a city in the north of England for some years. She was a 'teaching midwife' and always had a student. I was a rarity for that area in that I was a registered nurse who had done Part One Midwifery (ask your mother) in London. Mrs Silver was not used to 22-year-old registered nurses. I'm not sure that she thought she would get on with such a young snob, but fate had flung us together and she did her best with me.

Every morning she would ring me. Having understood her directions of where to meet her, I would hang up. The phone would ring again immediately. 'You'll have to do better than that', she remonstrated, 'I like a good chat in a morning, there's no point me putting myself out to have a student if I can't get a good chat.' Years later I realised that through all the seeming aimlessness, she was subtly testing me to see if I had noticed things about her clients and their grubby families.

For visits, Mrs Silver drove a seemingly random path around endless council estates. She would screech to a halt outside a house and in we would go. The children would be running around wearing only a vest. No pants or nappy, they wee'd where they stood in the garden. Well, it was summertime. The latest baby would be propped up on the settee drinking grey milk out of a bottle, perhaps inexpertly held by a big brother or sister. When I queried the colour of the milk, Mrs Silver would explain that it was tea. The mother, who was only slightly older than me, looked ancient and had no teeth. She was expecting her fifth child and this visit, which I had thought was postnatal, was actually an antenatal visit. Gently, over the weeks, Mrs Silver demonstrated to me that Pauline was a 'good enough' mother given her circumstances and the house was clean, if threadbare.

The day came that Pauline went into labour. The drill was that the midwife would phone the ambulance station who would tell the student where to go. The bags were kept in the nurses' home so the student had to clank up the long drive with four bags: a delivery bag, a postnatal bag, and two sets of inhalational analgesia. I delivered twenty-five women in their own homes, and not one of them would oblige me by asking for, or even accepting, any form of pain relief. However, I had high hopes of Pauline who was making lots of noise as we arrived. Mrs Silver said 'She'll not be long, she never is.' Resolutely, I got out the paraphernalia to give the reluctant client some Trilene. Mrs Silver sat on the edge of the bed wearing a paper facemask around which she puffed on her Park Drive tipped cigarette. I made sympathetic noises and invited Pauline to breathe deeply into the rubber mask at the next contraction. She did. She reared back in horror yelling '**** me! That stuff dunt arf **** stink, gerrit away!' It was hard to tell whether Mrs Silver was smirking, choking or just smoking behind her mask. The baby was born in the next half hour. 'Good job too', said Pauline. 'It's my Bingo night.'

After each delivery Mrs Silver would ask to look in my bag. She made nice noises about my shiny instruments, which I laboriously cleaned, polished and boiled up after every outing. She said, sadly, that it seemed a shame that I had 'all them lovely instruments' but never got to use them. What use were my shiny stitch scissors when no one ever had any stitches? Then she brightened up. We got into the car and screeched to a halt outside a different house. It was her own home. Inside we found the cat, languishing after its neutering operation. With enormous good will Mrs Silver let me use my pristine scissors to remove the cat's stitches. We were all delighted.

Mrs Silver rides again

Sandy Kirkman

When I was a student in northern England, my midwife, Mrs Silver (pseudonym) was a real character. She used considerable interpersonal skills to teach me vastly important lessons about giving the clients the service that they deserved and needed, rather than allowing me to be judgemental. Once, on the way upstairs behind me, she thought she saw me run my finger along a ledge for dust and she smacked my legs!

I was charmed by her ways in the bedroom where the baby was to be born. None of the women would tolerate any form of pain relief and we nearly always 'forgot' to send for the GP until it was far too late. One young man did come puffing up the stairs to find Mrs Silver perched on the edge of the bed, paper facemask lifted at the corner to allow her to smoke her cigarette. The woman lay on her back, legs akimbo, naked. It was high summer. The young GP stood at the end of the bed and peered into the vulva. At this, the woman gave a mighty heave and the membranes ruptured with a whoosh, soaking the GP and extinguishing Mrs Silver's fag. The GP left without a word and Mrs Silver stared sadly at her ruined smoke as I delivered the baby.

Mrs Silver wasn't saintly to all her clients. One family (let's call them the Smiths) were a real trial to her. Mrs Smith had eight daughters and was pregnant for the ninth time. She intended to keep going until she had a son. She had gross anaemia and we had to visit to give iron injections. (Remember, this was a long, long time ago.) At each visit we would take a delivery pack into the house, and every time we went back it had gone. We could never keep a piece of soap in the house either, and the kitchen stove was about an inch thick in burnt-on grease and food. Inevitably the family kept a greyhound which enjoyed the best of everything and lay across the end of the bed throughout the ninth labour, which I attended.

Mrs Silver and I had arrived together in response to a labour call at about 9pm. Alongside the recumbent form of Mrs Smith in the double bed lay her husband, flat on his back with his cloth cap pulled down over his eyes. He never moved or spoke all night. The greyhound lay across the bottom of the bed and lifted its lip menacingly every time I went near Mrs Smith. Mrs Silver took in the situation at a glance and, squinting through the smoke of her own cigarette, she pronounced. 'I'm off!' I quickly gathered my four bags together to accompany my midwife down the stairs when Mrs Smith called from the bed to me. 'Aye, go on then, but if tha' duz, this'll be the sixth bairn born after the midwife had gone 'ome.' Mrs Silver turned to me and said 'Suit yerself, I'll be back in the morning'. And with that, was gone.

It was a strange night. I had thrown my smart navy blue cardigan on top of a wardrobe when I arrived. As it grew cooler, I pulled it down only to find it transformed into a thickly furred version of itself, completely covered in fluff, dirt and cobwebs. The Smiths slept all night, someone had spirited away all the daughters but I could hear strange rustling noises from the direction of the kitchen. I didn't dare investigate for two reasons: firstly I thought it might be mice or rats, secondly the greyhound eyed me evilly every time I moved. I was trapped. Towards morning, almost simultaneously two things happened. Mrs Silver reappeared and Mrs Smith woke up and proceeded to push. Her ninth daughter was very soon born. When we went downstairs to make a drink we found that the previously filthy stove was gleaming. 'It'll be the neighbours crept in likely', said Mrs Silver. 'They'd take the chance to clean up for the sake of the new babby.'

Mrs Silver was and is my heroine. How did she know all she knew? How did those poor women who failed every test of suitability for home delivery ever have such short, healthy labours? Why did no woman ever require analgesia when their sisters in the hospital up the road had normal levels of medication? Why did I never get to use any of my shiny instruments except on the cat? How did she ever put up with me without howling with laughter at my 'hospital ways'? A genius! A saint!

I have a dream...

Jilly Rosser

Everybody is doing it. This year, December feels not so much like the season of goodwill as the season for proclaiming visions of the future. In this, the last issue of the millennium, *The Practising Midwife* thought it apt to look dispassionately at where we are, take stock and dream of how it could be better. Here is our vision for the maternity services of the future.

What is wrong with what we have?

Quite a lot. The maternity services are not, for the most part, a very nice place to work. Midwives are leaving in droves, and those who are staying feel stressed, undervalued and frustrated. There are barely enough midwives practising for the service to be maintained, and the more who leave, the worse it is for those who remain. The working environment is not conducive to innovation of any kind. Few women are getting the quality of care that they need and that midwives are capable of delivering. Choice remains an elusive ideal, evidence is used erratically to guide practice and many women have a horrible experience of pregnancy and childbirth. The more socially or psychologically needy the woman, the less likely she is to have her needs met. Despite the rhetoric, the maternity services are entirely medically orientated. Normal birth is rare and becoming rarer. There appears to be plentiful funding to buy any amount of technological equipment and to pay technicians to use it routinely, but not to provide good, basic care to women postnatally. There are few places for student midwives to learn about midwifery-led care. Some of the best students leave, unable to bear the discordance between the content of their lectures and the reality of the labour ward.

What are the opportunities?

They have never been better. Every recent Government paper is on the side of the angels – the NHS is to become more community based with a public health focus. The emphasis is on the tackling of inequalities, starting with mothers and babies. *Making a Difference*[1] urges midwives to take the initiative and set up services and projects which fulfil the new Government agenda. The maternity services are likely to become more polarised; 'high dependency' care will be concentrated in fewer acute units. These will leave huge geographical areas with a vacuum. Women, GPs and midwives want care that is locally based, at least for low-dependency maternity care. GPs will, in their new Primary Care Groups or trusts, have enormous financial clout. With the evidence consistently demonstrating that care in midwifery-led units is safe,[2] it all adds up to the development of free-standing birth centres, whether in large cities, towns or rural areas.

What are the constraints?

Mostly our belief – in ourselves and in our ability to bring about change. We think small – trying to make do with an ever-decreasing midwifery budget, not believing we have access to people in positions of power and influence. Most of them – particularly those in public health – would love it if a couple of midwives approached them and said 'We think we can fulfil a whole swathe of the Government's new NHS agenda, and here's how'. There is funding available to enact the NHS reforms. If we think strategically and start to see how we fit into the whole picture of improving the nation's health, we can find ways to get some of this money allocated to the midwifery services.

How does the future look?

The acute maternity services become concentrated in fewer, larger units (because of changes in the medical work force). The midwives working in these units are experts in high-dependency care and prefer the cut and thrust of a busy labour ward. They have excellent clinical skills for dealing with abnormality and are respected, much valued members of the team of clinicians who care for women with complicated pregnancies. These midwives rotate out of the unit for a short period every few months, to be reminded of the essential normality of birth and to ensure they remain understanding of, and empathic towards, their midwifery colleagues outside the unit. Student midwives have their placement on these units towards the end of their training, and always under the guidance of a mentor.

The focal point of maternity care is, however, the birth centres, where most women receive their care. These are based throughout the country according to local geography and population and aim to serve the local community. They may be in community hospitals, in old GP maternity units, in the new 'Healthy Living Centres' or free-standing in other buildings. This is where all the midwives in the locality are based. As well as rooms to give birth in there are facilities for groups to meet, spaces for exercise and relaxation and clerical/secretarial services.

The midwives have caseloads, or whichever organisation of workload suits them and the local situation best. Women from the locality book with the birth centre midwives and the midwives 'follow the women' wherever they give birth – at home, in the birth centre or in the acute unit. GPs are no longer directly involved in the provision of maternity care. There is strong midwifery leadership at each birth centre, which feeds into the local Primary Care Trust and also links in to the acute trust.

The ethos of care is woman centred and midwife friendly. There is continuity of midwifery care, an emphasis on choice and empowerment for women, and a strong commitment to keeping birth normal. Midwives can exercise their clinical judgement and normally expect to refer women with problems in pregnancy or labour to an obstetric registrar at least. Rule 40, which currently requires a midwife to refer care in the case of a 'deviation from the norm' has been changed so that midwives can ask for opinions (rather like GPs do now) about aspects of a woman's care, without necessarily handing over the

decision making. As well as being evidence based, care is informed by a thorough understanding of anatomy and physiology to maximise safety and effectiveness. Care is kind – women are treated with respect and gentleness and given time. Student midwives are based at a birth centre for most of their practical training and all their tutors work part time as clinical midwives at the birth centre.

The service is targeted to reach those women in most need – physically, socially and psychologically. The midwives are known in the community and respond to the women's priorities. There are effective strategies in place to recognise and help women who have problems such as poor housing, a violent partner, drug dependency and psychiatric illness. The midwives have professional links with social services, council housing departments, local schools and so on. The links with these and other agencies and organisations help to ensure that care for vulnerable women is holistic and continuous, for instance help with parenting skills is offered by referring women on to Sure Start.

By training and supervising local women to provide peer support in key areas such as breastfeeding – the so-called 'community capacity building' which the Government is keen to promote – the midwives multiply their effectiveness.

Some specialists from the acute unit visit the birth centre on an agreed basis, e.g. monthly visits by a consultant obstetrician. There are clear and rapid lines of communication with a range of clinicians: consultant obstetricians, paediatricians, diabetic nurses, radiologists and so on. When referral to the acute unit is required, the midwife can accompany the woman and continue to provide care.

There is ongoing audit of a range of birth centre activities. The midwives meet together regularly to update themselves, discuss their work and to reflect on unexpected outcomes through a process of peer review. At these meetings the midwives often pause to remember how they used to work, back in the 1990s, and how unsatisfactory their working lives had been. They wonder how they stuck it for so long and praise those pioneering midwives who, back at the turn of the century, decided the time had come to make their dreams become reality.

REFERENCES

1 Department of Health. Making a difference. Strengthening the nursing, midwifery and health visiting contribution to health and healthcare. London: DoH; 1999.

2 Campbell R, Macfarlane A, Hempsall V, et al. Evaluation of midwife-led care provided at the Royal Bournemouth Hospital. Midwifery 1999; 15(3):183–193.

Index